MATH SKILLS FOR ALLIED HEALTH CAREERS

Daniel L. Timmons

Alamance Community College

Catherine W. Johnson

Alamance Community College

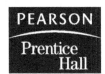

PEARSON

Prentice Hall

Upper Saddle River, New Jersey
Columbus, Ohio

Library of Congress Cataloging-in-Publication Data

Timmons, Daniel L.
   Math skills for allied health careers / Daniel L. Timmons, Catherine W. Johnson.
      p. cm.
   ISBN 0-13-171348-5
   1. Medicine—Mathematics.   2. Mathematics.   3. Medical sciences.   I. Johnson, Catherine W.   II. Title.
   R853. M3 T56 2008
   610.1'51—dc22

                                                                                2007000045

Editor in Chief: Vernon R. Anthony
Editor: Gary Bauer
Development Editor: Linda Cupp
Production Editor: Kevin Happell
Production Coordination: GGS Book Services
Design Coordinator: Diane Ernsberger
Production Manager: Pat Tonneman
Director of Marketing: David Gesell
Senior Marketing Manager: Leigh Ann Sims
Marketing Coordinator: Alicia Dysert

This book was set in Times Ten Roman by GGS Book Services. It was printed and bound by Edwards Brothers Malloy. The cover was printed by Edwards Brothers Malloy.

Pearson Education Ltd.
Pearson Education Singapore Pte. Ltd.
Pearson Education Canada, Ltd.
Pearson Education—Japan

Pearson Education Australia Pty. Limited
Pearson Education North Asia Ltd.
Pearson Educación de Mexico, S.A. de C.V.
Pearson Education Malaysia Pte. Ltd.

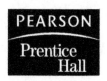

16 17 18 19 20
ISBN–13: 978-0-13-171348-2
ISBN–10:   0-13-171348-5

PREFACE

Our goal in writing *Math Skills for Allied Health Careers* is to get students to think of mathematics as a useful tool in the allied health professions. To provide students with a solid mathematical foundation, it is necessary to present clear explanations of the mathematical concepts required of health care workers. This book addresses this need with understandable discussions that are supported with many examples and over 2000 questions and problems for students to work in order to practice the concepts that are presented here.

The authors realize that calculators are used within professional health care environments. Therefore, this text not only presents the manual way of calculating answers but also includes clear information on the use of calculators to do the same calculations.

Math Skills for Allied Health Careers is written and designed for students in a two-year associate in arts health care curriculum. We have written the book in nonthreatening mathematical language so that students who have previously been fearful of or intimidated by mathematics will be able to comprehend the concepts.

The text begins with a review of mathematical and algebraic concepts necessary for success in the allied health field. Problems in these chapters specifically target several different health care areas. The various measurement systems used in allied health fields are covered in Chapter 3. Chapter 4 introduces students to medication labels, prescriptions, and syringe calculations. Chapter 5 models applications in various health occupation fields. It is designed so that instructors may omit sections not applicable to their health area without compromising content. Chapter 6 addresses calculations used in basic IV therapy. Chapter 7 covers the fundamentals of descriptive statistics with a brief look at standard deviation and control charts. An introduction to the mathematical concept of logarithms and their use in relation to pH and ionic solutions is presented in Chapter 8.

Key features include:

- Answers to odd-numbered problems in the back of the book
- Chapter reviews and practice tests with all of the answers provided in the back of the book
- Chapter summaries and lists of key terms and formulas at the end of each chapter
- Calculator lessons interspersed throughout the book
- Clear step-by-step examples presented in each section
- Dosage calculations presented using ratio and proportions, formulas, and dimensional analysis methods

An online Instructor's Manual and a computerized test bank (TestGen) are also available to instructors through this title's catalog page at **www.prenhall.com**. Instructors can search for a text by author, title, ISBN, or by selecting the appropriate discipline from the pull down menu at the top of the catalog home page. To access supplementary materials online, instructors need to request an instructor access code. Go to **www.prenhall.com**, click the **Instructor Resource Center** link, and then click Register Today for an instructor access code. Within 48 hours of registering you will receive a confirming e-mail including an instructor access code. Once you have received your code, go to the site and log on for full instructions on downloading the materials that you wish to use.

We welcome any comments, criticisms, or suggestions from users of this text. Our purpose is to provide the very best book that we can for our colleagues and their students. We have attempted to provide a book that will promote student understanding. We have not avoided the difficult topics, but have tried to present them in an understandable and digestible manner.

We have taken every reasonable precaution intended to ensure that the instructions contained in this text are current and accurate. We make no specific or implied warranties with respect to material included in this text. All examples and problems are intended for instructional purposes only and are not intended to represent actual dosages, prescription amounts, etc. The rendering of specific medical services or the prescription and administration of drugs should be left to trained medical practitioners.

Acknowledgments

There have been many whose assistance has brought us to this point. We are indeed grateful to them for their help, encouragement, and suggestions. Without their support, this book would not have been possible. We would particularly like to thank:

Kaye Acton, Department Head, Medical Assisting, Alamance Community College

Sandra Hinton, Instructor, Nursing Assistant Program, Alamance Community College

Tyler Johnson, Math Editor

Rhonda Pierce, Department Head, Nursing Assistant Program, Alamance Community College

Susan Reed, Instructor, Nursing, Alamance Community College

Cindy Thompson, Instructor, Medical Assisting, Alamance Community College

We would also like to thank the reviewers of this book: Gordon DeSpain, San Juan College; Gwen English, Sinclair Community College; Rob Farinelli, Community College of Alleghany County; and Jan Hoeweler, Cincinnati State Technical and Community College.

CONTENTS

BASIC ARITHMETIC COMPUTATIONS IN HEALTH APPLICATIONS

Objectives for Chapter 1

After completing this chapter, the student should be able to:

1. Understand the Roman numeral system.

2. Do calculations with numbers written as fractions.

3. Do calculations with numbers written as decimals.

4. Work with numbers expressed as percents.

5. Convert decimals to percents and to fractions.

6. Convert fractions to decimals and to percents.

7. Convert percents to decimals and to fractions.

8. Apply knowledge of decimals, fractions, and percents to problems in the allied health field.

SECTION 1.1   INTRODUCTION TO MATHEMATICS AS USED IN THE ALLIED HEALTH FIELD

As the demand for health care workers grows each year, the study of mathematics becomes increasingly important for students pursuing careers in the allied health field. Mathematics is an essential skill for health care workers whether they are in the field of nursing, medical assisting, radiology, pharmacy technology, dental assisting, surgical technology or any other related medical field. Accuracy of computation is important in health care as you calculate medical dosages, take inventory, or report patient intake and output. Mathematical errors can have serious repercussions in patient care. The presentation of topics in this book is designed to assist you in becoming more accurate and efficient in the mathematics required for allied health careers.

Many of the arithmetic topics that you learned early in your mathematical studies are used in allied health careers. One of the topics that is specific to health care is the use of **Roman numerals**. In our everyday lives, we use the Hindu-Arabic numerals 0–9 and combinations of these numerals to complete required mathematical calculations. However, doctors sometimes use Roman numerals in writing prescriptions and in medical records and charts. This is because one measurement system used in prescribing dosages of medication is the apothecary system. Until the late nineteenth century, pharmacies were called apothecary shops. Occasionally, you will see a pharmacy with that term in its title even today. The apothecary system of measurement uses units such as *grain* in combination with the Roman numeral number system to indicate dosage amounts.

Generally, lowercase Roman numerals are used for the numbers 1 to 10. Uppercase letters are used when smaller numerals are part of a number over 30 such as 33 (XXXIII

Table 1.1 Roman Numerals

1 = i or I	9 = ix or IX
2 = ii or II	10 = x or X
3 = iii or III	$\frac{1}{2}$ = ss
4 = iv or IV	50 = L
5 = v or V	100 = C
6 = vi or VI	500 = D
7 = vii or VII	1000 = M
8 = viii or VIII	

not xxxiii). Table 1.1 lists many of the notations used for Roman numerals. Note that there is no Roman numeral to represent a value of 0, nor for any other fraction except $\frac{1}{2}$.

Combinations of the letters in Table 1.1 are used without commas to create different values in the Roman numeral system. To create some numbers, we string the letters together to add up to the number required. For example, iii = 3, vi = 6, and XXVI = 26. The rule is to use the biggest numeral possible at each stage, so xv is used to represent 15 instead of vvv or xiiiii. In these cases, numerals are always listed from left to right in descending order. However, if this were the only rule for Roman numerals, there could be some very long strings used to represent some values. For example, using this rule, 49 would be XXXXVIIII. To avoid this, another rule that involves subtracting a smaller value to the left of a larger value was developed. So the number 9 becomes ix (10 − 1) instead of viiii.

There are three important things to keep in mind when using the rule that pertains to creating values using subtraction of a smaller value from a larger value.

1. The numeral to the left that is being subtracted must be I, X, or C. The numerals V, L, D, and M cannot be subtracted.

2. The subtracted number must be no less than a tenth of the value of the number it is subtracted from. For example, X can be placed to the left of C or L, but not to the left of D or M. The letter I can be placed in front of V and X only.

3. Normally, only one number can be placed to the left of the larger value. For example, while 9 = IX, 7 is not written IIIX.

For examples of writing numbers as Roman numbers and changing Roman numerals to Hindu-Arabic numerals, look at the illustrations in Examples 1 and 2.

EXAMPLE 1: Interpreting Roman Numerals

Write the given values expressed in Roman numerals as Hindu-Arabic numerals.

1. xiii = 10 + 1 + 1 + 1 = 13
2. xxvss = 10 + 10 + 5 + $\frac{1}{2}$ = $25\frac{1}{2}$
3. XL = 50 − 10 = 40
4. xxix = 10 + 10 + (10 − 1) = 29
5. LXXXIX — when working with long Roman numerals, separate them into groups for easier analysis:

$$\text{LXXXIX} = \quad \text{L} \quad \text{XXX} \quad \text{IX}$$

$$50 \; + \; 30 \; + \; (10 - 1) = 89$$

EXAMPLE 2: Writing Roman Numerals from Hindu-Arabic Numerals

Write the given values expressed in Hindu-Arabic numerals in Roman numerals.

1. $17 = 10 + 7 = $ xvii
2. $120 = 100 + 10 + 10 = $ CXX
3. $419 = 400 + 10 + 9 = $ CD $+$ X $+$ IX $= $ CDXIX
4. $24\frac{1}{2} = 10 + 10 + 4 + \frac{1}{2} = $ xxivss

Mathematical skills such as addition of whole numbers, multiplication of whole numbers, and estimation are important as health care workers monitor a patient's food and fluid intake and output during a 24-hour period. Intake includes water, juices, or other foods and fluids consumed by a patient. Output is the food and fluid eliminated by the patient. It may be in the form of urine, diarrhea, suction material, or wound drainage. Normally, total fluid output should be approximately the same as total fluid input. By comparing daily input and output values, the health care professional can determine if a fluid imbalance exists. Steps can then be taken to prevent dehydration or over hydration of the patient.

Most facilities currently use the metric unit cubic centimeter (cc) to record a patient's intake of fluids and food. One cubic centimeter (cc) is equal to 1 millimeter (mL) or $\frac{1}{1000}$ of a liter. An ounce (oz) in the U.S. customary system is equal to 30 cc. Therefore, if a patient drinks an 8-oz glass of milk, he has consumed $8 \times 30 = 240$ cc of milk. This is the amount that will be recorded in the Intake and Output Record in his chart. Most Intake and Output Records will have a listing of standard items used at the facility and the corresponding number of ounces or cubic centimeters each contains. Look at the estimation guide from one hospital's Intake/Output form.

Standard Measurements:

1 oz = 30 cc

Carton milk = 240 cc

Juice carton = 120 cc

1 cup jello = 120 cc

1 soup bowl = 150 cc

Ice cream/sherbet = 120 cc

Popsicle = 90 cc

EXAMPLE 3: Determining Intake

Mrs. Pierce had one bowl of soup, one 6-oz cup of coffee, and an 8-oz glass of water for lunch. Determine her total intake in cubic centimeters (cc).

Solution

Using the hospital estimation guide:

1 bowl soup =		150 cc
1 cup of coffee = 6 oz $\times$ 30 cc/oz	=	180 cc
1 glass of water = 8 oz $\times$ 30 cc/oz	=	+240 cc
Total Intake		570 cc

The Institute for Safe Medication Practices publishes a list of error-prone medical abbreviations that are reported as frequently being misinterpreted, resulting in harmful medication errors. The abbreviation for cubic centimeters (cc) is included on this list and it is recommended that all measurements be given in milliliters (mL). Since these unit labels indicate equal amounts of volume, they are interchangeable (25 cc = 25 mL). Some hospitals are moving toward standardization of these units. However, many facilities still use both in their records.

EXAMPLE 4: Discovering Fluid Imbalances

During the past 24 hours, Ms. Hinton has consumed 3 cups of jello, four 8-oz glasses of water, two 6-oz glasses of ginger ale, and one popsicle. Her output includes urine output of 250 mL, 200 mL, 300 mL, 275 mL, 200 mL, 225 mL, and 295 mL. Determine this patient's fluid balance or imbalance.

Solution

Using the estimation chart, we compute the following intake:

$$
\begin{array}{lll}
\text{3 cups of jello} & = 3 \times 120 \text{ cc} & = 360 \text{ cc} \\
\text{4 glasses} \times 8 \text{ oz} = 32 \text{ oz} \times 30 \text{ cc/oz} & = 960 \text{ cc} \\
\text{2 glasses} \times 6 \text{ oz} = 12 \text{ oz} \times 30 \text{ cc/oz} & = 360 \text{ cc} \\
\text{1 popsicle} = & \underline{+ 90 \text{ cc}} \\
& \text{Total Intake} & 1770 \text{ cc or } 1770 \text{ mL}
\end{array}
$$

Total output is the urine total.

$$250 \text{ mL} + 200 \text{ mL} + 300 \text{ mL} + 275 \text{ mL} + 200 \text{ mL} + 225 \text{ mL}$$
$$+ 295 \text{ mL} = 1745 \text{ mL or } 1745 \text{ cc}$$

Intake − Output = 1770 cc − 1745 cc = 25 cc (25 mL) fluid retention

Because the intake and output amounts are approximately equal, there is not a reportable difference here.

Inventory is an important clerical function in a doctor's office, dental office, hospital, residential care facility, or pharmacy. Supply technicians, medical assistants, nursing assistants, pharmacy technicians, or other staff may be assigned to complete this task. Keeping accurate records of inventory is important to reduce overstocking and to ensure adequate supplies to meet demand. Health care workers must use addition, subtraction, multiplication, and division of whole numbers to count supplies and determine the number needed to restock the inventory to acceptable levels.

EXAMPLE 5: Maintaining Inventory

A pharmacy tries to maintain a minimum inventory of 250 tablets of a particular medication. At the end of the day, there are 30 tablets left on the shelf. How many bottles of this medication must be ordered to meet the minimum inventory requirement? This medication is commercially available in a 60-tablet bottle.

Solution

Subtract to find the difference between the minimum requirement and the number of tablets on the shelf.

$$250 \text{ tablets} - 30 \text{ tablets} = 220 \text{ tablets}$$

Since these tablets must be ordered in bottles of 60, divide the number of tablets needed by 60 tablets/bottle to calculate the number of bottles to order.

$$220 \text{ tablets} \div 60 \text{ tablets/bottle} = 3.67 \text{ bottles}$$

Rounding to the nearest whole bottle, the order should be for 4 bottles.

Health care professionals use many basic math skills as part of their daily jobs, from the Roman numeral system and the skills of addition, multiplication, and estimation to the more advanced topics of algebra, ratio/proportion, and statistics. Throughout this book, we will examine the many applications of mathematics in the health care field. A complete knowledge of a variety of mathematical skills will help you as a health care provider to be successful in your career, regardless of the health care discipline that you enter.

PRACTICE PROBLEM SET 1.1

Convert the following values given in Roman numerals to Hindu-Arabic numerals.

1. xviii	8. xix	15. CD	22. MDCL
2. xxi	9. xxviii	16. CM	23. MDCIXss
3. xiiss	10. xxxii	17. LVII	24. DXCIss
4. xxss	11. xxiv	18. CXII	25. CLXXXIX
5. xv	12. xxix	19. LXXII	26. CDLXXIV
6. vii	13. XL	20. CLXI	
7. iv	14. XC	21. MMDC	

Convert the following values given in Hindu-Arabic numerals to Roman numerals.

27. 8	33. 19	39. 40	45. 450
28. 3	34. 24	40. 90	46. 950
29. 12	35. 69	41. 99	47. 390
30. 17	36. 64	42. 49	48. 209
31. $3\frac{1}{2}$	37. 29	43. 146	49. 1626
32. $10\frac{1}{2}$	38. 39	44. 193	50. 1429

Solve each of the following word problems.

51. Total the outputs for this patient given the following report: 1200 mL of urine, 350 mL of vomitus, and 535 mL of drainage.
52. Total the urine output for Mr. Thompson at the end of a 24-hour period:

$$350 \text{ mL}, 250 \text{ mL}, 300 \text{ mL}, 200 \text{ mL}, 300 \text{ mL}, 300 \text{ mL}, 250 \text{ mL}$$

Use the hospital estimation chart to estimate the total intake for a patient who eats and drinks the following items. Give your answers in cc's.

53. one 6-oz cup of coffee, one cup of sherbet
54. two 8-oz glasses of water, one popsicle, one bowl of soup
55. one cup of jello, two cartons of juice, one 6-oz cup of coffee
56. two 8-oz glasses of water, one carton of juice, one popsicle, two cups of jello

Determine the fluid balance or imbalance for each patient given these amounts recorded during a 24-hour period.

57. Mr. Neathery — intake: three cups of jello, four 6-oz glasses of water, two popsicles, one bowl of soup, one juice carton

   urine output: 200 cc, 300 cc, 250 cc, 350 cc, 300 cc, 250 cc

58. Mrs. Helms — intake: one carton milk, two bowls soup, two 8-oz cups of coffee, one cup of ice cream, one cup of jello, one juice carton

   urine output: 350 cc, 300 cc, 325 cc, 250 cc, 300 cc, 200 cc

59. At the beginning of the month, a dental office had 3524 latex examination gloves on hand. On the last day of the month, an inventory showed that 821 gloves remained. How many gloves were used during the month? If the office manager places an order for gloves so there will be a minimum of 3000 gloves on hand at the beginning of the next month, how many should be ordered? If gloves come in boxes of 250, how many boxes should be ordered?

60. A medical assistant needs to order file labels for a doctor's office. The inventory is to be kept at 1500 labels and a current count reports there are only 275 labels on hand. How many labels should be ordered? If labels come in boxes of 250 labels, how many boxes must be ordered?

61. The maximum inventory for ampicillin capsules is 1000. An inventory at the end of the week indicates there are 328 capsules in stock. How many capsules should the pharmacy technician order to restock to the maximum level? If capsules are sold in bottles of 250, 100, and 25, how many of each bottle should be ordered?

62. A certain medication is to be maintained at a minimum inventory of 500 tablets and a maximum of 2000 tablets. If the number of tablets currently in stock at the end of the week is 182, how many are needed to meet the inventory minimum? If tablets come in bottles of 250, 100, and 25, how many bottles of each should be ordered to restock to an inventory level of at least 1000 tablets?

63. A certified nursing assistant is taking inventory at Oak Grove Skilled Nursing Facility. He records the following values while counting medicine cups: 345, 215, 181, 500, 28. How many medicine cups are currently in stock? If the facility wants to start a month with a minimum of 2000 medicine cups, how many should he order?

64. The certified medical assistant is taking inventory of the disposable syringes in the office at the end of the month. She counts two boxes in Exam Room 1, four boxes in Exam Room 2, three boxes in Exam Room 3, and nine boxes in Exam Room 4. If there are 50 syringes in a box, how many disposable syringes are in stock?

65. The total caloric intake of these patients must be calculated daily. Complete the chart using the values given.

Patient	Breakfast	Lunch	Dinner	Daily Total
Ray	375	625	982	
Nancy	280	520	1020	
John	525	60	1289	

66. The dosages of medication that patients receive in a day must be closely monitored by health care providers. If each patient receives the same dosage of medication each time the medication is administered, calculate the total amount of medication given in a 24-hour period.

Patient	Dosage	Number of Doses	Total Medication Received
P. Hall	150 micrograms	3 times a day	
S. Holt	200 milligrams	2 times a day	
T. Adams	25 milligrams	4 times a day	

An understanding of basic fractions is helpful to health care workers in the allied health field. Although many measurements in the medical field are given as decimals or percents, some values, such as measurements in the apothecary system, are stated as fractions. For example, the apothecary measurement gr $\frac{3}{4}$ = 45 mg. Our review of fractional numbers begins with the terms **numerator** and **denominator**. In the fraction $\frac{1}{2}$, the top number, 1, is the *numerator* and the bottom number, 2, is the *denominator*. If the numerator is smaller than the denominator, the fraction is called a **proper fraction**. If the numerator is larger than the denominator, the fraction is called an **improper fraction**. If the answer to a problem is an improper fraction, it may be left in fractional form or converted to a mixed number depending on the requirements of the problem.

Reducing Fractions

The fractions $\frac{2}{3}$ and $\frac{6}{9}$ both represent the same numerical value. However, the fraction $\frac{2}{3}$ is in lowest terms because the only factor common to both the numerator and denominator is 1. On the other hand, the number 3 is a common factor to both the numerator and denominator of the fraction $\frac{6}{9}$. If the numbers 6 and 9 are both divided by 3, the resulting reduced fraction will be $\frac{2}{3}$.

EXAMPLE 6: Reducing Fractions to Lowest Terms

Reduce the following fractions to simplest form: a. $\dfrac{16}{24}$ b. $\dfrac{200}{75}$

Solution

a. Look for the largest number that will divide 16 and 24 evenly. Although these numbers are both divisible by 2, 4, and 8, we will use the largest common factor, 8, in order to reduce the fraction completely in one step.

$$\frac{16}{24} = \frac{16 \div 8}{24 \div 8} = \frac{2}{3}$$

b. The largest number that will divide 200 and 75 evenly is 25.

$$\frac{200}{75} = \frac{200 \div 25}{75 \div 25} = \frac{8}{3}$$

This fraction is reduced but remains an improper fraction. The mixed number form of this fraction is found by dividing 3 into 8 with the remainder being written in fraction form.

$$\frac{8}{3} = 8 \div 3 = 2\frac{2}{3}$$

Finding Least Common Denominators for Fractions

The **least common denominator (LCD)** is the smallest number or multiple that all denominators of the fractions in the problem will divide evenly. This number may be one of the denominators in the problem, such as the 4 in the problem $\frac{1}{2} + \frac{1}{4}$. Or, you may need to examine the multiples of the largest denominator in order to find the least common denominator. Look at the following examples.

EXAMPLE 7: Finding the Least Common Denominator for Fractions

Find the least common denominator (LCD) for the following problems.

a. $\dfrac{1}{6} + \dfrac{2}{3} + \dfrac{1}{2} = ?$

Solution

The largest denominator of these terms is 6. Since it is divisible by 2 and 3, 6 is the least common denominator (LCD) for this problem.

b. $\dfrac{9}{10} - \dfrac{2}{25} = ?$

Solution

The largest denominator of these terms is 25. Since it is not divisible evenly by 10, we must find another number that is divisible by both 10 and 25. Consider 25, the largest denominator, and its multiples: $\{25, 50, 75, 100 \dots\}$. The number 50 is the smallest multiple of 25 that is divisible by 10. Therefore, 50 is the least common denominator (LCD) for the problem.

If the least common denominator is not obvious or easily calculated with the methods used in Example 7, another method, factoring each denominator into prime numbers, can be used to find it. Prime numbers are numbers greater than 1 having exactly two factors — the number itself and 1. Six is not prime because it can be factored into the product 2×3. However, 3 is prime because its only factors are 3 and 1. The first ten prime numbers are $2, 3, 5, 7, 11, 13, 17, 19, 23,$ and 29.

Let us use another method to find the least common denominator for the problem in Example 7b. The denominators are 10 and 25. The common denominator for any numbers must be a number that will divide both evenly. Therefore, the LCD must include the prime factorization of 10 and 25. We know that $10 = 2 \times 5$ and $25 = 5 \times 5$. To include all necessary factors, we need to include 5 twice and 2 once. Look at the illustration in Figure 1.1.

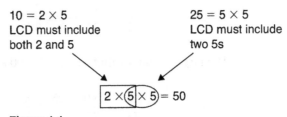

Figure 1.1

EXAMPLE 8: Finding the LCD Using Prime Factorization

Find the LCD for the fractions $\dfrac{1}{6}, \dfrac{1}{4},$ and $\dfrac{2}{15}$.

Solution

Factor each denominator into its prime factors to obtain the LCD.

$$4 = 2 \times 2 \qquad 6 = 2 \times 3 \qquad 15 = 3 \times 5$$

$$\text{LCD} = (2 \times 2 \times 3 \times 5) = 60$$

By multiplying these prime factors, we arrive at the LCD of 60.

## Chapter 1

Ordering Fractions

In health care fields, the comparison of fractions is necessary when sizes of medical items or pieces of equipment are being calculated. For example, if you need to place surgical instruments in order for a surgeon prior to surgery, you need to understand the size relationships of the instruments. This can be done using common denominators. Recall the mathematical symbols, $<$, $>$, and $=$. Look at how they are used in the following statements:

$$5 \text{ is less than } 15 \rightarrow 5 < 15$$

$$12 \text{ is greater than } 2 \rightarrow 12 > 2$$

$$\frac{100}{50} \text{ is equal to } 2 \rightarrow \frac{100}{50} = 2$$

If you are asked to determine the relationship among fractions with different denominators, find the least common denominator for the given fractions, convert them to equivalent fractions, and then determine their order using the values of the numerator. This process is demonstrated in Example 9.

EXAMPLE 9: Ordering Fractions

Determine the correct order of the given fractions in descending order.

$$\frac{3}{8}, \frac{3}{5}$$

Solution

The number 8 is the largest denominator but it is not divisible by 5. If we factor 8 into primes we have $2 \times 2 \times 2$. The number 5 is itself a prime number, so in order to build the LCD we will need all factors of 8 and the number 5. This gives us $2 \times 2 \times 2 \times 5 = 40$ as the least common denominator. Now find equivalent fractions for these numbers using 40 as the denominator.

$$\frac{3}{8} = \frac{3 \cdot 5}{8 \cdot 5} = \frac{15}{40} \qquad \frac{3}{5} = \frac{3 \cdot 8}{5 \cdot 8} = \frac{24}{40}$$

Comparing the numerators of the fractions having the common denominator 40, it is easy to see that $\frac{24}{40} > \frac{15}{40}$, so $\frac{3}{5} > \frac{3}{8}$.

Adding and Subtracting Fractions

When adding or subtracting fractions, the denominators of the fractions must be alike. For example, in order to add $\frac{1}{2}$ and $\frac{1}{4}$, both fractions must be expressed in fourths in order for them to be combined. Once the common denominators have been determined and equivalent fractions have been calculated, add or subtract *only* the numerators when completing the problem.

EXAMPLE 10: Addition and Subtraction of Fractions

a. Add $\frac{1}{2}$ and $\frac{3}{5}$ and simplify the final answer.

Solution

The smallest multiple of 5 that is divisible by 2 is 10, so this is the least common denominator (LCD).

$$\frac{1}{2} = \frac{1 \cdot 5}{2 \cdot 5} = \frac{5}{10}$$
$$+ \frac{3}{5} = \frac{3 \cdot 2}{5 \cdot 2} = \frac{6}{10}$$
$$\frac{11}{10} = 1\frac{1}{10}$$

b. Subtract $\frac{2}{3}$ from $\frac{3}{4}$ and simplify the final answer.

Solution

The smallest multiple of 4 that is divisible by 3 is 12, so 12 is the LCD.

$$\frac{3}{4} = \frac{3 \cdot 3}{4 \cdot 3} = \frac{9}{12}$$

$$-\frac{2}{3} = \frac{2 \cdot 4}{3 \cdot 4} = \frac{8}{12}$$

$$\frac{1}{12}$$

EXAMPLE 11: Addition and Subtraction of Mixed Numbers

    a. Add $5\frac{3}{4} + 3\frac{9}{10}$ and simplify if needed.

Solution

Using prime factors, $4 = 2 \times 2$ and $10 = 2 \times 5$, so the LCD is $2 \times 2 \times 5 = 20$. Now we find equivalent fractions and add the whole numbers together and the fractions together. In this problem, the resulting fraction is an improper fraction. To determine the final answer, we simplify the improper fraction and add the whole number to that answer.

$$5\frac{3}{4} = 5\frac{3 \cdot 5}{4 \cdot 5} = 5\frac{15}{20}$$

$$+ 3\frac{9}{10} = 3\frac{9 \cdot 2}{10 \cdot 2} = 3\frac{18}{20}$$

$$8\frac{33}{20} = 8 + 1\frac{13}{20} = 9\frac{13}{20}$$

    b. Subtract $4\frac{2}{3} - 1\frac{1}{2}$ and simplify if needed.

Solution

The LCD for prime numbers 3 and 2 is the number $2 \times 3 = 6$. Find the equivalent fractions. Then, subtract the fractions and subtract the whole numbers to get the final answer.

$$4\frac{2}{3} = 4\frac{2 \cdot 2}{3 \cdot 2} = 4\frac{4}{6}$$

$$-1\frac{1}{2} = 1\frac{1 \cdot 3}{2 \cdot 3} = 1\frac{3}{6}$$

$$3\frac{1}{6}$$

Subtraction of fractions sometime involves borrowing. Look at the two problems in Example 12.

EXAMPLE 12: Subtraction of Mixed Numbers Requiring Borrowing

    a. Subtract $5 - 2\frac{3}{5}$.

Solution

Since 5 is a whole number, we will need to borrow 1 from 5 and turn it into a fraction in order to subtract the $\frac{3}{5}$. Recall that $1 = \frac{2}{2}, \frac{3}{3}, \frac{4}{4}, \frac{5}{5}, \ldots$, so we will use the fractional equivalent that has the same denominator as the fraction in our problem, $\frac{5}{5}$.

$$5 = 4\frac{5}{5}$$
$$-2\frac{3}{5} = 2\frac{3}{5}$$
$$\overline{\quad\quad 2\frac{2}{5}}$$

b. Subtract $15\frac{1}{3} - 9\frac{5}{8}$ and simplify if needed.

Solution

The LCD for the 3 and 8 is 24. We will first write the problem with equivalent fractions.

$$15\frac{1}{3} = 15\frac{1\cdot 8}{3\cdot 8} = 15\frac{8}{24}$$
$$-9\frac{5}{8} = 9\frac{5\cdot 3}{8\cdot 3} = 9\frac{15}{24}$$

Because $\frac{15}{24}$ is larger than $\frac{8}{24}$, we will need to borrow 1 from the 15 in the form $\frac{24}{24}$ and combine it with $\frac{8}{24}$ in order to complete the problem.

$$15\frac{8}{24} = 14\frac{24}{24} + \frac{8}{24} = 14\frac{32}{24}$$
$$-9\frac{15}{24} = 9\frac{15}{24} \quad\quad = 9\frac{15}{24}$$
$$\overline{\quad\quad\quad\quad\quad\quad\quad\quad\quad 5\frac{17}{24}}$$

Multiplication and Division of Fractions

To multiply fractions, multiply the numerators together to get the new numerator and multiply the denominators together to get the new denominator. If the problem involves mixed numbers, convert the mixed numbers to improper fractions and then multiply. To divide fractions, use the property of reciprocals that tells us to multiply the first fraction by the **reciprocal**, or multiplicative inverse, of the second fraction, or divisor. Recall that the reciprocal of $\frac{2}{3}$ is $\frac{3}{2}$. If there is a whole number in the problem, make it into a fraction by using a 1 as the denominator of the fraction. The use of common denominators is not required for the operations of multiplication and division.

EXAMPLE 13: Multiplication and Division of Fractions

a. Multiply and simplify the final answer. $\dfrac{2}{3} \cdot 2\dfrac{3}{4} = ?$

Solution

Change the mixed number to an improper fraction, multiply, and then reduce and simplify the answer.

$$\frac{2}{3} \cdot 2\frac{3}{4} =$$

$$\frac{2}{3} \cdot \frac{11}{4} = \frac{22}{12} \qquad \text{Change mixed number to an improper fraction and multiply.}$$

$$\frac{22}{12} = \frac{22 \div 2}{12 \div 2} = \frac{11}{6} = 1\frac{5}{6} \qquad \text{Reduce and simplify the answer to a mixed number.}$$

b. Divide and simplify the final answer. $2\dfrac{4}{5} \div 10 = ?$

Solution

Change the mixed number, $2\frac{4}{5}$, to an improper fraction and put a 1 under the 10. Use the reciprocal of the divisor by inverting $\frac{10}{1}$ to $\frac{1}{10}$, multiply, and then reduce the answer.

$$2\frac{4}{5} \div 10 =$$

$$\frac{14}{5} \div \frac{10}{1} = \qquad \text{Change mixed number and whole number to fractions.}$$

$$\frac{14}{5} \cdot \frac{1}{10} = \frac{14}{50} \qquad \text{Use the reciprocal of the second fraction and multiply.}$$

$$\frac{14}{50} = \frac{14 \div 2}{50 \div 2} = \frac{7}{25} \qquad \text{Reduce the fraction.}$$

When multiplying fractions, many people use cancellation during the process to make multiplying fractions easier and quicker. To cancel during the multiplication process, divide one number in the numerator and a second number in the denominator by their greatest common factor. For example, you could work problem *a* in Example 13 using cancellation as follows.

$$\frac{2}{3} \cdot 2\frac{3}{4} = ?$$

$$\frac{2}{3} \cdot \frac{11}{4} = \qquad \text{Change mixed number to improper form.}$$

$$\frac{\overset{1}{\cancel{2}}}{3} \cdot \frac{11}{\underset{2}{\cancel{4}}} = \qquad \text{Use cancellation dividing by 2.}$$

$$\frac{1}{3} \cdot \frac{11}{2} = \frac{11}{6} = 1\frac{5}{6} \qquad \text{Multiply and simplify the improper fraction.}$$

Cancellation allows the reducing of the components of the multiplication problems resulting in smaller numbers to multiply and usually a completely reduced result. However, please note this potential error. Cancellation is *only* valid for multiplication problems—not for addition or subtraction. In division problems, cancellation should only be used after the second fraction has been reciprocated and the operation has been changed to multiplication.

Complex Fractions

A complex fraction is a fraction within a fraction. Nurses and pharmacy technicians use complex fraction to compute exact dosages. Examples of complex fractions are $\dfrac{\frac{1}{4}}{5}$ and $\dfrac{\frac{3}{4}}{\frac{2}{3}}$.

You should view these problems as division problems. For example, $\frac{\frac{1}{4}}{5} = \frac{1}{4} \div 5$ and $\frac{\frac{3}{4}}{\frac{2}{3}} = \frac{3}{4} \div \frac{2}{3}$.

EXAMPLE 14: Simplifying Complex Fractions

Simplify the complex fraction $\dfrac{\frac{1}{2}}{\frac{1}{100}}$ and reduce the answer.

Solution

Rewrite the fraction as a division problem, invert the divisor, and multiply.

$$\frac{\frac{1}{2}}{\frac{1}{100}} = \frac{1}{2} \div \frac{1}{100} = \qquad \text{Rewrite as a division problem.}$$

$$\frac{1}{2} \cdot \frac{100}{1} = \frac{100}{2} = 50 \qquad \text{Reciprocate, multiply, and reduce.}$$

Dosage calculations will require the use of complex fractions in problems with whole numbers and decimals. Look at this example of a more complicated calculation involving a complex fraction.

EXAMPLE 15: Problems Involving Complex Fractions

Complete the following problem: $\dfrac{\frac{1}{200}}{\frac{1}{100}} \times 25 = ?$

Solution

Rewrite the complex fraction as a division problem, simplify it, and then multiply by 25.

$$\frac{\frac{1}{200}}{\frac{1}{100}} \times 25 = \left(\frac{1}{200} \div \frac{1}{100} \right) \times 25 = \qquad \text{Write as a division problem.}$$

$$\left(\frac{1}{\underset{2}{\cancel{200}}} \times \frac{\overset{1}{\cancel{100}}}{1} \right) \times 25 = \qquad \begin{array}{l} \text{Reciprocate the second fraction} \\ \text{and use cancellation dividing by 100.} \end{array}$$

$$= \frac{1}{2} \times 25 = 12\frac{1}{2} \qquad \text{Multiply and simplify.}$$

Using Calculators for Problems Involving Fractions

Problems involving fractions can be easily done using scientific calculators. The fraction key on a calculator is labeled $\boxed{a^b/_c}$. When entering a fraction like $\frac{3}{4}$ into a calculator, enter 3 then the fraction key and then 4. The display will look like 3 ⌋ 4. If you need to reduce a fraction, you can enter the fraction into the calculator using the fraction key and press =. The resulting fraction will be the reduced answer. If the original fraction is improper, the result will be a mixed number. For example, if you enter $\frac{10}{9}$ into the calculator as 10 $\boxed{a^b/_c}$ 9 =, the display will read 1 ⌐ 1 ⌋ 9, indicating $1\frac{1}{9}$.

For long arithmetic calculations, the calculator is programmed to follow the order of operations. For example, to complete this problem using a calculator, follow the steps as indicated.

$$2\frac{1}{2} + \frac{3}{10} \times \frac{1}{4} = 2\;\boxed{a^b/_c}\;1\;\boxed{a^b/_c}\;2 + 3\;\boxed{a^b/_c}\;10 \times 1\;\boxed{a^b/_c}\;4 = 2\_23\rfloor40$$

This display represents the answer $2\frac{23}{40}$.

A complete understanding of operations with fractions will be an important asset to all health care providers. For example, exposure to X-rays is measured in units called *roentgens*. A patient might receive $\frac{1}{2}$ a roentgen for an X-ray exposure. Radiology assistants use fractions for exposure factors, that is, decreasing or increasing an exposure.

Nursing assistants use fractions to estimate the amount of a meal a resident consumes. Since many residents don't completely finish all items on their plates, the use of fractions is necessary to determine the amount to be recorded. For example, $\frac{1}{2}$ of a 3-oz serving of meat is $\frac{1}{2} \times 3$ oz $= 1\frac{1}{2}$ oz. An understanding of fractions is also important to medical assistants and nursing assistants who measure the heights and weights of patients before they see a doctor or the weights of residents in a nursing facility.

The preparation of medications by health care providers requires knowledge of fractions as dosages are calculated. Most drug dosage calculations involve a problem that contains from one to five common fractions. If a dosage is given using the apothecary system, it is not unusual for fractions to be used. For example, if a medication label reads gr $\frac{1}{8}$ and a dosage of gr $\frac{1}{4}$ is prescribed for the patient, division of fractions can be used to calculate the number of tablets needed ($\frac{1}{4} \div \frac{1}{8} = \frac{1}{4} \times \frac{8}{1} = 2$ tablets). A more complete explanation of dosage calculations will be given in Chapter 4.

EXAMPLE 16: Measuring Weight

Residents at White Oak Manor are weighed monthly. At the end of June, Mae weighed $110\frac{1}{2}$ lb. By the end of July, she had gained $2\frac{1}{4}$ lb. What was the weight recorded for Mae at the end of July?

Solution

Find a common denominator for the fractions and add.

$$110\frac{1}{2} = 110\frac{2}{4}\text{ lb}$$

$$+2\frac{1}{4} = +2\frac{1}{4}\text{ lb}$$

$$112\frac{3}{4}\text{ lb should be recorded as Mae's weight}$$

Though many measurements today are done with digital instruments giving values in decimals, the use of fractions in daily health care is still required. A thorough understanding of fractions and operations with fractions will make your work as a health care provider more efficient and accurate.

PRACTICE PROBLEM SET 1.2

Reduce the following fractions to lowest terms. Simplify improper fractions to mixed numbers.

1. $\dfrac{12}{16}$

2. $\dfrac{18}{24}$

3. $\dfrac{75}{175}$

4. $\dfrac{50}{225}$

5. $\dfrac{20}{19}$

6. $\dfrac{23}{21}$

7. $\dfrac{56}{18}$

8. $\dfrac{75}{60}$

Give the least common denominator (LCD) for the following sets of fractions.

9. $\dfrac{2}{5}, \dfrac{11}{25}$

10. $\dfrac{7}{18}, \dfrac{1}{6}$

11. $\dfrac{1}{2}, \dfrac{1}{5}$

12. $\dfrac{2}{3}, \dfrac{5}{8}$

13. $\dfrac{4}{5}, \dfrac{2}{3}, \dfrac{3}{10}$

14. $\dfrac{3}{4}, \dfrac{1}{9}, \dfrac{7}{12}$

Determine the correct order of the following fractions in descending order.

15. $\dfrac{1}{3}, \dfrac{1}{2}, \dfrac{1}{6}$

16. $\dfrac{1}{4}, \dfrac{1}{12}, \dfrac{1}{6}$

17. $\dfrac{2}{3}, \dfrac{2}{5}, \dfrac{3}{10}$

18. $\dfrac{5}{8}, \dfrac{4}{9}, \dfrac{1}{3}$

19. $\dfrac{1}{2}, \dfrac{3}{5}, \dfrac{1}{8}, \dfrac{3}{4}$

20. $\dfrac{1}{4}, \dfrac{2}{5}, \dfrac{3}{8}, \dfrac{1}{10}$

Perform the following operations with fractions and simplify the answers completely.

21. $\dfrac{5}{8} + \dfrac{3}{5}$

22. $\dfrac{2}{3} + \dfrac{3}{10}$

23. $\dfrac{5}{12} + \dfrac{7}{8}$

24. $\dfrac{5}{6} + \dfrac{13}{15}$

25. $11\dfrac{1}{3} + 2\dfrac{1}{2}$

26. $4\dfrac{2}{5} + 1\dfrac{1}{4}$

27. $6\dfrac{5}{6} + 3\dfrac{8}{9}$

28. $5\dfrac{3}{4} + 15\dfrac{7}{8}$

29. $7\dfrac{9}{10} + 5\dfrac{3}{4}$

30. $12\dfrac{2}{3} + 4\dfrac{4}{5}$

31. $\dfrac{11}{12} - \dfrac{2}{3}$

32. $\dfrac{7}{8} - \dfrac{1}{4}$

33. $\dfrac{13}{15} - \dfrac{3}{10}$

34. $\dfrac{17}{18} - \dfrac{5}{24}$

35. $7 - 3\dfrac{3}{4}$

36. $25 - 4\dfrac{9}{10}$

37. $9\dfrac{3}{8} - 2\dfrac{14}{15}$

38. $16\dfrac{1}{10} - 3\dfrac{11}{12}$

39. $\dfrac{3}{4} \times \dfrac{4}{9}$

40. $\dfrac{5}{6} \times \dfrac{3}{10}$

41. $\dfrac{7}{8} \times 21$

42. $\dfrac{4}{10} \times 36$

43. $1\dfrac{2}{3} \times 2\dfrac{7}{10}$

44. $5\dfrac{5}{8} \times 3\dfrac{2}{5}$

45. $\dfrac{5}{6} \div \dfrac{7}{12}$

46. $\dfrac{4}{5} \div \dfrac{8}{25}$

47. $2\dfrac{1}{4} \div 18$

48. $5\dfrac{3}{4} \div 2$

49. $1\dfrac{5}{8} \div 2\dfrac{1}{12}$

50. $3\dfrac{1}{3} \div 6\dfrac{5}{8}$

Complete the problems containing complex fractions and simplify the final answers.

51. $\dfrac{\frac{2}{3}}{\frac{5}{6}}$

52. $\dfrac{\frac{3}{8}}{\frac{11}{12}}$

53. $\dfrac{\frac{3}{125}}{5}$

54. $\dfrac{\frac{1}{100}}{25}$

55. $\dfrac{\frac{3}{200}}{\frac{1}{100}} \times 50$

56. $\dfrac{\frac{12}{25}}{\frac{1}{200}} \times 25$

57. $\dfrac{\frac{3}{50}}{\frac{6}{75}} \times 125$

58. $\dfrac{\frac{15}{200}}{\frac{1}{50}} \times 100$

Work each of the following word problems. Give answers in lowest terms.

59. Your job is to prepare medications to administer to the patients on the floor this morning. Each patient's dose of a particular medication is $1\dfrac{1}{4}$ oz and 16 patients are to receive this medication. How much total medication is needed?

60. As a medication aide, you need to administer 26 doses of a particular medication. Each dose is $1\frac{1}{3}$ oz. If you only have a 32-oz bottle of medication in stock, is there enough to administer all 26 doses?

61. As a nursing assistant, you record the intake of fluids for each patient during your shift. Mr. Hardison had $\frac{2}{3}$ of a 6-oz cup of coffee, $\frac{1}{2}$ of an 8-oz glass of water, and $\frac{3}{4}$ of a 4-oz juice carton. How many ounces of liquid did he consume during your shift? How many cc of liquid is this?

62. It is your job to chart the amount of food consumed by the residents on your hall. At dinner, Mrs. Dalton ate $\frac{1}{3}$ of a 3-oz serving of meat loaf, $\frac{3}{4}$ of a 3-oz serving of mashed potatoes, $\frac{3}{4}$ of a 1-oz serving of gravy, and $\frac{1}{4}$ of a 2-oz serving of green beans. She also ate $\frac{1}{2}$ of a 1-oz serving of bread and all of her 3-oz serving of cake. How many ounces of solid food did Mrs. Dalton consume at dinner?

63. As a dietary services worker, you are supposed to make the desserts for lunch. You are preparing four sheet cakes and a triple batch of brownies. How much cooking oil will you need if one cake requires $2\frac{1}{4}$ cups of oil and one batch of brownies requires $1\frac{1}{2}$ cups of oil?

64. Your job is to prepare the soup for lunch today. Each $\frac{1}{2}$ gallon of soup requires $2\frac{1}{4}$ cups of beef stock. How much beef stock will you use to make 6 gallons of soup?

65. It takes $1\frac{3}{4}$ teaspoons of cinnamon to make one batch of snickerdoodle cookies. You are preparing four batches for tomorrow's snack. How much cinnamon will you need?

66. To sweeten tea for the residents' supper, you use $\frac{3}{4}$ cup of sweetener per gallon. If you prepare 6 gallons of tea, how much sweetener will you use?

67. When Joshua came to Blackwell Nursing Facility at the beginning of May, he weighed 230 lb. At the end of May he had lost $3\frac{1}{4}$ lb. At the end of June he had gained back $1\frac{3}{4}$ lb and at the end of July he had lost another $2\frac{1}{2}$ lb. How much does Joshua weigh at the end of July?

68. A patient is put on a diet to lose 35 lb in six months. He loses $8\frac{3}{4}$ lb the first month, $5\frac{1}{2}$ lb the second month, and $6\frac{1}{4}$ lb the third month. How much more weight does he need to lose to meet his goal at the end of six months?

69. Nationally, there are about 1,375,000 people working as nursing assistants. About one-half of these work in nursing and personal care facilities. How many nursing assistants work in nursing and personal care facilities?

70. There are 250 American Dental Association accredited dental assisting education programs in the United States. If $\frac{3}{50}$ of those programs are located in North Carolina, how many accredited programs are in North Carolina?

SECTION 1.3 A REVIEW OF OPERATIONS WITH DECIMALS

Much of the work done in health care settings will involve the use of decimal numbers. Many instruments are digital and give decimal readouts as you monitor patients. Medication dosages measured in milligrams, micrograms, or milliliters may be given in decimal amounts. Updating patient records as well as billing and bookkeeping will also require the use of decimals. Therefore, it is important to be comfortable with calculations done using decimals.

Place Value

Decimal numbers are equivalent to fractions with denominators of 10, 100, 1000, etc. Look at the value of each digit in the decimal number in Figure 1.2. The whole number is found to the left of the decimal point and the fractional part of the number is to the right of the decimal point. In the number shown in Figure 1.2, 150 is the whole-number part of the decimal number, and 2785 ten-thousandths is the fractional part of the decimal number.

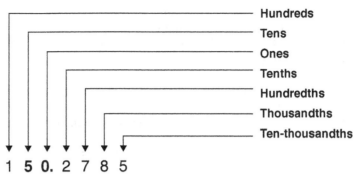

Figure 1.2 Place Value in Decimal Numbers

If a decimal number is less than 1, then a 0 is used in the ones place in front of the decimal to emphasize the fact that the number is a fraction. $\left(\dfrac{1}{2} = 0.5\right)$

Changing a Decimal to a Fraction

To find a fractional equivalent for a decimal number, note the place value held by the last digit in the number. Then use the number associated with that digit as the denominator for the fraction. For example, to change the decimal number 0.15 to a fraction, put 15 over 100 (5 is in the hundredths place) and reduce: $\dfrac{15}{100} = \dfrac{3}{20}$.

EXAMPLE 17: Changing Decimals to Fractions

Change these decimal numbers to fractions and simplify if needed.

a. 0.0125　　　　b. 0.003　　　　c. 25.02

Solution

a. The 5 is in the ten-thousandths place, so $0.0125 = \dfrac{125}{10000} = \dfrac{1}{80}$.

b. The 3 is in the thousandths place, so $0.003 = \dfrac{3}{1000}$.

c. The 2 is in the hundredths place. This decimal has a whole number (25) and a fractional part (.02), so the result will be the mixed number $25\dfrac{2}{100} = 25\dfrac{1}{50}$.

Operations Using Decimal Numbers

The addition and subtraction of decimals is a very straightforward process using the same operational rules that you used with whole numbers. The important thing to remember when adding or subtracting decimals is to line up the decimal points before you begin combining the numbers. Writing your problem vertically will make the problem easier to work. Remember that all whole numbers have an "invisible" decimal point located to the right of the ones place in the number.

To multiply decimal numbers, ignore the decimals and multiply the numbers in the same way you would multiply whole numbers. It is not necessary to line up the decimals when writing down the problem. To finish the problem, count the total number of decimal places contained in the two numbers being multiplied together. Using this total, count that number of places from right to left in the answer to locate the decimal point.

When dividing a decimal number by another decimal number, we must first make the divisor (the number that you are dividing with) into a whole number by moving the decimal point as many places to the right as is necessary to make it into a whole number. Then, in order to keep the values of the numbers equivalent, we must also move the decimal point in the dividend (the number that is to be divided) the same number of places to the right. Divide the numbers and place the decimal in the answer above its final location in the dividend. If you are dividing by a whole number, simply bring the decimal straight up in the answer and divide as usual.

For example, in the problem $1.25 \div 2.5$, the number 2.5 is the divisor. In order to make it into a whole number, we move the decimal one place to the right. The next step is to move the decimal in the dividend (1.25) one place to the right also.

$$2.5\overline{)1.25} = 25\overline{)12.5}$$

Continue the problem by dividing by 25. The decimal in the answer will then be located directly above its location in the 12.5 giving an answer of 0.5.

EXAMPLE 18: Operations with Decimal Numbers

Perform the following computations:

    a. $5 + 8.5 + 0.018 + 2.18 =$

    b. $2.57 - 1.003 =$

    c. $2.045 \times 13.18 =$

    d. $4.375 \div 1.25 =$

Solution

    a. Line up the decimals first and then add. Bring the decimal point straight down into the answer.

$$
\begin{array}{r}
5. \\
8.5 \\
0.018 \\
+2.18 \\
\hline
15.698
\end{array}
$$

    b. Line up the decimals first. Add enough zeros as placeholders after the last digit in the minuend (the number you are subtracting from) before subtracting. Then subtract the numbers the same way that you subtract whole numbers and bring the decimal straight down into your answer.

$$
\begin{array}{r}
2.57 \\
-1.003 \\
\hline
\end{array}
=
\begin{array}{r}
2.570 \\
-1.003 \\
\hline
1.567
\end{array}
\quad \leftarrow \quad \text{Add a 0 after the 7 as a placeholder.}
$$

    c. Multiply the numbers and count the total number of decimal places.

$$
\begin{array}{r}
2.045 \\
\times 13.18 \\
\hline
16360 \\
2045 \\
6135 \\
2045 \\
\hline
26.95310
\end{array}
\quad
\begin{array}{l}
\rightarrow \text{ 3 decimal places} \\
\rightarrow \text{ 2 decimal places} \\
\\
\\
\\
\\
\rightarrow \text{ 5 decimal places}
\end{array}
$$

    d. In division, move the decimal in the divisor and the dividend.

$$1.25\overline{)4.375} = 125\overline{)437.5} \quad \begin{array}{r} 3.5 \\ \hline \end{array}$$

$$\begin{array}{r} 3.5 \\ 125\overline{)437.5} \\ -\,375 \\ \hline 625 \\ -\,625 \\ \hline \end{array}$$

Move decimal two places to the right and divide.

Calculators will make your calculations speedier and often more accurate. However, since calculators are not always available, you should become familiar with these rules. If you do use a calculator, familiarity with these rules will also help you judge if your calculator has given you a reasonable answer.

Rounding Decimals

When working with decimals in health care, it is often necessary to round off numbers to make them more manageable. Whether you round to a whole number, tenths place, hundredths place, or thousandths place will depend on the requirements of the problem and the precision necessary. Here we will briefly review the arithmetic rules used for rounding decimals.

Rounding Rules

To round a number to a certain place:

1. Locate the digit in that place.
2. Look at the digit to the right of that place.
3. If the digit immediately to the right is 5 or more, round up; if the digit immediately to the right is 4 or less, drop the extra digits and do not round up.

EXAMPLE 19: Rounding Decimal Numbers

Round the following numbers:

a. 0.416 to hundredths place
b. 1.048 to tenths place
c. 248.546 to hundreds place

Solution

a. 0.416 to hundredths place
      ↑

Locate the digit 1 in the hundredths place. To the right of this number is 6. Since 6 > 5, we drop the 6 and round the 1 up to a 2. The correctly rounded answer is 0.42.

b. 1.048 to tenths place
     ↑

Locate the number 0 in the tenths place. To the right of this number is 4. Since 4 < 5, drop the extra digits and leave the 0 in the tenths place. The correctly rounded answer is 1.0.

The 0 is necessary in the rounded answer to indicate that rounding has been done to the tenths place. If you write 1, that indicates rounding has been done to the nearest whole number.

c. 2̣48.546 to hundreds

Locate the number 2 in the hundreds place (not hundred*ths*!). The number to the right of 2 is 4, so we will drop the 4 and all numbers to the right of the 4. The correctly rounded answer is 200.

Comparing Decimals

In health occupations, many different pieces of equipment used may give metric measurements. The metric system is based on powers of 10 and is, therefore, a decimal-based measurement system. Understanding the relationship among decimal numbers is important to determine which instrument or measurement is smaller or larger. To compare decimals accurately, write all decimals with the same number of decimal places by adding zeros to the end of each decimal number. This is equivalent to finding a common denominator since you will be expressing all numbers given in hundredths or thousandths. Look at the problem in Example 20.

EXAMPLE 20: Comparing Decimals

Which is larger, 0.082 or 0.12?

Solution

The first number has three decimal places and the second has only two decimal places. Therefore, in order to write both numbers with the same number of decimal places, we will add a 0 to the number 0.12. Now compare the numbers.

$$0.082 \rightarrow \text{eighty-two thousandths}$$

$$0.120 \rightarrow \text{one-hundred twenty thousandths}$$

It is easy to conclude that $0.12 > 0.082$.

Changing Fractions to Decimal Numbers

Calculations performed with decimal numbers are often much easier to do than calculations done with fractions. Therefore, it is a good idea to know how to change a fraction to its decimal equivalent. The bar in a fraction represents the operation of division, so in order to change a fraction to a decimal, we divide the numerator of the fraction by its denominator. Answers will either be exact decimals or repeating decimals. For example, $\frac{7}{8} = 7 \div 8 = 0.875$ and $\frac{1}{6} = 1 \div 6 = 0.16666\ldots$. Although changing a fraction to a decimal is a simple calculation, especially using a calculator, the following table gives several fraction/decimal equivalents that you should strive to remember. Knowing these equivalents can make your mental calculations as a health care worker easier when working with fractions and decimals.

Table 1.2 Fraction/Decimal Equivalents

$\frac{1}{5} = 0.2$	$\frac{2}{5} = 0.4$	$\frac{3}{5} = 0.6$	$\frac{4}{5} = 0.8$
$\frac{1}{4} = 0.25$	$\frac{2}{4} = \frac{1}{2} = 0.5$		$\frac{3}{4} = 0.75$
$\frac{1}{3} = 0.3333\ldots$		$\frac{2}{3} = 0.6666\ldots$	
$\frac{1}{2} = 0.5$			

In Section 1.5, we will examine more closely fraction/decimal equivalents and their relationship to numbers given as percents.

Many situations that a health care provider encounters daily will require the use of decimal numbers. This may include calculating your gross pay for a 35-hour workweek, administering certain dosages of medication, monitoring grams of fat in a meal, or reading a thermometer. Look at the operations using decimals in the following examples.

EXAMPLE 21: Calculating Wages

In Minnesota, the median wage for nursing assistants is $11.30 per hour. Nationally, the median wage is $9.59 per hour.

a. How much higher is the median wage in Minnesota than the national median average?

Solution

Since you are asked to find a difference, this is a subtraction problem.

$$\begin{array}{r} \$11.30 \\ -\ 9.59 \\ \hline \$\ 1.71 \end{array}$$

The median hourly wage in Minnesota is $1.71 more than the national median.

b. If a nursing assistant in Minnesota works 40 hours in a week and is paid $11.30 per hour, what is her gross pay for the week?

Solution

This is a multiplication problem. Count two decimal places in the answer.

$$40 \text{ hours} \times \$11.30/\text{hour} = \$452.00$$

Her gross pay for a 40-hour week is $452.00.

EXAMPLE 22: Calculating Medication Dosages

Mr. Queen receives 2.25 g of medication daily. Tablets come in 0.75 g dosages. How many tablets will he need to take each day?

Solution

Mr. Queen's total medication requirements are larger than the dosage in a single pill. So, it will take more than one pill to ensure the proper dosage is given. Therefore, we will divide the 2.25-g total by 0.75 g to determine how many tablets that size are required. (This problem is easily done with a calculator.)

$$2.25 \text{ g} \div 0.75 \text{ g/tablet} =$$

$$0.75\overline{)2.25} =$$

move the decimal

$$\begin{array}{r} 3 \\ 75\overline{)225} \\ -225 \\ \hline 0 \end{array}$$

Mr. Queen will take 3 tablets daily in order to receive 2.25 g of medication.

PRACTICE PROBLEM SET 1.3

Change these decimal numbers to fractions and simplify if needed.

1. 0.4	5. 0.113	9. 0.0025	13. 3.0001
2. 0.6	6. 0.007	10. 0.0125	14. 5.0003
3. 0.15	7. 0.825	11. 16.125	
4. 0.75	8. 0.375	12. 25.875	

Perform the following calculations.

15. $3.52 + 2.035 + 1.2$	21. $28.9 - 13.253$	27. $0.648 \div 2.7$
16. $5.6 + 3.871 + 2.36$	22. $55.12 - 32.275$	28. $0.396 \div 3.6$
17. $25.03 + 8 + 2.1152$	23. 3.75×2.006	29. $0.1344 \div 0.032$
18. $1.605 + 9.0001 + 3$	24. 5.0045×9.12	30. $0.1404 \div 0.052$
19. $16.03 - 2.5$	25. 25.1×0.35	
20. $15.287 - 12.33$	26. 35.2×0.002	

Round the numbers to the given place value.

31. 5.249	tenths	36. 2.30172	thousandths
32. 3.546	tenths	37. 10.613	whole number
33. 0.0267	hundredths	38. 15.751	whole number
34. 0.1208	hundredths	39. 1.998	tenths
35. 60.12574	thousandths	40. 5.975	tenths

Place the correct symbol, > or <, between the numbers.

41. 0.15	0.5	46. 6.05	6.035
42. 0.6	0.59	47. 0.33	0.3
43. 0.87	0.087	48. 0.85	0.805
44. 0.025	0.105	49. 3.98	3.89
45. 1.005	1.0008	50. 2.504	2.540

Solve the following word problems involving decimals.

51. The office checking account has a balance of $2143.57. In the mail, you receive payments of $210.50, $85.25, $126.75, $25.00, $198.56, and $28.25. What is the total amount of the deposit that you will make today using these payments? What is the new balance on the account after this deposit?

52. As the office manager, you pay the bills at the end of each week. The current balance in the checking account is $4529.56. You write checks to pay bills in the following amounts: $356.82, $76.93, $1250, $359.50. Find the total amount of the checks written. What is the new balance in the checkbook after you write these checks?

53. School cafeterias serve 1.9 million gallons of milk each day according to the American School Food Service Association. How many gallons of milk are served in school cafeterias during a five-day school week?

54. A sample of blood is collected from a patient. The pH of the blood is found to be 7.42. The same patient is tested the next day and his blood pH is then 7.38. What was the difference between the two blood pH measurements?

55. A patient is to receive 0.032 g of codeine sulfate. Each tablet contains 0.016 g of codeine sulfate. How many tablets should the patient be given?

56. A patient was given half of a gr 0.25 ephedrine sulfate tablet. How much medication did the patient receive?

57. A patient is to receive 0.025 g of medication 4 times a day. How many grams of medication will this patient receive in a seven-day period?

58. To give 0.5 mg of a medication using 0.25-mg tablets, how many tablets are needed?

59. If the pediatric dose of a certain medication is 1.5 mg for every 10 lb of body weight, how much medication should be given to a child who weighs 50 lb?

60. As a pharmacy technician, you are to measure 0.25 g of medication into unit dose oral containers. Your bulk container contains 350 g. How many containers can you prepare?

SECTION 1.4 A REVIEW OF OPERATIONS WITH PERCENTS

Knowledge of the meaning of percents can assist you in your health care profession. You will encounter percents in many areas, including, for example, the strengths of solutions for patient medication. The word **percent** means "out of 100." Any number written as a percent (%) means that many parts per 100 parts. For example, 12% means 12 parts per 100 parts. This can also be written $\frac{12}{100}$ or 0.12. The % symbol is a handy way to write fractions whose denominator is 100.

Conversions of percents to decimals or fractions may be necessary when carrying out calculations involving percents. Some calculators have percent keys, but the majority do not, so you will need to rely on your knowledge of equivalents to complete the required calculations. The following rules for conversions will assist you in your calculations.

Rule I: Changing a Percent to a Fraction

- Remove the % sign, multiply the number by $\frac{1}{100}$. (one-hundredth)
- Reduce the fraction.

$$5\% = 5 \times \frac{1}{100} = \frac{5}{100} = \frac{1}{20}$$

$$66\tfrac{2}{3}\% = 66\tfrac{2}{3} \times \frac{1}{100} = \frac{200}{3} \times \frac{1}{100} = \frac{2}{3}$$

Rule II: Changing a Percent to a Decimal

- Remove the % sign and multiply the number by 0.01. (one-hundredth)

$$2.5\% = 2.5 \times 0.01 = 0.025$$

$$0.001\% = 0.001 \times 0.01 = 0.00001$$

- The shortcut for this procedure is to remove the % sign and move the decimal two places to the left. Regardless of where the decimal is in the percent, it is moved exactly two places left when the % sign is removed. If the percent is a whole number, the decimal is understood to be to the right of the ones place.

$$0.005\% = 0.00005$$
$$125\% = 1.25$$

Rule III: Changing a Fraction or a Decimal to a Percent

- Multiply the fraction or decimal by 100 and add a % sign.

fraction to % : $\dfrac{3}{20} \times 100 = \dfrac{3}{20} \times \dfrac{100}{1} = \dfrac{300}{20} = 15\%$

decimal to % : $0.2 \times 100 = 20\%$

- Many times it is easier to change a fraction to a percent by first changing it to a decimal number and then multiplying it by 100. This is especially true when using a calculator for these conversions.

$$\frac{5}{8} = 5 \div 8 \times 100 = 0.625 \times 100 = 62.5\%$$

Remember that the % sign is very important in determining the value of the number. The percent symbol means "number of parts per 100." Don't confuse percents containing decimals with their decimal equivalents. Look at the differences in values of these three numbers.

$$2\% = \frac{2}{100} = 0.02 \qquad (2 \text{ out of } 100)$$

$$0.2\% = \frac{0.2}{100} = \frac{2}{1000} = 0.002 \qquad (0.2 \text{ out of } 100 \text{ or } 2 \text{ out of } 1{,}000)$$

$$0.02\% = \frac{0.02}{100} = \frac{2}{10000} = 0.0002 \qquad (0.02 \text{ out of } 100 \text{ or } 2 \text{ out of } 10{,}000)$$

Medications are manufactured in both pure and diluted forms. A pure drug contains only the drug with no diluting agent, but many drugs are in solution form, which is made by diluting some of the pure drug in a liquid. The percent strength of this solution gives the amount of pure drug per 100 parts of solution. The key to understanding the strength of any solution is to remember the definition of percents: parts per hundred. Pure drugs may be in the form of a solid or a liquid. Therefore, if a pure drug is in the form of a solid, a 1% solution means 1 part per 100 parts or 1 g of pure drug in 100 mL of solution. If the pure drug is in liquid form, a 1% solution means 1 mL of pure drug in 100 mL of solution.

Of course, you do not always have volumes of 100 mL. Therefore, knowledge of fractions and their conversions to percents will assist in determining the percent strength of a particular medication. Look at the following examples.

EXAMPLE 23: Finding the Strength of a Solution

Give the concentration or strength of a solution in percent form if the solution contains 15 parts solute in 75 parts total solution.

Solution

Remember, when setting up a ratio involving a solution, the denominator always represents the total volume of the solution. Rule III tells us to set up a fraction relating the parts and multiply by 100, adding a % sign to the answer. Either method of Rule III that you use for conversion of the fraction to a percent will give the correct percent concentration.

$$\text{Method 1:} \quad \frac{15 \text{ parts}}{75 \text{ parts}} \times 100 = \frac{1500}{75} = 20\%$$

$$\text{Method 2:} \quad \frac{15 \text{ parts}}{75 \text{ parts}} = 15 \div 75 \times 100 = 20\%$$

Therefore, a solution containing 15 parts solute in 75 parts solution has a concentration, or strength, of 20%.

EXAMPLE 24: Finding the Strength of a Medication

Give the % strength or concentration of a medication containing 15 mL of pure drug mixed with 35 mL of water.

Solution

This solution contains 15 mL of pure drug in 50 mL total solution (15 mL of the drug + 35 mL of water = 50 mL total solution). Now convert the fraction $\frac{15 \text{ mL}}{50 \text{ mL}}$ to a percent using Rule III for fractions.

$$\text{Method A:} \quad \frac{15 \text{ mL}}{50 \text{ mL}} = \frac{15}{50} \times \frac{100}{1} = 30\%$$

$$\text{Method B:} \quad \frac{15 \text{ mL}}{50 \text{ mL}} = 15 \div 50 \times 100 = 30\%$$

Therefore, a solution of 15 mL of pure drug mixed with 35 mL of water results in a medication having a strength, or concentration, of 30%.

In the next chapter we will examine the use of ratios and proportions to adjust the volumes of medications while retaining the proper strength. For example, if 25 mL of a particular 8% solution are needed, we will use our definition of percents and the properties of proportions to help us determine how many grams of solute will be required.

PRACTICE PROBLEM SET 1.4

Change each percent to a fraction. Reduce it to lowest terms.

1. 35%	3. 5%	5. $3\frac{1}{2}\%$
2. 65%	4. 2%	6. $25\frac{3}{4}\%$

Change each percent to a decimal.

7. 6%	10. 40%	13. 0.0012%	16. 6.25%
8. 9%	11. 0.04%	14. 0.00015%	17. 145%
9. 75%	12. 0.25%	15. 1.5%	18. 250%

Change each fraction or decimal to a percent.

19. $\dfrac{5}{8}$ 22. $\dfrac{5}{6}$ 25. 0.2 30. 0.000001

20. $\dfrac{1}{25}$ 23. $\dfrac{5}{4}$ 26. 0.1 31. 1.5

21. $\dfrac{1}{3}$ 24. $\dfrac{3}{2}$ 27. 0.375 32. 3.15

28. 0.005

29. 0.00125

Give the percent strength of each of the following solutions.

33. 100 total parts containing 12.5 parts pure drug
34. 100 mL containing 0.5 mL pure drug
35. 0.01 g pure drug in 10 mL of solution
36. $\frac{1}{2}$ mL of pure drug in 20 mL of total solution
37. 1 mL pure drug in 30 mL total solution
38. 2 mL pure drug in 15 mL total solution
39. 50 mL total solution containing 0.025 g of pure drug
40. 25 mL total solution containing 0.2 g of pure drug
41. 15 mL pure drug + 85 mL water
42. 5 mL pure drug + 20 mL water
43. 30 mL of pure drug mixed with 45 mL of water
44. 0.5 mL of pure drug mixed with 9.5 mL of water
45. What would be the concentration of a saline solution that contains 5 g of salt in 150 mL of water?
46. Two milliliters of acetic acid are mixed with 38 mL of water. What is the concentration of the resulting solution?
47. One gram of potassium permanganate solution is diluted in 20 mL of solution. What is the strength of this solution?
48. Forty grams of magnesium sulfate is diluted to make 200 mL of solution. What is the strength of this solution?

SECTION 1.5   CONVERSIONS AMONG FRACTIONS, DECIMALS, AND PERCENTS

To accomplish their daily tasks, health care workers must rely on a variety of mathematical skills. For example, medical dosage calculation requires knowledge of whole numbers, fractions, decimals, and percents. The ability to convert easily among these types of numbers will benefit workers in all areas of the allied health field.

In previous sections we have examined the properties of and operations with fractions, decimals, and percents. In this section, we will look at the relationships among these three types of numbers. Start by reviewing the rules given in Table 1.3.

Table 1.3 Rules for Conversion

To Change:	Use This Method:
Decimals to Fractions	Remove the decimal and place the number over a denominator equal to the place value of the last digit in the decimal.
Fractions to Decimals	Divide the numerator of the fraction by the denominator.
Decimals to Percents	Multiply the decimal by 100 and add the percent sign.
Fractions to Percents	Multiply the fraction by 100 and add the percent sign.
Percents to Decimals	Remove the percent sign and multiply by 0.01. The shortcut is to move the decimal two places left. Add zeros as placeholders if necessary.
Percents to Fractions	Remove the percent sign and put the number over 100. Reduce this fraction to lowest terms.

Familiarity with the rules of conversion will make mathematical calculations easier, especially when the numbers in a problem are given in different forms. For example, 1 kilogram (kg) equals approximately 2.2 lb. If a problem requires you to give the number of pounds equivalent to $2\frac{3}{4}$ kg, it would be easiest to write $2\frac{3}{4}$ kg as 2.75 kg and then multiply by 2.2 lb. Remembering those basic fraction/decimal equivalents listed in Section 1.3 can also make these problems quicker to complete.

Practice conversions between forms until you can complete the process accurately and easily. Using a calculator will make these conversions less tedious. However, a calculator can also be a fast way to get a wrong answer, because it cannot think for you. You must understand the rules in order to correctly calculate the equivalents even with a calculator. Look at the following examples of number conversions.

EXAMPLE 25: Finding a Fraction and a Percent Equivalent to a Given Decimal

Complete the table by filling in the correct fraction and percent equivalents.

FRACTION	DECIMAL	PERCENT
	0.02	

Solution

a. Change 0.02 into a percent by multiplying it by 100 and adding a % sign.

$$0.02 \times 100 = 2\%$$

b. Change 0.02 to a fraction by putting 2 over 100, since 2 is in the hundredths place. Then reduce the fraction.

$$\frac{2}{100} = \frac{2 \div 2}{100 \div 2} = \frac{1}{50}$$

Answers:

FRACTION	DECIMAL	PERCENT
$\frac{1}{50}$	0.02	2%

EXAMPLE 26: Finding a Fraction and a Decimal Equivalent to a Given Percent

Complete the table by filling in the correct fraction and decimal equivalents.

FRACTION	DECIMAL	PERCENT
		1.5%

Solution

a. Change 1.5% to a decimal number by removing the % sign and moving the decimal two places to the left. Add zeros as placeholders.

$$1.5\% = 01.5 = 0.015$$

b. Change 1.5% to a fraction by putting 1.5 over 100 and simplifying.

$$\frac{1.5}{100} = \frac{1.5 \times 10}{100 \times 10} = \frac{15}{1000} = \frac{15 \div 5}{1000 \div 5} = \frac{3}{200}$$

An alternative to this method is to use the decimal equivalent 0.015 to write the fraction $\dfrac{15}{1000}$ and reduce.

Answers:

FRACTION	DECIMAL	PERCENT
$\dfrac{3}{200}$	0.015	1.5%

EXAMPLE 27: Finding a Percent and a Decimal Equivalent to a Given Fraction

Complete the table by filling in the correct decimal and percent equivalents.

FRACTION	DECIMAL	PERCENT
$\dfrac{3}{20}$		

Solution

a. Change $\dfrac{3}{20}$ to a decimal by dividing 3 by 20.

$$3 \div 20 = 0.15$$

b. Change $\dfrac{3}{20}$ to a percent by multiplying it by 100 and adding the % sign.

$$\frac{3}{20} \times 100 = \frac{300}{20} = 15\%$$

Another way to easily find the equivalent percent is to use the decimal equivalent, 0.15, move the decimal two places to the right, and add the % sign.

Answers:

FRACTION	DECIMAL	PERCENT
$\dfrac{3}{20}$	0.15	15%

EXAMPLE 28: Conversions in Medical Applications

a. The National Center for Health Statistics reports that according to a recent study, 4 out of 10 visits to U.S. hospital emergency rooms were for an injury.

Write this number as a fraction and as a percent.

Solution

As a fraction, 4 out of 10 becomes the number $\dfrac{4}{10}$, or $\dfrac{2}{5}$.

Change the number $\dfrac{2}{5}$ to a percent by multiplying it by 100.

$$\frac{2}{5} \times 100 = \frac{200}{5} = 40\%$$

b. Some drugs have a suggested dosage based on the body surface area (BSA) of a patient. If a patient has a BSA of 0.85 m², write this number as a fraction.

Solution

Because this is a two-decimal-place number, we put the 85 over 100 and reduce.

$$0.85 = \frac{85}{100} = \frac{85 \div 5}{100 \div 5} = \frac{17}{20}$$

c. You are asked to prepare a 7.5% dextrose solution using D_5W and $D_{10}W$. Write this percent as an equivalent fraction and decimal.

Solution

$$\text{Fraction: } 7.5\% = \frac{7.5}{100} = \frac{7.5 \times 10}{100 \times 10} = \frac{75}{1000} = \frac{3}{40}$$

$$\text{Decimal: } 7.5\% = 0.075$$

Learning to do conversions of fractions to decimals, percents to decimals, or decimals to percents will make your work as an allied health care provider easier since you encounter numbers in all three forms throughout your daily activities.

PRACTICE PROBLEM SET 1.5

Convert the following numbers to an equivalent form as indicated in the table. Reduce all fractions to lowest terms and round decimals to the nearest hundredth if necessary.

	FRACTION	DECIMAL	PERCENT
1.		0.875	
2.		0.125	
3.	$\frac{2}{5}$		
4.	$\frac{3}{10}$		
5.			3.5%
6.			8.1%
7.		0.02	
8.		0.18	
9.	$\frac{1}{2}$		
10.	$\frac{3}{8}$		
11.			9%
12.			6%
13.		0.0001	
14.		0.0025	
15.	$\frac{1}{3}$		

	FRACTION	DECIMAL	PERCENT
16.	$\frac{1}{6}$		
17.			0.2%
18.			0.05%
19.	$2\frac{1}{4}$		
20.	$1\frac{3}{100}$		

21. A drug is to be given at a dosage of 0.625 mg/kg. Write this dosage as a reduced fraction.
22. A doctor's order calls for 0.25 mg of a medication. Express this dosage as a reduced fraction.
23. A patient's morning medication dosage is gr $\frac{1}{8}$. Write this dosage as a decimal number.
24. A child dosage of a certain medication is gr $\frac{1}{150}$. Write this dosage as a decimal number.
25. A single X-ray picture or radiograph exposes a patient to $\frac{1}{2}$ roentgen. Write this fraction as a decimal.
26. A patient receives three X-rays, which exposes him to $\frac{3}{2}$ roentgens. Write this number in decimal form.
27. Calcium comprises about 1.75% of the weight of an adult's body. Write this percent as an equivalent fraction and equivalent decimal number.
28. A 4.25% boric acid solution is prepared from boric acid crystals. Write this percent as an equivalent fraction and equivalent decimal number.
29. Sodium chloride crystals are used to prepare a 0.9% saline solution. Write this percent as an equivalent fraction and equivalent decimal number.
30. A $\frac{1}{4}$% solution of bichloride mercury is prepared using pure bichloride of mercury liquid. Write this percent as an equivalent decimal number and as a fraction.

Chapter Summary

In this chapter you reviewed your basic math skills in the areas of Roman numerals, fractions, decimals, and percents. The numbers you encounter in your work in the allied health field will involve numbers in many different forms. The ability to complete accurate calculations with all forms of numbers is an important skill for a health care worker. Understanding the conversions of one form of a number to another will be very useful to you as you try to understand prescriptions, calculate dosages of medications based on patients' weights, or do many other health-related tasks.

Important Terms and Rules

denominator

improper fraction

least common denominator (LCD)

numerator

percent

place value

proper fraction

reciprocal

Roman numeral

Rounding Rules

To round a number to a certain place:

1. Locate the digit in that place.
2. Look at the digit to the right of that place.
3. If the digit immediately to the right is 5 or more, round up; if the digit immediately to the right is 4 or less, drop the extra digits and do not round up.

Chapter Review Problems

Convert the following values given in Roman numerals to Hindu-Arabic numerals.

1. xxvii
2. xiv
3. xxviss
4. XLV
5. CXXXIV

Convert the following values given in Hindu-Arabic numerals to Roman numerals.

6. 6
7. 19
8. 38
9. 150
10. $9\frac{1}{2}$

Reduce the following fractions to lowest terms. Simplify improper fractions to mixed numbers.

11. $\dfrac{14}{49}$

12. $\dfrac{18}{48}$

13. $\dfrac{50}{1250}$

14. $\dfrac{35}{6}$

Determine the correct order of the following fractions in descending order.

15. $\dfrac{1}{3}, \dfrac{1}{4}, \dfrac{1}{6}$

16. $\dfrac{1}{8}, \dfrac{1}{3}, \dfrac{1}{6}$

17. $\dfrac{2}{3}, \dfrac{2}{5}, \dfrac{3}{10}$

Perform the following operations with fractions and simplify the answers completely.

18. $\dfrac{5}{6} + \dfrac{2}{5}$

19. $3\dfrac{2}{3} + 2\dfrac{1}{4}$

20. $\dfrac{7}{8} - \dfrac{5}{24}$

21. $16 - \dfrac{7}{12}$

22. $35\dfrac{1}{2} - 18\dfrac{7}{12}$

23. $\dfrac{3}{5} \times \dfrac{3}{9}$

24. $1\dfrac{5}{12} \times 3\dfrac{2}{3}$

Complete the problems containing complex fractions, simplifying the final answers.

25. $\dfrac{\frac{1}{3}}{\frac{5}{9}}$

26. $\dfrac{\frac{9}{100}}{\frac{1}{200}} \times 250$

Change these decimal numbers to fractions and simplify if needed.

27. 0.125
28. 0.06
29. 0.0015
30. 0.00001

Perform the following calculations.

31. $4.562 + 2.0235 + 1$
32. $5.06 + 23.871 + 0.36$
33. $18.65 - 13.153$
34. $5.12 - 2.175$
35. 3.075×0.006
36. 5.45×1.1
37. $0.258 \div 0.6$
38. $0.18891 \div 0.9$

Round the numbers to the given place value.

39. 255.249   hundredths
40. 38.246   tenths
41. 0.0267   thousandths
42. 0.0065   hundredths

Place the correct symbol, > or <, between the numbers.

43. 0.45   0.5   44. 0.06   0.059

Change each percent to a fraction. Reduce it to lowest terms.

45. 55%   46. 6.5%   47. 0.005%

Change each percent to a decimal.

48. 2.5%   49. 0.09%   50. 5%

Change each fraction or decimal to a percent.

51. $\frac{1}{8}$ 53. $\frac{2}{3}$ 55. 0.575

52. $\frac{3}{25}$ 54. 0.003

Give the percent strength of each of the following solutions.

56. 15 parts in 100 total parts
57. 3.5 parts in 10 total parts
58. 35 mL pure drug + 65 mL water

Convert the following numbers to an equivalent form as indicated in the table. Reduce all fractions to lowest terms and round decimals to the nearest hundredth if necessary.

	FRACTION	DECIMAL	PERCENT
59.		0.005	
60.			2.5%
61.	$\frac{4}{5}$		

Complete the following word problems. Reduce all fractional answers to lowest terms.

62. Mrs. Allison—intake: one carton milk, two bowls soup, one 8-oz cup of coffee, one cup of ice cream, two cups of jello, two juice cartons
    urine output: 300 cc, 325 cc, 325 cc, 200 cc, 325 cc, 250 cc

    Calculate the fluid balance or imbalance for this patient. (Use the hospital estimation guide in Section 1.1.)

63. At the beginning of the month, a medical office had 2275 latex examination gloves on hand. On the last day of the month, an inventory showed that 525 gloves remained. How many gloves were used during the month? If the office manager places an order for gloves so there will be a minimum of 3000 gloves on hand at the beginning of the next month, how many should be ordered? If gloves come in boxes of 250, how many boxes should be ordered?

64. An estimate for the measure of an adult's wrist is $\frac{1}{4}$ of the waist size. If Jerry has a 36-in. waist, estimate the size of his wrist.

65. A doctor orders gr $\frac{1}{8}$ of a medication. The nurse has gr $\frac{1}{6}$ in stock in the medicine cabinet. Should the patient be given more or less of the dosage on hand?

66. A pharmacy has six 1-g vials of medication. How many $\frac{1}{2}$-g doses are available?

67. For a 150-lb person, walking an hour at a rate of 4 mph will burn approximately 330 calories. If June weighs 150 lb and walked $\frac{1}{2}$ hr each day for five days last week, estimate the number of calories she burned.

68. An estimate for an adult's waist measurement is found by dividing the neck size measured in inches by 0.5. Porky's neck measures 18.5 in. Estimate his waist size.

69. A patient received 2.25 g of medication daily. Tablets are available in 0.75-g dosages. How many tablets should this patient be given?

70. The office checking account has a balance of $8145.57. In the mail, you receive payments of $110.50, $85.00, $125.75, $225.00, $250.00, and $25.75. What is the total amount of the deposit that you will make today using these payments? What is the new balance on the account after this deposit?

71. What is the percent concentration of a solution containing 12 g of NaCl (salt) in 150 mL of water?

72. The recommended amount of potassium per day for an adult is 3000 milligrams. The nutrition label of a particular cereal states that 440 milligrams of potassium will be consumed by eating one serving with skim milk. What percent of the daily allowance of potassium will be provided by eating one serving of this cereal with skim milk? (Round to the nearest tenth.)

73. In 2002, health benefits for 29% of all U.S. employees were provided by a health maintenance organization (HMO). (*Source:* William M. Mercer, Inc.) What fractional part of Americans were covered by HMOs? What fractional part were covered by other types of health plans?

74. According to the accompanying table from the Red Cross, what fractional part of the population has A Rh-positive blood? Write this number as a decimal and a fraction.

Distribution of Blood Types in Blood Donors

Blood Type	Percent of Population
O Rh-positive	37%
O Rh-negative	7%
A Rh-positive	36%
A Rh-negative	6%
B Rh-positive	9%
B Rh-negative	1%
AB Rh-positive	3%
AB Rh-negative	1%

Source: American Red Cross Biomedical Services.

75. What percent of the population has Type O blood? Write this percent as an equivalent fraction and equivalent decimal.

76. If a survey of 300 people in a nursing facility revealed that 20 had AB Rh-positive blood, would this be unusual based on the Red Cross statistics?

Chapter Test

Convert the following values given in Roman numerals to Hindu-Arabic numerals.

1. xviii

2. xivss

3. XCV

4. MCCXXI

Convert the following values given in Hindu-Arabic numerals to Roman numerals.

5. $4\frac{1}{2}$

6. 29

Determine the correct order of the following fractions in descending order.

7. $\frac{1}{5}, \frac{3}{4}, \frac{5}{6}$

8. $\frac{7}{10}, \frac{1}{3}, \frac{5}{12}$

Perform the following calculations. Reduce all fractions to lowest terms.

9. $\frac{3}{4} + \frac{5}{12} + \frac{1}{3} =$

10. $2\frac{2}{3} + 6\frac{3}{4} + \frac{1}{6} =$

11. $5\frac{9}{100} - 2\frac{3}{10} =$

12. $\frac{5}{8} \times 1\frac{3}{25} =$

13. $\frac{3}{4} \times 48 =$

14. $\frac{9}{10} \div \frac{3}{5} =$

15. $\frac{7}{12} \div 49 =$

16. $0.025 + 1.85 + 3 =$

17. $16.85 - 1.0025 =$

18. $35.28 \times 0.25 =$

19. $0.00275 \times 1.2 =$

20. $0.375 \div 0.5 =$

21. Round 23.985 to the tenths place.

22. Put these decimal numbers in order from highest value to lowest value.

$$0.152, 0.1, 0.2152, 0.2, 0.015$$

23. Give the percent strength of a solution with 3 parts solute in 20 mL of water.

Convert the following numbers to an equivalent form as indicated in the table. Reduce all fractions to lowest terms and round decimals to the nearest hundredth if necessary.

	FRACTION	DECIMAL	PERCENT
24.			0.9%
25.		0.025	
26.	$\frac{5}{6}$		

27. The maximum inventory for ampicillin capsules is 1500. An inventory at the end of the week indicates there are 493 capsules in stock. How many capsules should the pharmacy technician order to restock to the maximum level? If capsules are sold in bottles of 250, 100, and 25, how many of each bottle should be ordered?

28. A child takes a $\frac{1}{12}$-fluid-oz dose of medication. How many doses can be prepared from 5 oz?

29. A child is to receive a dose of 0.5 fluid oz of cough medicine every 4 hr. The bottle contains 12 fluid oz. If you give the child a dose every 4 hr, how many days will this bottle last?

30. According to Princeton Survey Research, 46% of Americans eat pasta 1 or 2 times a week. Write this number as an equivalent decimal and an equivalent reduced fraction.

2

A REVIEW OF ALGEBRA

Objectives for Chapter 2

After completing this chapter the student should be able to:

1. Solve basic algebraic equations.

2. Solve problems involving ratios and proportions.

3. Solve problems involving the use of percentages.

4. Perform the calculations necessary in medical formulas.

SECTION 2.1   SIGNED NUMBERS AND THE ORDER OF OPERATIONS

We begin our review of algebra with a short discussion of **signed numbers**. Signed numbers include all positive numbers, negative numbers, and the number 0. Negative numbers represent values that are less than 0. For example, an overdrawn bank account or a temperature in °C that is below freezing can be represented with negative numbers. Numbers written in scientific notation require the use of negative numbers as exponents when representing numbers with values between 0 and 1. Signed numbers are also called directed numbers and can be used to represent losses or gains. For example, a weight loss of 2 lb would be -2 lb, and an increase of 1.5° in a patient's temperature could be represented as $+1.5°$. Briefly review the rules for operations with signed numbers.

Operations with Signed Numbers

Addition:

- If the numbers have the same sign, add the numbers and use the same sign for the answer.
- If the numbers have different signs, find the difference between the numbers and use the sign of the number with the larger absolute value as the sign of the sum. (Recall: $|-5| = 5$, $|5| = 5$, $|0| = 0$.)

Subtraction:

- To subtract two integers, add the opposite of the second number to the first number.

Multiplication/Division:

- Multiply or divide the two numbers.
  - If the signs are alike, the answer is positive.
  - If the signs are different, the answer is negative.

The definition of subtraction refers to the **opposite** of a number. Two numbers that are the same distance from 0 on the number line, but on the opposite sides of it are called **opposites**. For example, -5 is the opposite of $+5$ and $+1$ is the opposite of -1. (Zero is its own opposite.) Parentheses are used when trying to find the opposite of a negative number. For example, $-(-7)$ is read "the opposite of negative seven" and its value is 7. Look at the problems in Example 1 that illustrate the rules for operations involving signed numbers.

EXAMPLE 1: Operations with Signed Numbers

Perform each calculation using the rules for signed numbers

a. $-6 + (-8) = -14$

The numbers have the same sign so they are added and the answer has the same sign as the addends.

b. $-15 + 7 = -8$

Since the numbers have opposite signs, we take the difference of the numbers $(15 - 7 = 8)$ and make the answer negative since $|-15| > |7|$.

c. $-7 - (-3) = -7 + 3 = -4$

The -3 is being subtracted so it is changed to its opposite, $+3$, and then it is combined with the -7 using the rules for addition.

d. $(-10)(-8) = 80 \qquad -16 \div (-2) = 8 \qquad (9)(3) = 27 \qquad 8 \div 4 = 2$

In multiplication and division problems, if the signs are alike, the answer will be positive.

e. $(5)(-3) = -15 \qquad -20 \div 4 = -5$

In multiplication and division problems, if the signs are different, the answer will be negative.

EXAMPLE 2: Using Signed Numbers

Mr. Bailey's temperature has been high for several hours. After receiving some medication at 8 PM to reduce fever, the nurse's aide noted the following reductions in his fever: $-0.5°$ at 9 PM and $-0.8°$ at 10 PM. How many degrees has Mr. Bailey's temperature dropped since he was given his medication?

Since both numbers are negatives, we add: $-0.5° + -0.8° = -1.3°$

His fever has dropped $1.3°$ since taking his medication at 8 PM.

EXAMPLE 3: Balancing a Check Register

Mary is balancing the check register to determine if she is overdrawn at the bank. Use the information in the register to determine her balance. Remember to add deposits to her balance and subtract the amount of the checks that have been written.

Check No.	Date	Check Issued to or Deposit	Amount of Check	Amount of Deposit	Balance 249.85
215	5/10	Williams Medical Supplies	99.25		
216	5/10	CWS Pharmacy	40.00		
	5/11	Deposit from insurance		150.00	
217	5/12	Merry Hill Medical Clinic	85.00		
218	5/12	Stewart Physical Therapy	178.50		

$$\$249.85 - \$99.25 = \$150.60$$
$$\$150.60 - \$40.00 = \$110.60$$
$$\$110.60 + \$150.00 = \$260.60$$
$$\$260.60 - \$85.00 = \$175.60$$
$$\$175.60 - \$178.50 = -\$2.90$$

Because the balance is negative, this indicates that the account is overdrawn by $2.90.

One important topic in mathematics is the **order of operations** that is used when doing several calculations in a single problem. Many formulas have several variables and involve a combination of operations such as multiplication and addition. If these calculations are not done in the proper order, an incorrect result will be obtained. Suppose that you are to find the numerical value of the following expression:

$$8 + 5(3)$$

There are two possible results, depending upon which operation, addition or multiplication, is performed first. If the addition is done first, then the result will be as follows:

$$8 + 5(3) = 13(3) = 39$$

If the multiplication is done first, then the result will be different:

$$8 + 5(3) = 8 + 15 = 23$$

The order in which operations are performed does make a difference. So, which is correct? We can easily find out if we first study the rules for the order of operations.

The Order of Operations

1. If any operations are enclosed in parentheses, do those operations first.
2. If any numbers have exponents (or are raised to some power), do those next.
3. Perform all multiplication and division in order from left to right.
4. Finally, perform all addition and subtraction in order from left to right.

In the problem $8 + 5(3)$, there are two operations, addition and multiplication. Following the order of operations, we should multiply first and then add the resulting numbers. Therefore, the correct result is 23.

This rule becomes very easy to remember with a little practice. The order of operations is an important part of many algebra problems and formulas, so you should practice problems using the correct order of operations until you can successfully complete them without difficulty. As an aid to remembering the rule, this silly statement is often used in mathematics classrooms to assist students' memories:

"Please Excuse My Dear Aunt Sally."

The first letter of each word (PEMDAS) corresponds to part of the rule for the order of operations. P stands for parentheses, E for exponents, MD for multiplication/division, and AS for addition/subtraction.

EXAMPLE 4: Using the Order of Operations

Find the value of each of the following expressions by following the order of operations.

$$
\begin{aligned}
1.\quad 3(6 - 8) = &\qquad \text{parentheses} \\
3(-2) = &\qquad \text{multiplication} \\
-6 &
\end{aligned}
$$

2. $(5^2 + 3) - 2 =$ exponent inside the parentheses
   $(25 + 3) - 2 =$ addition inside the parentheses
   $28 - 2 =$ addition and subtraction (from left to right)
   26

3. $-3[5 + (-3 + 2)] =$ parentheses
   $-3[5 + (-1)] =$ brackets
   $-3[4] =$ multiplication
   -12

4. $24 \div 4 \cdot 3 + 4^2 =$ exponent
   $24 \div 4 \cdot 3 + 16 =$ division (left to right)
   $6 \cdot 3 + 16 =$ multiplication (left to right)
   $18 + 16 =$ addition
   34

If a problem contains a complicated fraction with several operations in either the numerator or denominator or both, then you must evaluate the numerator and denominator as if they were two separate expressions and then divide last. For example, look at the problem $\dfrac{3(-4)^2}{2(3) + 6}$. To evaluate this expression, start with the numerator and follow the order of operations until you arrive at the answer (48). Do the same for the denominator (12). Then, divide the numerator by the denominator (48 ÷ 12) to arrive at the final value.

$$\frac{3(-4)^2}{2(3) + 6} = \frac{3(16)}{6 + 6} = \frac{48}{12} = 4$$

A scientific calculator will perform several operations at once and is able to follow the order of operations automatically. Just be careful to enter all of the operations, numbers, and symbols in the correct order. Your calculator manual can give you specific information about the correct entries needed for your model. For example, to enter a negative number, some calculators require that you enter the number first, followed by the negative sign. Other calculators are direct-entry calculators and require that you enter the negative sign followed by the number. When entering a problem like $\dfrac{20 + 35}{5}$ into your calculator, besure to enter 20 ⊞ 35 ⊟ ÷ 5. If you do not enter the = sign, the calculator will only divide 35 by 5 and then add 20. It is following the order of operations!

PRACTICE PROBLEM SET 2.1

Evaluate each of the following by applying the appropriate rule for basic operations with signed numbers.

1. $5 + (-2)$
2. $-8 + 5$
3. $16(-85)$
4. $-15(24)$
5. $0 \div (-67)$
6. $0 \div 25$

7. $-567 \div 0$
8. $37 \div 0$
9. $-1\frac{1}{3} + \frac{7}{8}$
10. $\frac{5}{8} - \left(-\frac{2}{3}\right)$

11. $\frac{5}{6} \div \left(-\frac{3}{10}\right)$

12. $-\frac{8}{9} \div \frac{4}{21}$
13. $7.5 - (-2.1)$

14. $-3.6 - 9.4$
15. $(-0.12)(-0.5)$
16. $(0.25)(-3.5)$

Evaluate each of the following expressions, being careful to follow the order of operations.

17. $7 \cdot 3 - 2 \cdot 13$

18. $(-3)(5) - (-8)(2)$

19. $\dfrac{27}{(-24 + 21)}$

20. $\dfrac{16}{-3 - (-2)}$

21. $8 - (-6)(4 - 7)$

22. $40 - (-2)[8 - 3(-1)]$

23. $\dfrac{2(-6 + 6)}{23 - 97}$

24. $\dfrac{6(-5) - 10}{-7 - (-2)}$

25. $(-8)^2 - 7(8) + 5$

26. $(-6) - (-3)^2 + 4$

27. $\dfrac{2^2 + 4^2}{5^2 - 3^2}$

28. $\dfrac{3^3 - 1^3}{2^3 - 6}$

29. $\dfrac{3^3 - 2^3}{-4(-3 + 1)}$

30. $\dfrac{5^2 - 3(2)^2}{3(-2 + 1)}$

31. $-3^2 + 3(6 - 5)^2$

32. $-(8 + 5)^2 + (3 - 7)^2$

33. $2.5 + \dfrac{7.5}{0.3} + (0.5)^2$

34. $3.75 + (0.25)^2 + 0.14 \div 0.2$

35. $-4[(-2.1)(6) - 7.5]$

36. $-6[(5)(-2.3) - 8.1]$

37. $(3 - 8)(-2) - 10$

38. $-20 - (-1)(-7 - 11)$

39. $\dfrac{5(-8 + 3)}{13(-2) + (-6 - 1)(-4 + 1)}$

40. $\dfrac{16(-7 + 4)}{15(-3) + (-7 - 4)(-9 + 6)}$

SECTION 2.2 A REVIEW OF SOLVING LINEAR EQUATIONS

In our review of equation solving procedures, we will make extensive use of the properties of real numbers. The principles used are designed to result in what are called **equivalent equations**. For example, are $x + 3 = 5$ and $x = 2$ equivalent equations? If x is replaced with the number 2 in both equations, then both equations can be seen to be true mathematical statements. Because of this, they are equivalent equations. The properties of equality that we study in algebra are very important in the process of solving equations. These properties are briefly reviewed in this section.

The Addition/Subtraction Properties of Equality

For any real numbers a, b, and c,

$$\text{if } a = b, \text{ then } a + c = b + c$$
$$\text{and}$$
$$\text{if } a = b, \text{ then } a - c = b - c$$

These properties simply say that the same number may be added to or subtracted from both sides of an equation and the new equation will be equivalent to the original equation.

EXAMPLE 5: Solving a Linear Equation Using the Subtraction Property of Equality

Solve the equation $x + 15 = 28$ for the value of x.

To solve this, or any, equation you must isolate the variable on one side of the equal sign. To do this here, the 15 must be removed. Since it is added, we can remove it by subtracting 15 from both sides of the equation.

$$x + 15 - 15 = 28 - 15$$
$$x + 0 = 13$$
$$x = 13$$

Check this answer by substituting 13 for x in the original equation.

$$\text{Check:} \quad x + 15 = 28$$
$$13 + 15 = 28$$
$$28 = 28 \checkmark$$

The Multiplication/Division Properties of Equality

For any real numbers a, b, and c,

$$\text{if } a = b, \text{ then } ac = bc$$
$$\text{and}$$
$$\text{if } a = b, \text{ then } \frac{a}{c} = \frac{b}{c} \quad (c \neq 0)$$

This property states that if we multiply or divide both sides of an equation by the same number, the new equation will be equivalent to the original one. The object of this property is to change the coefficient of the variable to a 1.

EXAMPLE 6: Solving Linear Equations Using the Multiplication Property of Equality

Solve $3y = 36$ for the value of y.

The coefficient of the variable in this equation is 3, not 1. If we multiply by the reciprocal of 3, or divide both sides by 3, then the resulting coefficient of the variable will equal 1. So, using the multiplication/division property of equality, we divide both sides of the equation as follows:

$$3y = 36$$
$$\frac{3y}{3} = \frac{36}{3}$$
$$y = 12$$

Check your answer by substituting 12 for y in the original equation.

$$3y = 36$$
$$3(12) = 36$$
$$36 = 36 \checkmark$$

Often several steps will be required to solve a particular equation involving several terms. One of the properties of real numbers that is quite useful in algebra when simplifying each side of an equation is the **distributive property**. This property allows us to remove parentheses in an equation so the properties of equality can be applied in order to find the solution.

The Distributive Property

For all real numbers a, b, and c,

$$a(b + c) = ab + ac$$

Using this property, we will multiply each term inside the parentheses by the number on the outside of the parentheses. It is very important that the number in front of the parentheses multiplies *all* terms inside the parentheses. Remember that parentheses must be removed first in the solving process if at all possible. Simplify each side completely and then apply the properties of equality.

The following general procedure is a step-by-step process for solving linear equations. There may be several ways to approach different equations, but this procedure will be useful as a general guideline. Remember that your goal is to isolate the variable and find its value in the form $x = a$, where a is a real number.

General Procedure for Solving Linear Equations

1. Use the distributive property to remove any parentheses in the equation.
2. If the equation contains fractions, multiply both sides of the equation by the least common denominator (LCD) in order to eliminate all fractions from the equation.
3. Combine like terms on both sides of the equation.
4. Use the addition/subtraction property of equality to isolate the variable on one side of the equation with all constants on the other side of the equation. You may need to do this process twice in order to get the equation to the form $ax = b$, where a and b are real numbers.
5. Solve for the variable by dividing both sides of the equation by the coefficient of the variable.

EXAMPLE 7: Solving a Linear Equation Using the Distributive Property

Solve $3(x - 2) = 18$ for the value of x.

$$3(x - 2) = 18$$
$$3x - 6 = 18 \qquad \text{distributive property}$$
$$3x - 6 + 6 = 18 + 6 \qquad \text{addition property of equality}$$
$$3x = 24 \qquad \text{simplify}$$
$$\frac{3x}{3} = \frac{24}{3} \qquad \text{division property of equality}$$
$$x = 8 \qquad \text{solution}$$

Check your answer by substituting 8 for x in the original equation. Follow the order of operations to evaluate this expression.

$$\text{Check:} \quad 3(x - 2) = 18$$
$$3(8 - 2) = 18$$
$$3(6) = 18$$
$$18 = 18 \checkmark$$

EXAMPLE 8: Solving a Linear Equation Containing Fractions

Solve the equation $\frac{1}{3}x - 3 = \frac{1}{2} + 3x$.

The easiest way to solve an algebraic equation containing fractions is to first multiply the entire equation by the least common denominator (LCD) of the fractions in the equation. This will result in an equivalent equation with only integer coefficients. The LCD of this equation is 6, so we will multiply all terms by 6.

$$\frac{1}{3}x - 3 = \frac{1}{2} + x$$

$$6\left(\frac{1}{3}x\right) - 6(3) = 6\left(\frac{1}{2}\right) + 6(x) \qquad \text{multiply each term by LCD}$$

$$2x - 18 = 3 + 6x \qquad \text{simplify}$$

$$2x - 18 - 6x = 3 + 6x - 6x \qquad \text{subtraction property of equality}$$

$$-4x - 18 = 3 \qquad \text{simplify}$$

$$-4x - 18 + 18 = 3 + 18 \qquad \text{addition property of equality}$$

$$-4x = 21 \qquad \text{simplify}$$

$$\frac{-4x}{-4} = \frac{21}{-4} \qquad \text{division property of equality}$$

$$x = -\frac{21}{4} \qquad \text{solution}$$

EXAMPLE 9: Solving a Linear Equation Containing Decimals

Solve the equation $5.7x - 3.1(x + 5) = 5.3$.

$$5.7x - 3.1x - 15.5 = 5.3 \qquad \text{distributive property}$$

$$2.6x - 15.5 = 5.3 \qquad \text{combine like terms}$$

$$2.6x - 15.5 + 15.5 = 5.3 + 15.5 \qquad \text{addition property of equality}$$

$$2.6x = 20.8 \qquad \text{simplify}$$

$$\frac{2.6x}{2.6} = \frac{20.8}{2.6} \qquad \text{division property of equality}$$

$$x = 8 \qquad \text{solution}$$

PRACTICE PROBLEM SET 2.2

Solve each of the following linear equations.

1. $x - 6 = -4$
2. $x + 9 = -2$
3. $k - 76.98 = -3.56$
4. $y - 2.5 = 0.75$
5. $x + \frac{1}{2} = \frac{3}{4}$
6. $y - \frac{2}{3} = -\frac{7}{8}$
7. $-5x = 15$
8. $6x = -24$
9. $3x + 7 = x$
10. $5x + 6 = 2x$
11. $2a - 8 = 64$
12. $2x - 5 = -7$
13. $5x + 9 = 6$

14. $2x = 15 - 3x$
15. $-5x = 21 - 2x$
16. $28 - 8x = 4x$
17. $35 - 3x = 5$
18. $5 = 3 - 4x$
19. $\frac{2}{5}x - 12 = 6$
20. $2 = \frac{2}{5}f + 3$
21. $\frac{3x}{4} = \frac{4}{7} + 1$
22. $2 - \frac{2}{3}x = \frac{1}{4}$
23. $-4.1x = -4x + 4.5$
24. $5.75x = 2.25x - 10.5$
25. $7 - 3x = 9 - 5x$

26. $3x + 9 = 42 + 2x$
27. $3d - 9 = -9d + 15$
28. $8 - 3c = 2c + 8$
29. $8x + 19 = 3x + 4$
30. $-3x - 5 = 5 + 2x$
31. $3x + 5 = -5x - 19 + 2x$
32. $2x + 6 - 5x = 6x - 12$
33. $5x - 2 + x = -6 + 2x$
34. $7x - 5 + 2x = -3x - 41$
35. $-7(2x + 3) = -7$
36. $3(x - 2) = 12$
37. $5(2x - 3) = 35$
38. $-2(x - 4) = -16$
39. $5x - 3(1 - 2x) = 4(2x - 1)$

40. $8x + 40 = 2(5x + 2)$ 44. $2p + 4(p - 3) = 5p - 1$ 48. $6 + 2(3x - 8) = 2x + 18$

41. $7a - (a - 5) = -10$ 45. $4(3 - x) + 2x = -12$ 49. $\frac{3}{4}(4 - x) = 3 - x$

42. $3s + 5(s - 3) + 8 = 0$ 46. $3 - 2(x - 4) = 3(3 - x)$ 50. $3(x - 5) + 1 = \frac{1}{4}(2x - 8)$

43. $3(x - 5) - 5x = 2x + 9$ 47. $3(x - 2) + 7 = 5 + 4x$

SECTION 2.3   A REVIEW OF RATIOS AND PROPORTIONS

We use ratios to make comparisons between things that are measured in the same units. A **ratio** of two values is usually written as a fraction, with a colon, or using the word *to*. Look at these forms of the ratio of 1 mL to 10 mL.

1. Written as a reduced fraction: $\frac{1}{10}$

2. Written using a colon as the ratio symbol: 1:10

3. Written using the word *to*: "1 to 10"

Often, ratios are fractions that represent a part-to-whole relationship. A ratio should be written in the same order as the words expressing it are written. If the nurse-to-patient ratio in the Intensive Care Unit is one nurse to every two patients, the ratio is 1:2, or 1 to 2. If we state that there are two patients per nurse, then the ratio is 2:1, or 2 to 1.

A **proportion** is a statement that two ratios are equal. Although the numbers that make up the two ratios will be different, their relative values will be the same. In the health care profession, there are many applications of proportions. For example, they provide an easy, straightforward method for calculating measurement conversions, medication dosages, and supply orders.

An example of a proportion is $\frac{2}{5} = \frac{4}{10}$. Another way to write this is 2:5::4:10, which is read, "2 is to 5 as 4 is to 10." We know that this is a true proportion because if we reduce $\frac{4}{10}$, the result will be $\frac{2}{5}$. Another way to verify proportions is to use the **cross-multiplication property**.

Cross-Multiplication Property

To solve a proportion, we use the property of proportionality that states:

The cross products of any true proportion are equal.

If $\frac{a}{b} = \frac{c}{d}$, then ad = bc, where $b \neq 0$ and $d \neq 0$.

We can see that this property is true by looking at the preceding example and noting that $(4)(5) = (2)(10)$.

We can also use the cross-multiplication property to solve problems involving proportions. In Example 10 we will use this property to solve a proportion.

EXAMPLE 10: Solving Proportions Using the Cross-Multiplication Property

$$\frac{3}{x} = \frac{10}{75}$$

$(3)(75) = (10)(x)$ cross-multiplication property

$225 = 10x$ simplify

$\dfrac{225}{10} = \dfrac{10x}{10}$ division property of equality

$22.5 = x$

We can verify our answer by substituting the value for x into the proportion and solving.

$$\frac{3}{x} = \frac{10}{75}$$

$$\frac{3}{22.5} = \frac{10}{75}$$

$$(3)(75) = (10)(22.5) \qquad \text{cross-multiplication property}$$

$$225 = 225 \quad \checkmark \qquad \text{Solution checks.}$$

Using the cross-multiplication property and the algebraic properties of equality, direct proportions are quickly and easily solved. To solve application problems using direct proportions, look at the following list of steps.

Solving Application Problems Using Proportions

1. Let the unknown quantity be represented by a variable.
2. Use the given information to set up a ratio of known values on the left side of the equation. On the right side of the equation, set up a ratio using the variable and the other given quantity. Be sure that the same units are in the same positions in each ratio. For example, a correctly labeled proportion might be $\frac{\text{mg}}{\text{dL}} = \frac{\text{mg}}{\text{dL}}$.
3. Drop the units from each ratio and use the cross-multiplication property to solve for the unknown.
4. Answer the question that was asked.

Often in a chemistry lab we are asked to prepare a specific volume of solution with a given concentration. Using a proportion to calculate the parts needed to prepare the solution will make the preparation easy. Three of the four values of the proportion must be given. Use the steps previously stated to set up the proportion and solve. Look at this process as demonstrated in Example 11.

EXAMPLE 11: Preparing a Solution

If there are 3 g of solute in 25 mL of solution, how many grams would be in 125 mL of this solution?

Set the given ratio equal to the unknown ratio and use the cross-multiplication property to solve for the missing value. Be sure the given ratio and the unknown ratio are written in the same order and are in the same units.

$$\text{Given ratio: } \frac{3 \text{ g}}{25 \text{ mL}}$$

$$\text{Unknown ratio: } \frac{x \text{ g}}{125 \text{ mL}} \text{ (how many grams?)}$$

Given ratio = Unknown ratio

$$\frac{3 \text{ g}}{25 \text{ mL}} = \frac{x \text{ g}}{125 \text{ mL}}$$

$$(3)(125) = (25)(x) \qquad \text{cross-multiplication property}$$

$$375 = 25x \qquad \text{simplify}$$

$$\frac{375}{25} = \frac{25x}{25} \qquad \text{division property of equality}$$

$$15 = x$$

Therefore, there would be 15 g of solute in 125 mL of solution.

Proportions are used in many aspects of health care. Nutritionists can use proportions in calculating the amount of protein, fats, or carbohydrates that are in particular foods. They can also calculate the amount of nutrients in foods, such as calcium, using proportions. Proportions are also used quite often in dosage calculations. If a doctor orders a drug for your patient and the drug isn't available in the correct strength, you can use proportions to calculate the right amount of the drug to administer. Look at the following examples.

EXAMPLE 12: Proportions in Nutrition Calculations

Baked beans contain 33 g of carbohydrates in a $\frac{1}{2}$-cup serving. How many grams of carbohydrates are in 6 cups of baked beans?

Known ratio = Unknown ratio

$$\frac{33 \text{ g}}{\frac{1}{2} \text{ cup}} = \frac{x \text{ g}}{6 \text{ cups}}$$

$(33)(6) =$ cross-multiplication property $\frac{1}{2} x$

$198 = \frac{1}{2} x$ \quad simplify

$2(198) = 2 \left(\frac{1}{2} x \right)$ \quad multiplication property of equality

$396 = x$

Therefore, in 6 cups of baked beans there are 396 g of carbohydrates.

EXAMPLE 13: Determining the Correct Amount of Insulin Using Proportions

A vial of insulin marked U40 has 40 units of insulin per cubic centimeter (cc) of fluid. How much insulin should a patient be given if she needs 12 units of U40?

Known ratio = Unknown ratio

$$\frac{40 \text{ units}}{1 \text{ cc}} = \frac{12 \text{ units}}{x \text{ cc}}$$

$(40)(x) = (1)(12)$ \quad cross-multiplication property

$40x = 12$ \quad simplify

$$\frac{40x}{40} = \frac{12}{40}$$ \quad division property of equality

$x = 0.3$

Therefore, 0.3 cc of U40 insulin should be administered to the patient.

PRACTICE PROBLEM SET 2.3

Use the cross-multiplication property to determine if the following proportions are true or false.

1. $\dfrac{9}{10} = \dfrac{27}{30}$

2. $\dfrac{15}{30} = \dfrac{9}{16}$

3. $\dfrac{3}{8} = \dfrac{4.5}{12}$

4. $\dfrac{16}{40} = \dfrac{1.2}{3}$

5. $\dfrac{0.1}{2.5} = \dfrac{0.02}{0.5}$

6. $\dfrac{6.5}{100} = \dfrac{3.5}{50}$

Use the cross-multiplication property to solve the following problems.

7. $\dfrac{2}{3} = \dfrac{x}{9}$

8. $\dfrac{3}{5} = \dfrac{x}{75}$

9. $\dfrac{x}{24} = \dfrac{3}{8}$

10. $\dfrac{x}{16} = \dfrac{15}{48}$

11. $\dfrac{6}{x} = \dfrac{54}{12}$

12. $\dfrac{15}{x} = \dfrac{45}{6}$

13. $\dfrac{9}{25} = \dfrac{27}{x}$

14. $\dfrac{15}{63} = \dfrac{5}{x}$

15. $\dfrac{0.01}{5} = \dfrac{x}{2.5}$

16. $\dfrac{0.5}{1} = \dfrac{x}{0.25}$

17. $\dfrac{x}{0.5} = \dfrac{1}{2.5}$

18. $\dfrac{x}{0.1} = \dfrac{0.25}{0.5}$

19. $\dfrac{1.5 \text{ mg}}{2 \text{ capsules}} = \dfrac{4.5 \text{ mg}}{x \text{ capsules}}$

20. $\dfrac{600 \text{ mg}}{1 \text{ capsule}} = \dfrac{x \text{ mg}}{3 \text{ capsules}}$

21. $\dfrac{8 \text{ mg}}{2.5 \text{ mL}} = \dfrac{4 \text{ mg}}{x \text{ mL}}$

22. $\dfrac{0.3 \text{ mg}}{1 \text{ tablet}} = \dfrac{6 \text{ mg}}{x \text{ tablets}}$

23. $\dfrac{0.25 \text{ mg}}{0.8 \text{ mL}} = \dfrac{0.125 \text{ mg}}{x \text{ mL}}$

24. $\dfrac{10 \text{ mg}}{1 \text{ mL}} = \dfrac{2.5 \text{ mg}}{x \text{ mL}}$

25. $\dfrac{350 \text{ mg}}{2 \text{ tablets}} = \dfrac{x \text{ mg}}{6 \text{ tablets}}$

26. $\dfrac{0.1 \text{ g}}{2 \text{ tablets}} = \dfrac{x \text{ g}}{3 \text{ tablets}}$

Read each problem and set up an appropriate proportion. Use the cross-multiplication property to solve and label your final answers with the correct units.

27. One tablet contains 325 mg of medication. How many tablets contain 975 mg of this medication?

28. Two tablets of a certain drug contain 350 mg of medication. How many milligrams are in five tablets?

29. How much insulin (in cc) should be given from a bottle marked U40 if a patient needs 35 units?

30. How much insulin (in cc) should be given from a bottle marked U100 if a patient needs 26 units?

31. A doctor's order calls for you to administer 0.1 mg of epinephrine S.C., but the only epinephrine in stock is a 1-mL ampule that contains 1 mg of epinephrine. Calculate the volume needed for this injection.

32. A dosage of 20 mg of a medication has been ordered. The dosage strength available is 25 mg in 1.5 mL. How many mL of the available medication should be administered?

33. If the available strength of a certain medication is 1.5 g per cc, how many cc will a 5-g dosage require?

34. How many milliliters of the medication on hand will be needed if the doctor's order prescribes 600 mcg of this medication and the available strength is 750 mcg/3 mL?

35. If 1.25 mg of medication is to be given for 10 lb of body weight, how many milligrams of medication should be given to a child that weighs 52 lb?

36. For each kilogram (kg) of a person's weight, 0.5 mg of an antibiotic is to be administered. If Joan weighs 63 kg, how much medication should she be given?

37. One glass of milk contains 280 mg of calcium. How much calcium is in $3\frac{1}{2}$ glasses of milk?

38. One cup of fat-free milk contains 115 mg of sodium. How much sodium is in $2\frac{1}{2}$ cups of fat-free milk?

39. There are 9 calories in 1 g of fat. How many calories are in 15 g of fat?

40. There are 4 calories in 1 g of protein. How many calories are in 540 g of protein?

41. There are 90 calories in 1 cup of fat-free milk. How many calories are in 4 cups of fat-free milk?

42. One slice of American cheese contains 70 calories. How many calories are in a package of 16 slices?

43. One tablespoon of mayonnaise contains 12 g of fat. How many tablespoons of mayonnaise would contain 54 g of fat?

44. One slice of American cheese contains 3 g of saturated fat. How many grams of saturated fat are in a package of 16 slices?

45. There are 41 g of carbohydrates in one $\frac{3}{4}$-cup serving of rotini pasta. How many grams would there be in $2\frac{1}{2}$ cups of rotini pasta?

46. A $\frac{1}{2}$-cup serving of canned peaches contains 15 g of sugar. How much sugar is in the $1\frac{1}{2}$-cup can?

47. Four out of six children receive fluoride treatments after their dental cleaning. If 132 children had their teeth cleaned this month, how many received fluoride treatments?

48. Last year at the local hospital, statistics showed that 5 out of every 52 babies born were premature. If 1862 babies were born at the hospital last year, how many were premature?

49. According to the National Center for Health Statistics, the infant mortality rate in the United States in the year 2000 was 6.9 deaths for every 1000 births. Based on this ratio, how many infant deaths would a hospital expect if, on average, there are 1250 births at the hospital each year?

50. During the year 2000, $31.70 out of every $100 spent on health care in the United States was spent on hospital care. (*Sources*: National Center for Health Statistics.) Based on this ratio, if $950,000 was spent on health care in this county last month, how much of that total was spent on hospital care?

SECTION 2.4   SOLVING PERCENTAGE PROBLEMS

In Chapter 1, we defined **percent** as parts per hundred. A percent is also defined to be a ratio with a denominator of 100. You can easily solve many percent problems by expressing a given percent as a ratio and using the cross-multiplication property for proportions. The basic model for solving a percent problem using the ratio/proportion method is stated here.

Using Proportions to Solve Percentage Problems

$$\frac{r}{100} = \frac{P}{B}$$

where r is the rate, P is the percentage, and B is the base.

To use this formula, we must determine the correct values for P (the percentage), B (the base), and r (the rate or percent). Another version of this formula can help you when trying to determine which number to put into each location in the proportion. It is a variation of the previous formula.

$$\frac{\%}{100} = \frac{\text{is (the part)}}{\text{of (the whole or total)}}$$

The number with the percent sign is always put over 100 since a percent is a comparison of a number to 100. The base is the whole or total and follows the words "% of" in the problem. For example, when you leave a tip at a restaurant, you customarily leave 15% of the amount of your bill. In this sentence, "the amount of your bill" follows the words "% of," so the amount of your bill is the base (B) in this problem. The percentage represents a quantity and is usually beside the word "is" in a problem. In the problem, 5% of 15 is 0.75, the base is the number 15 (follows "% of"), and the number 0.75 is the percentage (the amount that follows "is").

EXAMPLE 14: Setting Up Percentage Problems as Proportions

Set up the following percentage problems as proportions. Then solve each one.

a. What is 15% of 85?

The 15 represents the variable r (rate) and the 85 represents the B (base or total amount) since it follows the "% of." The percentage (P) is the missing number in this problem.

Setup: $$\frac{r}{100} = \frac{P}{B}$$

$$\frac{15}{100} = \frac{x}{85}$$

Solution: $(15)(85) = 100x$ cross-multiplication property

$1275 = 100x$ simplify

$$\frac{1275}{100} = \frac{100x}{100}$$ division property of equality

$12.75 = x$

b. 25% of what number is 18?

The 25 represents the variable r (rate) and the 18 represents the P (percentage) since it follows the "is." The base (B) is the missing number in this problem.

Setup: $$\frac{r}{100} = \frac{P}{B}$$

$$\frac{25}{100} = \frac{18}{x}$$

Solution: $(25)(x) = (100)(18)$ cross-multiplication property

$25x = 1800$ simplify

$$\frac{25x}{25} = \frac{1800}{25}$$ division property of equality

$x = 72$

c. What % of 250 is 37.5?

The 37.5 represents the P (percentage) since it follows the "is," and the 250 represents the B (base or total amount) since it follows the "% of." The rate (r) is the missing number in this problem.

Setup: $$\frac{r}{100} = \frac{P}{B}$$

$$\frac{x}{100} = \frac{37.5}{250}$$

Solution: $(250)(x) = (100)(37.5)$ cross-multiplication property

$250x = 3750$ simplify

$$\frac{250x}{250} = \frac{3750}{250}$$ division property of equality

$x = 15$, so the missing percent is 15%

Transactions in your daily life, such as department store discounts or restaurant tips, involve the use of percentages. In health care, when calculating dosages, looking at nutrition labels, or mixing solutions, you may encounter problems that involve percentages. Remember, if a pure drug is in the form of a solid, a 1% solution means 1 part per 100 parts, or 1 g of pure drug in 100 mL of solution. If the pure drug is in liquid form, a 1% solution means 1 mL of pure drug in 100 mL of solution.

EXAMPLE 15: Calculating a Percent Concentration Using a Proportion

A solution contains 15 mL of alcohol in 250 mL of solution. What is the percent concentration of the alcohol?

We are asked to find the percent concentration, so r is the unknown. The base (B) or total amount of solution is 250 mL, and the 15 mL of alcohol is the percentage (P).

$$\frac{r}{100} = \frac{P}{B}$$

$$\frac{r}{100} = \frac{15}{250} \qquad \text{substitute values}$$

$$250(r) = (100)(15) \qquad \text{cross-multiplication property}$$

$$250r = 1500 \qquad \text{simplify}$$

$$\frac{250r}{250} = \frac{1500}{250} \qquad \text{division property of equality}$$

$$r = 6$$

Therefore, the concentration of alcohol in this solution is 6%.

EXAMPLE 16: Solving an Application Problem Using Percents

A patient receives 500 mL of a 10% glucose solution. How many grams of glucose does the patient get out of the 500 mL of solution?

A 10% glucose solution is a ratio of

$$\frac{10 \text{ g glucose}}{100 \text{ mL of total solution}}$$

In this problem, the base (B) is the 500 mL of solution. Use a proportion to set up the problem and solve.

$$\frac{r}{100} = \frac{P}{B}$$

$$\frac{10 \text{ g}}{100 \text{ mL}} = \frac{x \text{ g}}{500 \text{ mL}} \qquad \text{substitute values}$$

$$(500)(10) = (100)(x) \qquad \text{cross-multiplication property}$$

$$5000 = 100x \qquad \text{simplify}$$

$$\frac{5000}{100} = \frac{100x}{100} \qquad \text{division property of equality}$$

$$50 = x$$

Therefore, 500 mL of a 10% glucose solution contains 50 g of glucose.

We can also solve percent problems by translating the problem into an algebraic equation and solving for the missing variable. Understanding a few key terms relating to mathematics can help you solve percent problems easily. One of these terms is the word *of*, which, in mathematics, means "multiply." Another is the word *is*, which, in mathematics, means "equal to." To find a percent of a number using an equation, change the percent to a decimal and then multiply it times the original quantity, which is called the *base*. The answer to this problem is called a *percentage*. For example, 25% of 350 is solved by the computation $0.25 \times 350 = 87.5$. In this problem, the 0.25 is the rate (the percent), the 350 is the base (the original total quantity), and the 87.5 is the percentage (the answer to the percent problem). The basic equation is given in the box below.

Using Equations to Solve Percentage Problems

$$r \cdot B = P$$

where *r* is the rate (% written as a decimal), *P* is the percentage (answer), and *B* is the base (original total amount).

Given any two of the three parts of this equation, you can easily solve for the third variable. Look at the following example, which uses the same problems that were demonstrated in Example 14.

EXAMPLE 17: Setting Up Percentage Problems as Algebraic Equations

Set up the following percentage problems as equations. Then solve each one.

a. What is 15% of 85?

The 15 represents the variable *r* (rate) and will be written in decimal form as 0.15. The 85 represents the *B* (base or total amount) since it follows the "% of." The percentage (*P*) is the missing number in this problem, represented by "what."

$$\text{Setup: } r \cdot B = P \text{ or } P = r \cdot B$$
$$\text{Solution: } x = 0.15 \cdot 85$$
$$x = 12.75 \qquad \text{simplify}$$

b. 25% of what number is 18?

The 25 represents the variable *r* (rate) and will be written in decimal form as 0.25. The 18 represents the *P* (percentage or answer) since it follows the "is." The base (*B*) is the missing number in this problem.

$$\text{Setup: } r \cdot B = P$$
$$0.25 \cdot x = 18$$
$$\text{Solution: } 0.25x = 18$$
$$\frac{0.25x}{0.25} = \frac{18}{0.25} \qquad \text{division property of equality}$$
$$x = 72$$

c. What % of 250 is 37.5?

The 37.5 represents the *P* (percentage) since it follows the "is," and the 250 represents the *B* (base or total amount) since it follows the "% of." The rate (*r*) is the missing number in this problem.

$$\text{Setup: } r \cdot B = P$$
$$x \cdot 250 = 37.5$$
$$\text{Solution: } 250x = 37.5$$
$$\frac{250x}{250} = \frac{37.5}{250} \qquad \text{division property of equality}$$
$$x = 0.15, \text{ so writing this decimal in percent form tells us}$$
$$\text{that the missing percent is } 15\%$$

When solving a problem involving a percent, you may use either the proportion method or an algebraic equation. Decide which method to use based on your understanding of each process and the one that seems easiest for a given problem. For example, in a problem asking you to calculate the amount required if you leave a 15% tip for a $25 meal, it may be easiest to multiply 0.15×25. But, if a problem directs you to calculate the percent concentration of a solution given its parts, you may find it more convenient to use the proportion method.

EXAMPLE 18: Calculating Target Heart Rates

Many gyms post charts that give target zones for heart rates of their members during exercise. Its purpose is to guide a person's exercise workout by keeping the intensity level between an upper and lower heart rate limit. There are various suggested target zones that correspond with a specific exercise goal. Each person's maximum heartbeat is calculated based on gender and age. Then, using this chart, each individual can calculate his target heart rate zone during exercise.

IDEAL FOR	BENEFIT DESIRED	INTENSITY LEVEL (% MAXIMUM HEART RATE)
Light exercise	Maintain healthy heart/get fit	50–60
Weight management	Lose weight/burn fat	60–70
Aerobic base building	Increase stamina and aerobic endurance	70–80
Optimal conditioning	Maintain excellent fitness condition	80–90
Elite athlete	Maintain superb athletic condition	90–100

a. If you are a 40-year-old woman, your age-adjusted maximum heart rate is 186 bpm (beats per minute). If you are exercising for weight management, what is the range of your optimal target heart rate during exercise?

The upper and lower target heart rates will be found by taking 60% and 70% of the maximum heart rate. We will set this problem up using the proportion method: $\dfrac{r}{100} = \dfrac{P}{B}$. The 186 bpm is the base.

Minimum: $\dfrac{60}{100} = \dfrac{x}{186}$

$(60)(186) = (100)x$ cross-multiply

$11,160 = 100x$ simplify

$\dfrac{11,160}{100} = \dfrac{100x}{100}$ division property of equality

$111.6 = x$

Maximum: $\dfrac{70}{100} = \dfrac{x}{186}$

$(70)(186) = (100)x$ cross-multiply

$13,020 = 100x$ simplify

$\dfrac{13,020}{100} = \dfrac{100x}{100}$ division property of equality

$130.2 = x$

Therefore, the target heart rate during exercise for a 40-year-old woman should be between 112 and 130 beats per minute.

b. If you are a 45-year-old man, your age-adjusted maximum heart rate is 175 bpm (beats per minute). If you are exercising to maintain a healthy heart and get fit, what is the range of your optimal target heart rate during exercise?

The upper and lower target heart rates will be found by taking 50% and 60% of the maximum heart rate. We will set this problem up using the algebra method: $r \cdot B = P$. The 175 bpm is the base.

$$\text{Minimum:} \ 0.50 \cdot 175 = P$$
$$87.5 = P$$
$$\text{Maximum:} \ 0.60 \cdot 175 = P$$
$$105 = P$$

Therefore, the target heart rate during exercise for a 45-year-old man should be between 88 and 105 beats per minute.

Many times we are interested in the percent increase or decrease of quantities that have changed over time. For example, if a health care worker makes $15.50 an hour and receives a $0.31 per hour increase, we can calculate the percent raise received using the following formula.

% Increase/Decrease

$$\% \text{ Increase/Decrease} = \frac{\text{New value} - \text{Original value}}{\text{Original value}} \cdot 100$$

If the new salary is $15.81 per hour and the original salary was $15.50 per hour, we calculate the percent change in salary as follows:

$$\% \text{ Increase/Decrease} = \frac{\text{New value} - \text{Original value}}{\text{Original value}} \cdot 100$$
$$= \frac{15.81 - 15.50}{15.50} = \frac{0.31}{15.5} \cdot 100 = 2\%$$

So, this employee has received a 2% increase in his salary. The % increase/decrease formula can be used to calculate % gains and losses in a patient's weight, % increases and decreases in the prices of goods and services, and in other similar types of problems.

EXAMPLE 19: Calculating Percent Loss of Weight

Joanna's weight on January 1 was 205 lb. She began a low-carbohydrate diet and by the end of February, she weighed 188 lb. Calculate her percent weight loss during these two months.

$$\% \text{ Loss} = \frac{\text{New value} - \text{Original value}}{\text{Original value}} \cdot 100 = \frac{188 - 205}{205} \cdot 100$$
$$= \frac{-17}{205} \cdot 100 = -0.0829268 \cdot 100 = -8.29\%$$

Therefore, Joanna has lost a little over 8% of her original weight.

PRACTICE PROBLEM SET 2.4

Use proportions to solve Problems 1–10.

1. Find 15% of 85.
2. Find 20% of 2510.
3. 25% of what number is 25.5?
4. 48% of what number is 148.8?
5. What percent of 450 is 157.5?

6. What percent of 150 is 3.75?
7. 1.5% of what number is 2.85?
8. 0.25% of what number is 8.75?
9. What percent of 175 is 87.5?
10. What percent of 2300 is 34.5?

Use an algebraic equation to solve Problems 11–20.

11. Find 12% of 850.
12. Find 52% of 250.
13. 50% of what number is 29.5?
14. 85% of what number is 246.5?
15. What percent of 65 is 1.95?

16. What percent of 150 is 3.6?
17. 1.75% of what number is 10.5?
18. 0.15% of what number is 3.675?
19. What percent of 275 is 9.625?
20. What percent of 2520 is 40.32?

Calculate the percent increase or decrease for the following changes.

21. original value: 25; new value: 30
22. original value: 160; new value: 180
23. original value: 1.50; new value: 1.35
24. original value: 27.5; new value: 22.0

25. original value: 1.10; new value: 1.00
26. original value: 55.20; new value: 57.96
27. original value: 0.550; new value: 0.536
28. original value: 0.025; new value: 0.105

Use one of the methods presented in this section to answer the following problems.

29. According to health charts, a woman with a "normal" body type and weight should have between 22% and 25% body fat. If Jean's body fat has been measured at 23% and her weight is 125 lb, how much of her total weight is body fat?
30. If a woman's body fat measures more than 32%, she is considered to be obese. If Marie's body fat is measured at 35% and her weight is 275 lb, how much of her total weight is body fat?
31. The average adult body fat for males is 15% to 18%. If Juan's body fat is determined to be 17% and his weight is 180 lb, how much of his weight is lean body mass (bone, muscle, organ tissue, blood, and everything else)?
32. Male athletes usually have between 6% and 13% body fat. Marty is a marathon runner and his body fat is 7%. If his weight is 160 lb, how much of his weight is lean body mass (bone, muscle, organ tissue, blood, and everything else)?
33. For a 30-year-old woman, the age-adjusted maximum heart rate is 196 bpm (beats per minute). If she desires to lose weight and burn fat through exercise, she should exercise so that her heartbeat is 60% to 70% of her maximum heart rate for at least 30 minutes a day, 3 days a week. Give the range of beats per minute for this level of exercise.
34. If you are a 35-year-old man, your age-adjusted maximum heart rate is 185 bpm (beats per minute). If you desire to maintain excellent fitness conditioning, you should exercise so that your heartbeat is 80% to 90% of the maximum heart rate for at least 30 minutes a day, 3 days a week. Give the range of beats per minute for this level of exercise.
35. What is the percent concentration of a salt solution containing 15 g of salt in 250 mL of water?
36. What is the concentration of a glucose solution containing 25 g of glucose in 500 mL of water?
37. There are 8 g of pure drug in 25 mL of solution. What is the percent strength of this medication?

38. There are 15 mL of alcohol in 250 mL of solution. What is the percent concentration of the alcohol?
39. How many grams of sodium chloride are there in 250 mL of a 0.4% saline solution?
40. How many grams of glucose would be required to make 75 mL of a 4% solution?
41. There are 9 mL of pure drug in 100 mL of a solution. How many milliliters of pure drug are in 40 mL of this solution?
42. A doctor has ordered a 5% saline solution. How many grams of sodium chloride are in 125 mL of solution?
43. How many grams of pure drug are in 500 mL of a 0.5% solution?
44. A 1% hydrocortisone cream is a compound that contains 1 g of hydrocortisone per 100 g of cream. How many grams of hydrocortisone are in 250 g of a 1% cream?
45. A certain medication is packaged 120 mg/0.8 mL. How many milliliters do you give in order to administer 80 mg?
46. A certain medication is supplied in the form of 10 mg in a 2-mL vial. How many milliliters do you give in order to administer 2.5 mg?
47. Mike's health insurance premium for last year was $1440. If he paid $1512 this year, what is the percent of increase on his health insurance premium?
48. As office manager you are responsible for buying some new furniture for the office. The original price of a sofa was $1500. The store manager is willing to give you a business discount and sell it for $1440. What is the percent decrease in the price?
49. Lydia weighed 150 lb at the beginning of November. After Christmas, she weighed 161 lb. Find the percent of increase in her weight.
50. Sal joined the local gym in order to lose weight. His current weight is 240 lb. If he loses 36 lb, what percent decrease in weight will this loss represent?

SECTION 2.5   USING FORMULAS

A **formula** is a statement of a fact, rule, principle, or other logical relation that typically has a real-life application. Formulas are often written in the form of an algebraic equation. We can think of a formula as a "recipe" for solving a particular type of problem. There are many standard formulas available that will help us solve problems. For example, in the area of health care there are formulas that are used for measurement conversions, dosage calculations, calculations of body fat, and preparing working solutions from stock solutions, to name a few. It is important when using formulas to identify the meaning of each of the variables in the formula and the units that each represents. Substitute the given values into the formula, and use the order of operations and rules of algebra to complete the calculations.

EXAMPLE 20: Using a Simple Formula

The formula $H = 1.36gs$ can be used to determine how much oxygen is in the hemoglobin of a blood sample, where H represents the milliliters of oxygen in the hemoglobin from 100 mL of whole blood, g is the number of grams of hemoglobin in 100 mL of whole blood, and s is the oxygen concentration, in decimal form, in the hemoglobin. A blood test tells you that a 100-mL sample contains 12.0 g of hemoglobin and the hemoglobin is 91% oxygen. Determine how much oxygen is in this sample.

Given $g = 12.0$ and $s = 91\% = 0.91$, substitute these values into the formula.

$$H = 1.36gs$$
$$H = 1.36(12.0)(0.91)$$
$$H = 14.8512 \text{ mL of oxygen}$$

EXAMPLE 21: Using a Conversion Formula

Temperature is commonly measured in degrees Fahrenheit and degrees Celsius. To convert degrees Fahrenheit to degrees Celsius, we use the conversion formula $C = \frac{5}{9}(F - 32)$. Convert 38°F to degrees Celsius.

Substitute the given value into the formula. Follow the order of operations by completing the subtraction in the parentheses and then multiplying the remaining numbers.

$$C = \frac{5}{9}(F - 32)$$

$$C = \frac{5}{9}(38 - 32)$$

$$C = \frac{5}{9}(6)$$

$$C = \frac{30}{9} = 3.33°$$

EXAMPLE 22: Using a Formula Involving Several Operations

In a hospital, the doctor frequently orders a specific volume of IV fluid to be given over a specific period of time in hours. The orders may be written in "cc per hour" and must be converted to "drops per minute" in order to determine how to adjust the drip set to administer the desired amount of fluid during the prescribed amount of time. The formula for this conversion is

$$D = \frac{A \cdot S}{T}$$

where D is drops per minute to be infused

A is amount of fluid ordered by the doctor

S is the drip set

T is the time in minutes

You are asked to infuse 1000 cc of D_5W to be given over an 8-hour time span and the hospital uses a 15-drop-per-cc drip set. How many drops per minute should the IV supply to the patient?

Substitute the given values into the formula. Complete the operations in the numerator, and then divide that result by the denominator. Since T represents time in minutes and the order is for 8 hours, we must convert 8 hours to minutes before substituting into the formula (8 hr · 60 min/hr = 480 min).

$$D = \frac{A \cdot S}{T}$$

$$D = \frac{1000 \cdot 15}{480} = 31.25 \text{ drops per minute}$$

So, the IV should be set to administer 31 drops per minute.

EXAMPLE 23: Calculating Body Mass Index Using a Formula

Body Mass Index (BMI) is a tool for determining the weight status of adults. It is a measure of weight in pounds based on height in inches. For adults over 20 years old, BMI falls into one of these categories:

BMI	WEIGHT STATUS
Below 18.5	Underweight
18.5–24.9	Normal
25.0–29.9	Overweight
30.0 and above	Obese

The formula used to calculate Body Mass Index is

$$\text{BMI} = \frac{W}{H^2} \cdot 703$$

where $\quad W$ = weight in pounds and H = height in inches

Mark wants to determine if he is overweight based on his BMI. He weighs 220 lb and is 6 ft, 3 in. tall.

In the formula, H is height in inches, so we must convert 6 ft, 3 in. to inches in order to substitute into the formula.

$$6 \text{ ft} \cdot 12 \text{ in./ft} + 3 \text{ in.} = 72 \text{ in.} + 3 \text{ in.} = 75 \text{ in.}$$

Now substitute these values into the formula and calculate his BMI.

$$\text{BMI} = \frac{W}{H^2} \cdot 703$$

$$\text{BMI} = \frac{220}{75^2} \cdot 703$$

$$\text{BMI} = \frac{220}{5625} \cdot 703$$

$$\text{BMI} = 0.03911 \cdot 703 = 27.5$$

Therefore, based on the chart, with a BMI of 27.5, Mark is overweight.

Many times we may need to rearrange a formula to answer the question asked. We do this by rewriting the given formula, solving for a specified variable. For example, in the formula for IV fluids, $D = \dfrac{A \cdot S}{T}$, we can rewrite this formula solving for T, giving $T = \dfrac{A \cdot S}{D}$. To solve a formula for a given letter, we must isolate that variable on one side of the equal sign. All other variables will be on the other side. We follow the same algebraic rules and principles that we have used to solve equations in the past in order to accomplish this revision. Look at the following example.

EXAMPLE 24: Rewriting a Temperature Formula

Solve the formula $F = \frac{9}{5}C + 32$ for the variable C.

$$F = \frac{9}{5}C + 32 \qquad \text{given formula}$$

$$5(F) = 5\left(\frac{9}{5}C\right) + 5(32) \qquad \text{multiply both sides by 5}$$

$$5F = 9C + 160 \qquad \text{simplify}$$

$$5F - 160 = 9C + 160 - 160 \qquad \text{subtraction property of equality}$$

$$5F - 160 = 9C \qquad \text{simplify}$$

$$\frac{5F - 160}{9} = \frac{9C}{9} \qquad \text{division property of equality}$$

$$\frac{5F - 160}{9} = C$$

The same relationship is maintained among the variables but the formula has been rewritten to solve for the value of C. By factoring out $\frac{5}{9}$ on the left side of the equation, we see the more commonly used version of this formula:

$$\frac{5}{9}(F - 32) = C$$

EXAMPLE 25: Rewriting a Formula for Making Solutions

Often a new solution is made by the addition of more solvent to a stock solution kept on hand in a laboratory. The formula $V_1 C_1 = V_2 C_2$ expresses the relationship between the stock solution and the solution being made. V_1 represents the volume of the stock solution that is needed to make the new solution; C_1 represents the concentration of the stock solution on hand; V_2 is the amount of solution that is being made; and C_2 is the desired concentration of the new solution. Solve $V_1 C_1 = V_2 C_2$ for V_1, and then calculate the volume of 12% stock solution needed to make 50 mL of a 8% solution.

$$V_1 C_1 = V_2 C_2 \qquad \text{given equation}$$

$$V_1 = \frac{V_2 C_2}{C_1} \qquad \text{rewritten formula using the}$$
$$\text{division property of equality}$$

Now substitute the given values: $V_2 = 50$ mL, $C_2 = 8\%$, $C_1 = 12\%$.

$$V_1 = \frac{50 \text{ mL} \cdot 8\%}{12\%} = 33.33 \text{ mL}$$

This result tells us that we should take 33.33 mL of stock solution and add a diluting agent such as water to increase the volume to a final volume of 50 mL. The resulting 50-mL solution will have a concentration of 8%.

Most formulas are short ways of writing mathematical rules or relationships. They were created by someone who figured out the relationships among the variables and created a model for everyone to follow when doing the necessary calculations. You can find many formulas by looking in reference books or handbooks related to your job. It is not necessary to memorize all formulas, but you must be familiar with the mathematical operations necessary to use them. Always be sure that you understand what each of the variables represents and that you pay attention to the measurement units being used in the problem. You would agree that 31 drops *per minute* and 31 drops *per hour* represent two different outcomes for a patient!

PRACTICE PROBLEM SET 2.5

Evaluate each formula using the given values of the variables.

1. Conversion of Fahrenheit to Celsius: $C = \dfrac{5}{9}(F - 32)$ if $F = 68°$

2. Conversion of Fahrenheit to Celsius: $C = \dfrac{5}{9}(F - 32)$ if $F = 23°$

3. Conversion of Celsius to Fahrenheit: $F = \dfrac{9}{5}C + 32$ if $C = 100°$

4. Conversion of Celsius to Fahrenheit: $F = \dfrac{9}{5}C + 32$ if $C = -10°$

Use this formula for the approximation of a child's dose of medication for Problems 5–10:

Formula: $c = \dfrac{w}{150} \cdot d$, where c = child's dosage, w = child's weight, and d = adult dosage.

5. $w = 50$ lb, $d = 10$ mg
6. $w = 90$ lb, $d = 0.35$ mg
7. $w = 60$ lb, d = 5.5 grains

8. $w = 45$ lb, $d = 0.125$ grains
9. $w = 75$ lb, $d = 1$ teaspoon
10. $w = 80$ lb, $d = 2$ teaspoons

Use the formula in Example 22 to find the drip rates for IVs, given the following information.

11. You are asked to administer 1000 cc of normal saline using a 15-drop-per-cc set during a 24-hour period.
12. You are asked to administer 500 cc of normal saline over a 2-hour period using a 15-drop-per-cc set.
13. Calculate the flow rate for an infusion of 500 cc in 5 hours with a drip set calibrated at 10-drop-per-cc.
14. Calculate the flow rate for an infusion of 1200 cc during a 10-hour period with a drip set calibrated at 20-drop-per-cc.

Use the formula for calculating BMI in Example 23 to determine if each of the following individuals is overweight.

15. Anne is 5 ft 2 in. and weighs 110 lb.
16. Dustin is 5 ft 10 in. and weighs 178 lb.
17. Jamal is 6 ft 1 in. and weighs 205 lb.

18. Roberta is 5 ft 9 in. and weighs 141 lb.
19. Maria is 5 ft $4\frac{1}{2}$ in. and weighs 131 lb.
20. Chad is 6 ft and weighs 160 lb.

Rewrite the following formulas, solving for the specified variables.

21. $H = 1.36gs$, for g
22. $V_1C_1 = V_2C_2$, for C_2
23. $C = \dfrac{5}{9}(F - 32)$, for F
24. $c = \dfrac{w}{150} \cdot d$, for d

25. $\text{BMI} = \dfrac{W}{H^2} \cdot 703$, for W
26. $D = \dfrac{A \cdot S}{T}$, for T

Use the formulas in each problem to answer the questions.

27. A person's thiamine requirement is related to his caloric intake. The formula that approximates the minimum daily requirement of thiamine is $T = \dfrac{c}{1000} \cdot 0.22$ mg, where c represents caloric intake. What is the approximate minimum daily requirement of thiamine for an intake of 1850 calories?

28. Using the formula in Problem 27, what is the approximate minimum daily requirement of thiamine for an intake of 2200 calories?

29. A person's *vital capacity* is the amount of air that can be exhaled after one deep breath. An estimate of the vital capacity for men can be obtained using the formula

$$C = (21.78 - 0.101a) \cdot h$$

where $a =$ age, $h =$ height in centimeters, and C is vital capacity in cc

If John is 184 cm tall and is 40 years old, find his vital capacity.

30. Using the formula in Problem 29, find Martin's vital capacity if he is 52 years old and 176 cm tall.

31. The BMR formula uses the variables of height, weight, age, and gender to calculate the Basal Metabolic Rate (BMR) for men and women. This is more accurate than calculating calorie needs based on body weight alone. The formula for women is: BMR $= 655 + (4.35 \times$ weight in pounds$) + (4.7 \times$ height in inches$) - (4.7 \times$ age in years$)$. Calculate the BMR for a woman who weighs 165 lb, is 5 ft 9 in. tall and is 50 years old.

32. Using the formula in Problem 31, calculate the BMR for a 28-year-old woman who is 5 ft 4 in. and weighs 135 lb.

33. The formula to calculate the BMR for men is BMR $= 66 + (6.23 \times$ weight in pounds$) + (12.7 \times$ height in inches$) - (6.8 \times$ age in years$)$. Calculate the BMR for a man who weighs 225 lb, is 6 ft tall, and is 36 years old.

34. Using the formula in Problem 33, calculate the BMR for a 60-year-old man who is 5 ft 10 in. tall and weighs 195 lb.

The Harris Benedict Equation is a formula that applies an activity factor to your BMR to determine your total daily energy expenditure (calories). To determine your total daily calorie needs to maintain your current weight, multiply your BMR by the appropriate activity factor, as follows:

    a. If you are sedentary (little or no exercise): Calorie calculation = BMR × 1.2.

    b. If you are lightly active (light exercise/sports 1–3 days/week): Calorie calculation = BMR × 1.375.

    c. If you are moderately active (moderate exercise/sports 3–5 days/week): Calorie calculation = BMR × 1.55.

    d. If you are very active (hard exercise/sports 6–7 days a week): Calorie calculation = BMR × 1.725.

    e. If you are extra active (very hard exercise/sports and physical job or 2x training): Calorie calculation = BMR × 1.9.

35. Use the Harris Benedict Equation to determine your total daily calorie needs if your BMR is 1745 and you are sedentary.

36. Use the Harris Benedict Equation to determine your total daily calorie needs if your BMR is 1650 and you are extra active.

37. Use the Harris Benedict Equation to determine your total daily calorie needs if your BMR is 1805 and you are moderately active.

38. Use the Harris Benedict Equation to determine your total daily calorie needs if your BMR is 1795 and you are lightly active.

Use the formula in Example 25 to solve Problems 39–44.

39. How much of a 25% stock solution would be needed to produce 250 mL of a 10% solution?
40. How much of a 10% stock solution would be needed to produce 150 mL of a 7.5% solution?
41. How much 25% alcohol is needed to make 500 mL of 15% alcohol?
42. How much 9% solution is needed to make 50 mL of a 2% solution?
43. You can make 75 mL of a 20% solution from 25 mL of what percent stock solution?
44. You can make 90 mL of a 0.5% solution from 3 mL of what percent stock solution?
45. For women who are 5 ft or taller, insurance companies in the past used a rule that said that a woman 60 in. tall should weigh 100 lb and for those taller, an additional 5 lb should be added for every inch over 60 in. In equation form, $w = 100 + 5(h - 60)$. If a woman is 5 ft 8 in., what is the ideal weight of this woman using this old insurance formula?
46. Rewrite the insurance formula in Problem 45 and solve it for h. Using this rewritten formula, what is the projected height for a woman who weighs 155 lb?

SECTION 2.6   MODELING MEDICAL APPLICATIONS

When we use a mathematical equation to represent real phenomena, we create a **mathematical model**. This may be done by applying the correct formula to a situation or by creating an algebraic equation that is specific to our particular problem. Mathematical models can also be given in the form of charts or graphs. By gathering statistical data over a period of time, charting it, and then graphing it, we can identify trends and make predictions about the future. Changes in policy or treatment may also result from the trends illustrated by graphical models.

EXAMPLE 26: Interpreting a Graphical Model

The National Heart, Lung and Blood Institute provides leadership and support for research in cardiovascular, lung, and blood diseases. It publishes a *Chart Book* that contains information on the progress being made in the fight against these diseases. The graph contained in the 2002 *Chart Book* and shown in Figure 2.1 illustrates the percent of

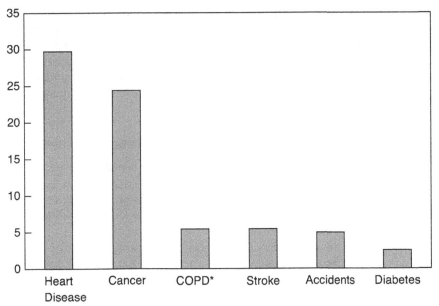

Percent of All Deaths

Figure 2.1 Leading Causes of Death, White Males, U.S., 2000
*COPD and allied conditions.

deaths attributable to various causes. Statisticians, medical researchers, and politicians alike can use this visual model to determine that the leading causes of death in white males are heart disease and cancer. Decisions about funding of programs and research can then be made based on this mathematical model.

Figure 2.2 is a graph of infant mortality rates for respiratory distress syndrome, also known as SIDS, from the 2002 *Chart Book*. It is easy to see that the trend during the past 26 years has been toward a much lower death rate. According to this graph, the death rate decreased steeply from 1974 to 1981 and has continued to decrease at a slower pace every year, with the exception of 1989. This model can support both research into the causes of SIDS and successful procedures and treatments that may have led to this decrease.

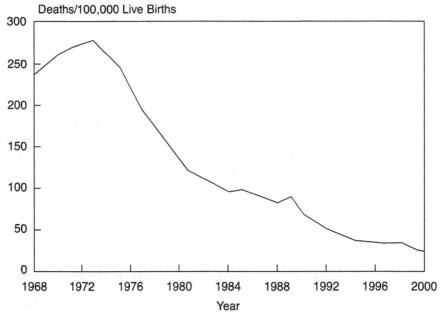

Figure 2.2 Infant Mortality Rate* for Respiratory Distress Syndrome, U.S., 1968–2000
*Under age 1.

To be successful in solving mathematical models that are in equation form, you must have a firm knowledge of the fundamental rules of algebra and be able to exercise some common sense. *Common sense* is a way of saying that it takes experience to become proficient at solving word problems. How do you acquire that needed experience? There's only one way. You must practice solving problems and look for patterns and similarities between types of problems. Many problems in the health care field can be solved using formulas, so you must read

---

Solving Application Problems

1. Read the problem carefully at least twice to make sure that you understand it.
2. If the problem calls for a specific formula, write down the formula, noting the meaning of each of the variables. Then, substitute the given values into the formula, paying special attention to the measurement units in the formula. Complete the calculations required using the correct order of operations.
3. If there is no formula applicable to this problem, determine which quantity you are being asked to find and choose a variable to represent that quantity. Write the words of the problem as an equation, and solve the problem using the properties of algebra.
4. Using your calculated value, answer the question posed by the problem.
5. Check your answer to be sure that it is a sensible answer and that the units are appropriate.

the problems carefully to ascertain the necessary formula to help you complete the problem. Use the general steps shown in the box on p. 62 when trying to solve an application problem.

Here is a list of key words to look for in solving word problems. These words indicate mathematical operations that are part of the problem.

Add	Subtract	Multiply	Divide
sum	difference	times	divided by
plus	less	of	per
more than	minus	product	
	less than	twice	

There are other key words in problems that will tell you what the problem expects you to do. Some examples are *calculate*, *compute*, *draw*, *write*, *show*, *identify*, *graph*, *evaluate*, and *state*.

EXAMPLE 27: Choosing the Correct Formula

Find the pediatric dosage of a medication if a child weighs 60 lb and the normal adult dosage of the medication is 25 mg.

There are several formulas used to calculate pediatric dosages. Each requires a different set of data in order to complete the calculation.

Young's Rule: $p = \dfrac{aA}{12 + a}$ where a = child's age in years, A = normal adult dosage, p = pediatric dosage

Clark's Rule: $p = \dfrac{wA}{150}$ where w = child's weight in pounds., A = normal adult dosage, p = pediatric dosage

Fried's Rule: $p = \dfrac{mA}{150}$ where m = child's age in months, A = normal adult dosage, p = pediatric dosage (generally used for children less than 1 yr)

Since the information we are given is the normal adult dosage (25 mg) and the weight of the child in pounds (60 lb), we will choose Clark's Rule for our calculation.

$$p = \frac{wA}{150}$$

$$p = \frac{60 \cdot 25 \text{ mg}}{150} = \frac{1500}{150} = 10 \text{ mg}$$

The pediatric dosage for this child is 10 mg.

It is important to choose the correct formula based on the facts of the problem. That is why reading the problem carefully is so important. Clark's Rule can also be written as $p = \dfrac{wA}{68.2}$, where w represents the child's weight in kilograms. If you do not pay attention to the units of weight that are given in the problem, you can use the wrong formula, thereby incorrectly calculating the pediatric dosage. This could cause you to overmedicate or undermedicate the child.

In some problems, you are asked to use a known formula or relationship and expand it to fit the problem. For example, in Example 25 you were introduced to a formula that is used to create new solutions from stock solutions: $V_1C_1 = V_2C_2$. In some problems, you may need to mix together two or more solutions to create a new solution of a given strength. Therefore, we must expand this formula to suit our problem.

EXAMPLE 28: Mixing Two Solutions to Create the Desired Strength Solution

How many milliliters of 20% alcohol and 50% alcohol should be mixed together to obtain 300 mL of 40% alcohol?

In this problem, we want to know how much of the 20% solution and how much of the 50% solution to mix together in order to produce 300 mL of a new solution with a concentration of 40%. We know that the total volume of our final solution is 300 mL, part of which is the 20% solution and part of which is the 50% solution. Therefore, we will assign the variable x to the volume of 20% solution (V_1) and $(300 - x)$ to the volume of 50% solution (V_2) because $x + (300 - x) = 300$ mL. Now recall the $V_1C_1 = V_2C_2$ formula. Since we are adding one stock solution to another, we will expand the formula to give

$$V_1C_1 + V_2C_2 = V_FC_F$$

In this equation, V_F represents the volume of the final solution, 300 mL, and C_F represents the concentration of the final solution, 40%. Substituting the values and variables into our equation gives

$$(x)(0.20) + (300 - x)(0.50) = (300)(0.40)$$
$$0.2x + 150 - 0.5x = 120$$
$$-0.3x + 150 = 120$$
$$-0.3x + 150 - 150 = 120 - 150$$
$$-0.3x = -30$$
$$\frac{-0.3x}{-0.3} = \frac{-30}{-0.3}$$
$$x = 100 \text{ mL of } 20\%$$
$$300 - x = 300 - 100 = 200 \text{ mL of } 50\%$$

Therefore, 100 mL of 20% solution mixed with 200 mL of 50% will produce 300 mL of a 40% solution.

Check: To check to be sure that you have calculated correctly, substitute all values into the equation to verify equality.

$$V_1C_1 + V_2C_2 = V_FC_F$$
$$(100)(0.20) + (200)(0.50) = (300)(0.40)$$
$$20 + 100 = 120$$
$$120 = 120 \checkmark$$

One type of problem that we encounter is adding a percent to a given amount or reducing a given amount by a percent. For example, if your meal including a 15% tip totaled $40.00, how much did the meal itself cost? Or, if you received a 5% wage increase and your new hourly rate is $15.75, what was your old rate? These questions can be modeled in a similar fashion. Look at the next example.

EXAMPLE 29: Determining an Original Value after a Percent Increase

Marilyn ordered 10 boxes of Steri-Strip™ Adhesive Skin Closures from the distributor. He informed her that his current price of $66.98 per box was a 1% price increase from her last order. What was the price she paid per box on the previous order?

Let x = the price per box on the previous order. The new price represents the old price plus 1% of the old price. Write this sentence as an equation and solve.

$$x + 0.01x = \$66.98$$
$$1.01x = \$66.98$$
$$\frac{1.01x}{1.01} = \frac{\$66.98}{1.01}$$
$$x = \$66.32$$

The previous price paid for a box of Steri-Strip™ Skin Closures was $66.32.

$$\text{Check: } x + 0.01x = \$66.98$$
$$\$66.32 + (0.01)(\$66.32) = \$66.98$$
$$\$66.32 + \$0.66 = \$66.98$$
$$\$66.98 = \$66.98 \checkmark$$

Each time that you are confronted with a math problem in a health care setting, you will need to analyze the problem based on the information given to you and the appropriate formulas or methods of solution available. **Pay attention to units of measure in your problems because incorrect units in results can have significant consequences in real-life applications.** Throughout the rest of this book, we will present various types of problems relating to the allied health field and methods of solution for those problems.

PRACTICE PROBLEM SET 2.6

1. The accompanying graph models blood flow through the kidneys for people of different ages.
   a. What does the graph tell us about the changing blood flow as one grows older?
   b. What percent normal flow does a 60-year-old have?

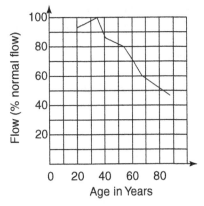

2. The accompanying graph models the normal head growth for a child. The vertical axis is the circumference of the head in centimeters and the horizontal axis is the age of the child.

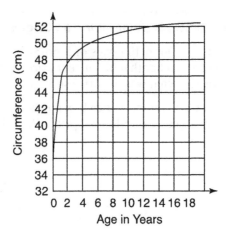

a. Based on this graphical model, give an explanation of the growth of a child's head from ages 0 to 5 years old.

b. Approximately what is the circumference for an average 8-year-old?

Choose the correct rule based on the information given and use it to calculate p, the pediatric dosage of medication, in Problems 3–12.

Young's Rule: $p = \dfrac{aA}{12 + a}$, where a = child's age, A = normal adult dosage

Clark's Rule: $p = \dfrac{wA}{150}$, where w = child's weight in lb, A = normal adult dosage

Clark's Rule: $p = \dfrac{wA}{68.2}$, where w = child's weight in kg, A = normal adult dosage

Fried's Rule: $p = \dfrac{mA}{150}$, where m = child's age in months, A = normal adult dosage

3. The child's weight is 45 lb and the normal adult dosage is 10 mg.
4. The child's weight is 94 lb and the normal adult dosage is 2 teaspoons.
5. The child's age is 6 years, and the normal adult dosage is 50 mg.
6. The child's age is 2 years 3 months and the normal adult dosage is 10 mL.
7. The child's age is 9 months and the normal adult dosage is 25 mL.
8. The child's age is 6 months and the normal adult dosage is 60 mg.
9. The child's weight is 10 kg and the normal adult dosage is 0.1 mg.
10. The child's weight is 34 kg and the normal adult dosage is 100 mg.
11. A doctor has ordered medication for an 8-year-old child. The adult dosage is 50 mg and the pharmacy carries 8-mg, 15-mg, and 25-mg tablets. What size tablets should you use and how many should the child be given for one dosage?
12. A doctor has ordered medication for a 38-lb child. The usual adult dosage is 100 mg. The drug label lists a supply dosage of 50 mg per tablet but does not list a pediatric dosage. Calculate the pediatric dosage and give the number of tablets that should be administered.
13. How much 7.5% solution can be made with 150 mL of 10% solution?
14. You could make 75 mL of 20% from 25 mL of what percent?
15. How much 9% solution is needed to make 50 mL of 10.5% solution?
16. How much 20% solution is required to make 200 mL of 3% solution?
17. What will be the concentration of a solution that is made by mixing 50 mL of an 11% solution and 25 mL of a 5% solution?
18. You mix 25 mL of 6% solution and 75 mL of 4% solution in a flask. What is the concentration of the final solution?
19. Twenty milliliters of 6% solution is mixed with 80 mL of another solution. The resulting mixture has a concentration of 3%. What is the concentration of the second solution that was used for the mixture?

20. Using 3 mL of a concentrated solution, you produce 90 mL of a solution having a concentration of 0.5%. What was the concentration of the original solution?
21. How much 9% HCl must be mixed with 4% HCl to produce 50 mL of 6% solution?
22. How much 15% HCl must be mixed with 8% HCl to produce 60 mL of 9% HCl?
23. The dental office ordered a case of earloop masks. The current cost of the case is $50.25, which represents a 1.5% increase from the cost last month. What was the price of a case last month?
24. The Urgent Care Clinic ordered a case of 12-cc syringes for $109.64. This price represents a 2% increase in the cost of a case from the last order placed. How much did the case cost before the price increase?
25. The lab ordered 25 boxes of blood collection tubes for $63.91. The advertisement for this distributor stated that this price was a 5% reduction from the original price. What was the original price?
26. The physical therapy department ordered a case of four dual-release light-weight walkers for $172.92. This price reflected a 4% discount the store was offering its customers in March. What was the original price of the case of four before the sale?
27. In Iowa, the median wage for nursing assistants (CNAs) in 2004 was $10.55 per hour based on an October 2004 report by the Iowa Caregivers Association. If a CNA earning $10.55 per hour receives a 4% raise, what is her new hourly rate?
28. Based on a 2004 report by the Iowa Caregivers Association, the median wage for a home care worker in 2004 was $9.65 per hour. If a home care worker receives a 2.5% raise, what is her new hourly rate?
29. A 2004 report by the Center for Heath Professions at the University of California, San Francisco, stated that the median hourly wage for medical assistants in the state of California is $12.61. This is approximately 5.6% higher than the national hourly wage. What is the national median hourly wage for medical assistants?
30. The national median hourly wage for full time DANB (Dental Assisting National Board) certified dental assistants was reported in their Fall 2004 newsletter as $15.48. This is approximately 11.4% higher than the national median for noncertified dental assistants. What is the hourly rate for non-DANB-certified dental assistants?
31. The cost model for producing manufactured goods includes an amount for fixed costs such as utilities, rent, employee wages, equipment costs, etc. and the per item cost of materials used to make the items being produced. If Thermo-Group manufactures thermometers at a fixed cost of $65,000 per month plus $3.50 per thermometer, write an algebraic model of this cost of production, and calculate the cost of producing 25,000 thermometers in a month.
32. A medical prosthetics company charges a $350.00 setup fee and $5.50 per piece to make a plastic brace for patients with sprained wrists. Write an equation to model this cost of production, and calculate the cost of producing 3000 braces.

Chapter Summary

In this chapter we have looked at the order of operations, some of the fundamental properties of algebra, and methods used to solve algebraic equations. We have used formulas and models to solve application problems in the allied health field. The most important thing about learning to solve algebraic equations is mastering the ability to think and work in a logical order. This skill will serve you well in your daily life and in your day-to-day workplace duties. When working practical problems, always be sure that your answers are sensible. Remember that just because a calculator gives a particular numerical result, that does not make it the correct answer. Common sense will help you distinguish between results that are realistic and those that are not.

Important Terms and Rules

cross-multiplication property	order of operations
distributive property	percent
equivalent equations	proportions
formula	ratio
mathematical model	signed numbers
opposite, opposites	

The Addition/Subtraction Properties of Equality: For any real numbers a, b, and c, if $a = b$, then $a + c = b + c$, and if $a = b$, then $a - c = b - c$.

The Multiplication/Division Properties of Equality: For any real numbers a, b, and c, if $a = b$, then $ac = bc$, and if $a = b$, then $\dfrac{a}{c} = \dfrac{b}{c}$ ($c \neq 0$).

The Distributive Property: For all real numbers a, b, and c, $a(b + c) = ab + ac$.

Cross-Multiplication Property: If $\dfrac{a}{b} = \dfrac{c}{d}$, then $ad = bc$, where $b \neq 0$ and $d \neq 0$.

Using Proportions to Solve Percentage Problems: $\dfrac{r}{100} = \dfrac{P}{B}$, where r is the rate, P is the percentage, and B is the base.

Using Equations to Solve Percentage Problems: $r \cdot B = P$, where r is the rate (% written as a decimal), P is the percentage (answer), and B is the base (original total amount).

% Increase/Decrease: $\dfrac{\text{New value} - \text{Original value}}{\text{Original value}} \cdot 100$

Chapter Review Problems

Evaluate each of the following expressions, being careful to follow the order of operations.

1. $7 \cdot 2 - 3 \cdot 3$

2. $(-4)(5) - (-10)(\frac{1}{2})$

3. $\dfrac{36}{(-2 + 12)}$

4. $4 - (-2)[6 - 3(-2)]$

5. $\dfrac{-6(-2) - 10}{-6 - (-2)}$

6. $(-5) - (-2)^2 + 14$

7. $\dfrac{2^3 - 3^3}{-(-2 + 1)}$

8. $3.5 + (0.5)^2 + 0.16 \div 0.8$

9. $-2[(5.1)(-0.3) - 8.6]$

10. $\dfrac{7(-6 + 5)}{5(-3) + (-1 - 4)(-2 + 6)}$

Solve each of the following linear equations.

11. $y - 3.5 = 0.65$

12. $x + \dfrac{1}{4} = \dfrac{3}{8}$

13. $2a - 6 = -36$

14. $x = 75 - 4x$

15. $\dfrac{2}{3}x - 8 = \dfrac{1}{4}$

16. $-4.2x = -5x + 4.8$

17. $5d - 8 = 9d + 12$

18. $-6x + 5 = -5x - 28 + 2x$

19. $-7(3x + 1) = 35$

20. $6x - 38 = 2(5x + 1)$

21. $5a - (a - 4) = -12$

22. $s + 3(s - 3) + 5 = 0$

23. $3(x - 5) - 5x = x - 18$

24. $8 - 2(x - 5) = 3(7 - x)$

25. $\frac{3}{4}(8 - x) = 2 - x$

Solve each equation for the specified variable.

26. $V_1C_1 = V_2C_2$, for C_1

27. $p = \dfrac{mA}{150}$, for m

Use the cross-multiplication property to solve the following problems.

28. $\dfrac{2}{5} = \dfrac{x}{125}$

29. $\dfrac{x}{16} = \dfrac{55}{176}$

30. $\dfrac{0.08}{15} = \dfrac{x}{2.5}$

31. $\dfrac{0.5}{1.5} = \dfrac{0.25}{x}$

32. $\dfrac{4 \text{ mg}}{2.5 \text{ mL}} = \dfrac{16 \text{ mg}}{x \text{ mL}}$

33. $\dfrac{50 \text{ mg}}{5 \text{ mL}} = \dfrac{25 \text{ mg}}{x \text{ mL}}$

34. $\dfrac{250 \text{ mg}}{2 \text{ tablets}} = \dfrac{x \text{ mg}}{3 \text{ tablets}}$

35. $\dfrac{7.5 \text{ mg}}{1 \text{ tablet}} = \dfrac{x \text{ mg}}{3 \text{ tablets}}$

Read each problem and set up an appropriate proportion. Use the cross-multiplication property to solve and label your final answers with the correct units.

36. One tablet contains 125 mg of medication. How many tablets contain 375 mg of this medication?

37. How much insulin (in cc) should be given from a bottle marked U40 if a patient needs 45 units?

38. A dosage of 120 mg of a medication has been ordered. The dosage strength available is 50 mg in 5 mL. How many milliliters of the available medication should be administered?

39. If the pediatric dosage of Ceclor® is 20 mg per 1 kg of body weight, how many milligrams of medication should be given to a child who weighs 24 kg?

40. Running burns 1360 calories in 2 hours. If you run for 45 minutes (0.75 hour), how many calories will you burn?

41. There are 90 calories in 1 cup of fat-free milk. How many calories are in 4 cups of fat-free milk?

42. A $\frac{1}{2}$-cup serving of canned peaches contains 20 g of sugar. How much sugar is in the $1\frac{1}{2}$-cup can?

Use proportions or algebraic equations to solve these percent problems.

43. Find 0.5% of 750.

44. 5% of what number is 255?

45. What percent of 150 is 2.5?

46. 2.5% of what number is 36?

47. What percent of 360 is 126?

48. Find 1.2% of 1250.

49. 0.85% of what number is 0.357?

50. What percent of 320 is 17.6?

Calculate the percent increase or decrease for the following changes.

51. original value: 125; new value: 130
52. original value: 75.20; new value: 69.94
53. original value: 5.5; new value: 5.36
54. original value: 25; new value: 105

Use one of the methods presented in this chapter to solve the following word problems.

55. What is the percent concentration of a salt solution containing 5 g of salt in 50 mL of water?
56. How many grams of sodium chloride are there in 500 mL of a 0.8% saline solution?
57. The U.S. Department of Agriculture's recommended daily allowance of potassium for the average adult is 3500 mg. One serving of a particular cereal provides 65 mg of potassium. What percent of the daily recommended allowance does one serving provide?
58. According to Red Cross statistics, 43% of the general population has Type A blood. If 275 people participate in a blood drive on Saturday, how many pints of Type A blood would you expect to be donated by the end of the blood drive?
59. Sickle-cell anemia occurs once in every 500 African-American births. What percent of these newborns would be expected to exhibit symptoms of sickle-cell anemia?
60. Researchers for a new medication reported that 30% of all patients who used the medication experienced adverse side effects. If the study involved 350 patients, how many of them did not experience adverse side effects?
61. Myra weighed 140 lb at the beginning of October. On New Year's Day, she weighed 152 lb. Find the percent of increase in her weight.
62. An estimate of the vital capacity for men can be obtained using the formula

$$C = (21.78 - 0.101a) \cdot h$$

where a = age, h = height in centimeters, and C is vital capacity in cc

If Daniel is 178 cm tall and is 35 years old, find his vital capacity.

63. Convert $-13°$ Fahrenheit to degrees Celsius using the formula $C = \frac{5}{9}(F - 32)$.

Choose the correct rule based on the information given and use it to calculate p, the pediatric dosage of medication, in Problems 64–66.

Young's Rule: $p = \dfrac{aA}{12 + a}$, where a = child's age, A = normal adult dosage

Clark's Rule: $p = \dfrac{wA}{150}$, where w = child's weight in lb, A = normal adult dosage

Clark's Rule: $p = \dfrac{wA}{68.2}$, where w = child's weight in kg, A = normal adult dosage

Fried's Rule: $p = \dfrac{mA}{150}$, where m = child's age in months, A = normal adult dosage

64. The child's weight is 45 kg and the normal adult dosage is 10 mg.
65. The child's weight is 44 lb and the normal adult dosage is 2 teaspoons.
66. The child's age is 6 months and the normal adult dosage is 50 mg.
67. The Center for Disease Control and Prevention published the following chart in its 2004 publication *Protecting Health for Life*. This model indicates that the percentage of U.S. high school students who reported that they smoked decreased from 1997 to 2003. What is the percent decrease in smoking among high school students reported from 1997 to 2003?

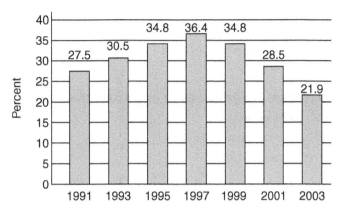

Percentage of U.S. High School Students who Reported Current Cigarette Smoking, 1991–2003

Source: CDC Youth Risk Behavior Survey.

68. The local high school has an enrollment of 1090 students. Based on the 2003 percentages given in the chart, approximately how many students at the high school smoke cigarettes?

69. How much 7.5% solution can be made with 100 mL of 12% solution?

70. You could make 150 mL of 2.5% from 25 mL of what percent?

71. You mix 75 mL of 5% solution and 25 mL of 1.5% solution in a flask. What is the concentration of the final solution?

72. The company that prints the office billing stationery charges a $50 setup fee and $0.001 per sheet. How much does an order of 2500 sheets of this stationery cost?

Chapter Test

Evaluate each of the following expressions, being careful to follow the order of operations.

1. $4 - (-2)[6 - 3(-2)]$

2. $3.5 + (0.5)^2 + 0.16 \div 0.8$

3. $-2[(5.1)(-0.3) - 8.6]$

4. $\dfrac{-2(-6 + 5)}{5(-2) + (4)(-2 + 6)}$

Solve each of the following linear equations.

5. $3a - 6 = -30$

6. $\dfrac{1}{5}x + 7 = \dfrac{7}{10}$

7. $-4.2x = -5x + 4.8$

8. $-6x + 5 = -x - 30 + 2x$

9. $-2(3x + 5) = 44$

10. $3(x - 5) - 5x = x - 18$

Use the cross-multiplication property to solve the following problems.

11. $\dfrac{20}{5} = \dfrac{x}{1.25}$

12. $\dfrac{200 \text{ mg}}{5 \text{ mL}} = \dfrac{80 \text{ mg}}{x \text{ mL}}$

Read each problem and set up an appropriate proportion. Use the cross-multiplication property to solve and label your final answers with the correct units.

13. One Zithromax® tablet contains 600 mg of medication. How many tablets would contain 900 mg of this medication?

14. Swimming burns 410 calories in 1 hour. If you swim for 20 minutes, how many calories will you burn?

Use proportions or algebraic equations to solve these percent problems.

15. Find 0.05% of 56.

16. 3.05% of what number is 14.64?

17. What percent of 685 is 51.375?

Solve the following word problems using the methods discussed in this chapter.

18. How many grams of salt are in 150 mL of a 0.75% saline solution?

19. The recommended daily allowance of sodium for an average person is 2400 mg or less. If a bran cereal has 80 mg of sodium per serving, what percent of the recommended daily allowance is this?

20. According to a hematology text, 38.5% of the general population has Type O blood. If 350 people participate in a blood drive on Saturday, how many pints of Type O blood would you expect to be donated by the end of the blood drive?

21. Cystic fibrosis occurs in North Carolina at a rate of 1 in every 2000 Caucasian births. If 123,250 Caucasian babies are born this year, predict the number of babies that will be diagnosed with cystic fibrosis.

22. The National Center for Health Statistics reported that the infant mortality rate in 2000 was 6.9 deaths per 1000 births. What percent of births does this ratio represent?

23. The cost of Jeremy's medication increased from $65.50 per month to $69.43. What percent increase in cost is this?

24. Convert −5° Celsius to Fahrenheit using the formula $F = \frac{9}{5}C + 32$.

25. How much 15% solution can be made with 10 mL of 25% solution?

SYSTEMS OF MEASUREMENT

Objectives for Chapter 3

After completing this chapter the student should:

1. Know the concepts related to measurements used in the allied health field, including volume, mass, weight, and temperature.

2. Be able to calculate using numbers written in scientific notation.

3. Be able to round answers to calculations that contain measurements using the rules for significant digits.

4. Be able to use the fundamental units of the metric system (SI), household units, and the apothecary system in making measurements and doing calculations related to allied health applications.

5. Be able to use common temperature scales and convert between scales when necessary.

SECTION 3.1   MEASUREMENT FUNDAMENTALS

How tall am I now mama? How much do you weigh? How do I get to your house? How much butter do I add to this cake mix? How much medicine do I take? Every day you make some kind of measurement or make a decision based on some other person's measurements. **Measurements** are common in our daily lives. They are also a vital part of all medical, scientific, technical, and business jobs that we may be doing to earn a living. It is easy to group measurements into a few simple categories like length, weight, volume, and time.

Let us start with *lengths*. **Length** describes an object's linear size or its distance from another object. My wife is 5 ft 2 in. tall. My house is 4.50 km from the college. This book is 18 cm wide. This patient has a 2.50-cm incision in his abdomen.

A second group of measurements includes what are called *weights* or *masses*. **Weight** is the force of gravitational attraction on an object exerted by some celestial body, like the gravitational pull of the earth in our case. I weigh 167 lb. This can of beans weighs 16 oz. **Mass** is a measure of the quantity of matter that an object contains. For example, my truck has a mass of 2200 kg. This multivitamin contains 60 mg of vitamin C.

The terms *mass* and *weight* are often used as if they mean the same thing. However, they do not. An object's mass is constant, no matter where the object is. The same object's weight is not constant. For example, if your weight on earth is 120 lb and you travel to the moon, your weight there would only be about 20 lb. This is because the force of gravity on the moon is approximately one-sixth that on the earth. However, your mass on both the earth and on the moon is 3.7 slugs = 54.5 kg. Your mass is the same in both places because your *mass* is a measure of the number of protons, neutrons, and electrons you are made of, not on how strong the pull of gravity may be.

A third group of measurements deals with *volumes*. **Volume** is used to measure the capacity of an object, that is, how much a container will hold or how much three-dimensional space an object takes up. My car's gas tank will hold 18 gal of gas. The volume of air in this room is 1800 ft^3. This prescription calls for 2.0 mL for an injection. This recipe calls for 3 cups of flour.

Time is also a commonly measured quantity. The basic units of time are the second, minute, hour, day, and year. At one time there was an effort made to develop new units for time measurements that would match the metric system, with the base time unit being the second and prefixes for the other time units. It was decided that this would be difficult and unpopular, so the idea was scrapped. Therefore, the units used for measurements of time will remain the traditional ones that have been used worldwide for centuries.

One thing about time that may be new to you is the use of **military time** in medical records. In many hospitals and other medical facilities, a 24-hour clock is used and the designations of A.M. and P.M. are not used. For example, if a medication were administered to a patient and the time were recorded as 2 A.M. on the standard clock, this same time would be recorded as 0200 (read as "two hundred hours") on the military clock; 2 P.M. would be recorded as 1400 ("fourteen hundred hours") on the military clock; a time of 7:15 P.M. on the standard clock would be 1915 (read as "nineteen-fifteen hours") on the military clock. Noon is 1200 hours, midnight is usually 0000 hours but some call it 2400 hours. Digital watches that are set to the 24-hour format will display midnight as 0000. Table 3.1 gives you the relationships between regular time and military time.

It should be noted that even though these times look like decimal numbers it is not possible to add or subtract times by carrying and borrowing as is done with decimal numbers.

Table 3.1

Regular Time	Military Time	Regular Time	Military Time
Midnight	0000	Noon	1200
1:00 A.M.	0100	1:00 P.M.	1300
2:00 A.M.	0200	2:00 P.M.	1400
3:00 A.M.	0300	3:00 P.M.	1500
4:00 A.M.	0400	4:00 P.M.	1600
5:00 A.M.	0500	5:00 P.M.	1700
6:00 A.M.	0600	6:00 P.M.	1800
7:00 A.M.	0700	7:00 P.M.	1900
8:00 A.M.	0800	8:00 P.M.	2000
9:00 A.M.	0900	9:00 P.M.	2100
10:00 A.M.	1000	10:00 P.M.	2200
11:00 A.M.	1100	11:00 P.M.	2300

A variety of units are used in allied health areas. Some of the units may be very familiar to you and others may be new to you. In many cases, several different units may be used to measure the same quantity. Also, units for several different measurement systems are commonly used and intermixed in the medical lab and office. One of the main goals of this text is to familiarize you with these unit systems so that you can deal with them in your application courses and at work sites.

PRACTICE PROBLEM SET 3.1

Write each of the following standard times in military time:

1. 4:00 A.M.   5. 2:35 P.M.   9. 12:15 A.M.
2. 6:00 A.M.   6. 7:48 P.M.   10. 12:45 P.M.
3. 3:00 P.M.   7. 12:00 A.M.
4. 5:00 P.M.   8. 12:00 P.M.

Write each of the following military times as standard times:

11. 0800 hours   15. 1820 hours   19. 0015 hours
12. 0900 hours   16. 2020 hours   20. 0035 hours
13. 1145 hours   17. 2400 hours
14. 1035 hours   18. 1200 hours

SECTION 3.2   SCIENTIFIC NOTATION

Sometimes the numbers used in the sciences, laboratory, or medical areas can be either extremely large, as in a white blood cell count, or very small, as the size of a virus. You may remember from your first chemistry class that 1 mole of oxygen contains 602,200,000,000,000,000,000,000 (Avogadro's number) oxygen atoms. A compact method of writing very large numbers like this one has been devised. This method or shorthand is called **scientific notation**.

Writing a number in scientific notation format requires that it be in the form $a \times 10^n$. The a is a number greater than or equal to 1 but less than 10 and the value of n is an integer. The exponent n will be positive for numbers larger than 10, negative for numbers less than 1. For numbers between 1 and 10, the n will be 0. Generally, only positive numbers are written in scientific notation format.

Don't panic. This all sounds pretty complicated but isn't really. Here are the basic steps needed to rewrite common decimal numbers into scientific notation format followed by some brief examples. With just a little practice, it will become very easy for you to write numbers in scientific notation and remove numbers from the notation.

The Steps for Writing Numbers in Scientific Notation Format

To write 350,000,000 in scientific notation:

1. Relocate the decimal point so that it is to the right of the first nonzero digit.

$$350,000,000 \quad \longrightarrow \quad 3.50000000$$
$$\wedge \qquad\qquad\qquad \wedge$$

2. Delete all meaningless or unnecessary zeros.

   In this case, all the zeros to the right of the 5 are meaningless. This gives us 3.5.

3. Count the number of places that you moved the decimal. Insert the symbol that indicates scientific notation is being used. This is $\times$ 10 (times-10). Give the 10 an exponent that is the same as the number of places that the decimal was moved.

   The decimal was moved 8 places.

$$3.5 \times 10^8$$

4. Now determine whether this exponent is a positive or a negative number by looking at the size of the original number. If that number is greater than 10, then the exponent is a positive number; if it is less than 1, the exponent will be a negative number; and if the number is between 1 and 10, the exponent will be 0.

   The exponent, 8, is positive here since the number 350,000,000 is larger than 10.

EXAMPLE 1: Writing Numbers in Scientific Notation Format

Write each number in scientific notation.

$$3,500 = 3.500 \times 10^3 = 3.5 \times 10^3 \quad \text{(the decimal moved 3 places)}$$
$$0.0097 = 0009.7 \times 10^{-3} = 9.7 \times 10^{-3} \quad \text{(the decimal moved 3 places)}$$
$$345 = 3.45 \times 10^2 \quad \text{(the decimal moved 2 places)}$$
$$6.2 = 6.2 \times 10^0 \quad \text{(the decimal moved no places)}$$

The Steps for Removing a Number from Scientific Notation Format

To rewrite 4.06×10^{-5} as a decimal number:

1. The exponent on the 10 will tell you how many places to move the decimal and in which direction to move it. If the exponent is positive, move the decimal to the right; if negative, move the decimal to the left; and if it is zero, don't move it at all.

    The negative 5 indicates that the decimal will move 5 places left.

2. Remove the $\times$ 10 notation.

    This leaves 4.06.

3. Move the decimal and insert zeros as placeholders.

    In this case 4 zeros are needed: 0.0000406.

Remember, if the exponent is positive, this indicates that the number is greater than 10 and the decimal should be moved to the right. If the exponent is negative, then the number is less than 1 and the decimal should be moved to the left.

EXAMPLE 2: Removing Numbers from the Scientific Notation Format

Write each of the following as decimal numbers:

4.76×10^4 (move the decimal 4 places right and add 2 zeros as placeholders) $= 47,600$
6.3×10^{-3} (move the decimal 3 places left and add 2 zeros as placeholders) $= 0.0063$
7.34×10^0 (move the decimal no places) $= 7.34$

Multiplication with Numbers in Scientific Notation

Numbers written in scientific notation may be multiplied just as they are. Multiply the numbers that are to the left of the $\times$ 10 notation and then add the exponents on the 10s. Be sure that the final answer is in correct scientific notation format.

EXAMPLE 3: Multiplying Numbers Using Scientific Notation

Multiply 3.2×10^4 by 2.7×10^{-6}.

Solution

$(7.2 \times 10^4)(2.7 \times 10^{-6})$

$(7.2 \times 2.7)(10^4 \times 10^{-6})$ Rearrange the problem.

$19.44 \times 10^{4+(-6)}$ Multiply the first two numbers.

19.44×10^{-2} Combine the exponents on the 10.

Since 19.44 is greater than 10, this answer is not in correct scientific notation format. Rewrite the 19.44 in correct scientific notation format and then combine the exponents on the 10s.

19.44×10^{-2}

$(1.944 \times 10^1) \times 10^{-2}$ Rewrite first number in scientific notation.

$1.944 \times (10^1 \times 10^{-2})$ Regroup problem.

1.944×10^{-1}, or 0.1944   Combine exponents on the 10 and simplify.

Division with Numbers in Scientific Notation

Divide the numbers that are to the left of the $\times 10$ and then subtract the exponents on the 10s following the usual algebraic subtraction process. The following example shows you how to proceed.

EXAMPLE 4: Dividing Numbers Using Scientific Notation

Divide $\dfrac{9.3 \times 10^4}{3 \times 10^{-2}}$.

Solution

$(9.3 \div 3) \times (10^4 \div 10^{-2})$ Rearrange the problem.

$3.1 \times 10^{4-(-2)}$ Divide the first two numbers.

$3.1 \times 10^{4+2}$ Subtract the exponents on the 10.

3.1×10^6, or 3,100,000   Simplify.

Using Calculators to Do Scientific Notation

Calculators have settings that allow you to do calculations using only scientific notation. When working problems that include numbers in both decimal notation and in scientific notation, the numbers given in scientific notation may be placed into the calculator using the appropriate key. This will be a key labeled "EE" or "exp" on most brands of calculators. This key alerts the calculator to the fact that the number you are entering is in scientific notation format. Although most calculators use very similar keys for this process, you may still need to refer to your calculator's instruction booklet or confer with your instructor. The basic steps are given here.

To enter 6.5×10^{-2} into your calculator, press 6.5   EE (or exp)   2   +/−.
The display should look similar to this: $\boxed{6.5 \quad ^{-02}}$.

The −02 is the exponent for the 10, which does not appear on your screen.

Examples of how to multiply or divide two numbers given in scientific notation with your calculator are given in Example 5.

EXAMPLE 5: Using Calculators to Multiply or Divide Numbers in Scientific Notation

    a. Multiply $(7.2 \times 10^{-3}) \times (1.28 \times 10^5)$.

Solution

Enter: 7.2   EE   3   +/−   ×   1.28   EE   5   =
You should see 921.6, or $\boxed{9.216\text{E}2}$, or $\boxed{9.216 \,^{02}}$ on your calculator. The answer shown is 9.216×10^2.

    b. Divide $\dfrac{6.8 \times 10^{-3}}{2 \times 10^4}$.

Solution

Enter: 6.8 EE 3 +/− ÷ 2 EE 4 =

You should see $\boxed{3.4E -7}$ or $\boxed{3.4^{-07}}$, which is 3.4×10^{-7}.

It is important to remember that you *do not enter the number 10* or multiply by 10 during this process. If you "times 10" with the multiplication key while using the EE or exp key, you will cause the answer to be incorrect. The EE key multiplies by 10 automatically.

When you use your calculator to work problems using scientific notation, the final answer may or may not be displayed in scientific notation automatically. Also, be sure to write down the × 10 that does not appear on your calculator screen. For example, $6.4^{-0.2}$ (or 6.4E −02) on your calculator's screen should be written as 6.4×10^{-2}. If you wish to have all of your answers given in scientific notation automatically, you will need to place your calculator in scientific notation mode using the directions supplied by the manufacturer of your particular brand of calculator.

PRACTICE PROBLEM SET 3.2

Write each of these numbers in scientific notation.

1. 8000
2. 5000
3. 0.0068
4. 0.0045
5. 234,000,000,000
6. 984,000,000,000
7. 236.6584

8. 706.3277
9. 0.2005
10. 0.4308
11. 4.65
12. 1.609
13. 5,000,000
14. 7,000,000

15. 458
16. 232
17. 0.03045
18. 0.002608
19. $\dfrac{3}{4}$
20. $\dfrac{1}{4}$

Write each of these numbers in decimal notation.

21. 8.5×10^{-1}
22. 7.1×10^{-4}
23. 4.25×10^{6}
24. 3.22×10^{7}
25. 7×10^{3}

26. 3×10^{4}
27. 8×10^{-5}
28. 4×10^{-3}
29. 4.52×10^{0}
30. 6.034×10^{0}

31. 6.457×10^{2}
32. 2.221×10^{3}
33. 2.15×10
34. 3.0026×10

Do the following problems involving scientific notation. Express each of the final answers in correct scientific notation.

35. $(1.8 \times 10^{-2}) \times (4.56 \times 10^{8})$
36. $(7 \times 10^{-4}) \times (3.12 \times 10^{5})$
37. $(2.35 \times 10^{6}) \times (3.88 \times 10^{3})$
38. $(6 \times 10^{2}) \times (5 \times 10^{3})$
39. $(5.4 \times 10^{-3}) \times (2.36 \times 10^{-2})$
40. $(7.1 \times 10^{-6}) \times (2.3 \times 10^{-3})$

41. $(3.21 \times 10^{-3}) \div (9.5 \times 10)$
42. $(7.23 \times 10^{4}) \div (6.03 \times 10^{-5})$
43. $\dfrac{5.4 \times 10^{-1}}{2.7 \times 10^{-1}}$
44. $\dfrac{2.36 \times 10^{3}}{1.2 \times 10^{2}}$

45. $\dfrac{(4.5 \times 10^{-3})(3 \times 10^4)}{7.5 \times 10^6}$

46. $\dfrac{(3.34 \times 10^4)(1.6 \times 10^{-1})}{1.6 \times 10^5}$

47. $\dfrac{3.56 \times 10^0}{3.56 \times 10^0}$

48. $\dfrac{1.2 \times 10^0}{2.4 \times 10^0}$

49. $\dfrac{2.8 \times 10^{-15}}{4 \times 10^{-18}}$

50. $\dfrac{1.2 \times 10^{-12}}{6 \times 10^{-6}}$

51. Three samples are weighed on an electronic scale and the following weights are obtained: 0.23698 g, 0.21567 g, and 0.22514 g. Write each of these weights in scientific notation.

52. What is the difference between the largest and smallest weight in Problem 51? Express your answer in scientific notation.

53. A certain thyroid medication is available in a 30-tablet supply. Each tablet contains a small amount of the medication, 0.00000025 g. Express this amount in scientific notation.

54. How many grams of thyroid medication are in the entire bottle of 30 tablets in Problem number 53? Express your answer in scientific notation.

55. Bacteria grow at a very fast rate. One type multiplies about every hour. If you started with 1 bacteria, after an hour there would be 2 bacteria; after another hour, they would become 4 bacteria ($2 \times 2 = 2^2 = 4$); and after another hour there would be 8 bacteria ($2 \times 2 \times 2 = 2^3 = 8$); and so forth. This growth rate can be expresses as follows: 2^n, where n = hours. How many bacteria will there be after 20 hr? Express your answer in scientific notation and as a standard number.

56. A soil sample is taken and is repeatedly diluted so that a bacteria count can be done. Each time the soil sample is diluted it is one-tenth of the original strength. So after one dilution the strength is $\frac{1}{10}$ the original. After the second dilution it is $\frac{1}{10} \times \frac{1}{10} = \frac{1}{100}$, or one-hundredth of its original strength. What would the strength be after 8 dilutions? Express your answer in scientific notation.

SECTION 3.3 SIGNIFICANT DIGITS AND ROUNDING

Any physical measurement that you make is only an **approximate** value. When counting objects such as the number of people in your class today, an **exact** answer can be obtained. Defined numbers such as 12 in. = 1 ft or 1 in. = 2.54 cm are also considered to be exact. However, no measurement is ever exact but is only an estimate. This is due to the limitations of the measuring devices used and how well they are used. If you make a measurement, the result that you write in a chart or report is bound by the precision of the test and sensitivity of the measuring instrument that is used. The number recorded should contain all the digits that are well known plus one digit that is estimated. These, then, are the **significant digits** (sometimes called significant figures) contained in the result.

A measurement recorded as the number 3.24 mL can be supposed to have a value greater than or equal to 3.235 mL but less than or equal to 3.244 mL. This means that we have assumed that the answer, 3.24 mL, may have been rounded from somewhere within this range of possible answers. The measurement just given is accurate to 3 significant digits.

The terms **accuracy** and **precision** both occur frequently in the use of measuring devices, whether they be rulers, graduated cylinders, micrometers, balances, or electronic scales. The term *precision* refers to the fineness of the measuring device used. For example, some common electronic scales will give weights to the nearest 0.1 g but other, more expensive, scales may give weights to the nearest 0.001 g. The latter scale would be said to be the most precise scale. The term *accuracy* refers to the closeness of a measurement to the actual value. The accuracy of a measurement (an approximate number) can be determined by counting the number of significant digits in that number.

Rules Defining Which Digits Are Significant in Written Measurements

1. In a written measurement, *all nonzero numbers* are significant.

    4.578 mL has 4 significant digits.

2. Zeros on the left-hand end of a measurement are never significant.

    0.00785 mg has 3 significant digits.

    4.5 mg (2 significant digits) can also be written as 0.0045 g. Both of these are the same measurement and thus both must have the same number of significant digits.

3. Zeros that lie between significant digits are significant.

    7005 mg has 4 significant digits.

    6.0035 mL has 5 significant digits.

4. Zeros on the right-hand end of a number that includes a written decimal point are significant.

    11.500 mL has 5 significant digits.

    1.0 mL has 2 significant digits.

    80. mL has 2 significant digits.

5. Zeros at the end of a number without a written decimal point are considered ambiguous and are *not* significant.

    10,000 mcg has 1 significant digit.

    650 mg has 2 significant digits.

When a whole number contains zeros that should be significant, a bar is placed over the rightmost significant zero. As an example, if there is a need to show two significant digits in the number 9000, it would be written as $9\bar{0}00$. The numbers to the right of the $\bar{0}$ are not significant. The number $900,\bar{0}00$ would have 4 significant digits.

As a result of doing calculations, answers may contain more digits than are justified by the rules for significant digits. The basic rules for rounding were given in the review of decimals in Chapter 1. They are stated here again for your convenience.

Basic Rules for Rounding Off Numbers

Rule 1: When the first digit after those you wish to retain is 4 or less, that digit and all others to its right are dropped. The last digit retained is not changed.

72.593 rounded to the nearest hundredth is 72.59 (the 3 is dropped).
5.00249 rounded to the nearest thousandth is 5.002 (the 4 and 9 are both dropped).

Rule 2: When the first digit after those you wish to retain is 5 or greater, that digit and all others to the right of it are dropped and the last digit to be retained is increased by one.

2.0468 rounded to the nearest thousandth is 2.047 (the 8 is dropped and the 6 is increased by one to 7).

Measurement numbers or the results of a calculation involving measurements should be rounded to the correct number of significant digits using the preceding rules. Exact numbers do not need to be rounded at all because they are not approximate numbers. Learning how to do this is confusing to many students, so pay close attention to the following rules for retaining significant digits after performing calculations.

Determining the Number of Significant Digits in Calculations

You have heard it said that "a chain is only as strong as its weakest link." This is true in the realm of measurements and the instruments that are used to make them. A calculated result, based on measurements, may not be more precise than the measurements used in the calculation. When a number that results from a measurement is used in a calculation, the results obtained may appear to be more precise (that is, have more significant digits) than they actually should. The answer you get with your calculator will often need to be rounded off in order to avoid reporting an overly precise answer.

Rounding Rule for Multiplying and/or Dividing Measurements

In calculations involving multiplication or division of measured amounts, the answer should contain the same number of *significant digits* as the measurement used in the calculation that has the least number of significant figures.

EXAMPLE 6: Rounding Products

Suppose that you make two length measurements to find the area of a rectangle. You measure the width (w) to be 3.46 cm long and the length (l) to be 7.114 cm long. Using the formula for the area of a rectangle,

$$A_{rectangle} = lw$$
$$A = (3.46 \text{ cm})(7.114 \text{ cm})$$
$$A = 24.61444 \text{ cm}^2$$

This 5-decimal-place answer does not result from very precise measurements but rather, the 5 decimal places result from the multiplication rules for decimal numbers. This answer needs to be rounded off by counting the significant digits in each measurement used in the calculation.

3.46 cm has 3 significant digits and 7.114 cm has 4 significant digits. By the rule for multiplying and/or dividing with measurements, our answer should contain only 3 significant digits. The final answer is $A = 24.6 \text{ cm}^2$.

EXAMPLE 7: Rounding Products and Quotients

Multiply the following, assuming that they all represent measured amounts. Round the answer to the correct number of significant digits.

$$\frac{(3.45 \text{ cm})(0.0053 \text{ cm})(11.87 \text{ cm})}{1500 \text{ cm}}$$

The result shown on the calculator is $0.0001446953 \text{ cm}^2$. Now determine the number of significant digits in each measurement:

Solution

3.45 cm has 3 significant figures.

0.0053 cm has 2 significant figures.

11.87 has 4 significant figures.

1500 has 2 significant figures.

The factors 1500 cm and 0.0053 cm contain the least number of significant digits (2) and therefore the calculated answer should be rounded off to two significant digits. The correctly rounded answer is 0.00014 cm^2.

Rounding Rule for Addition and/or Subtraction of Measurements

In adding or subtracting measured amounts, the final answer should be only as precise as (that is, contain the same number of *decimal places* as) the least precise measurement used in the calculation.

EXAMPLE 8: Rounding in Addition Problems

Add 345.17 g, 239.6 g, and 42.778 g and round off appropriately.

Solution

$$
\begin{array}{ll}
345.17 \text{ g} & \text{(precise to 2 decimal places)} \\
239.6 \text{ g} & \text{(precise to 1 decimal place)} \\
+\ 42.778 \text{ g} & \text{(precise to 3 decimal places)} \\
\hline
627.548 \text{ g} &
\end{array}
$$

Because 239.6 g is the least precise measurement, containing only 1 decimal place, the answer is rounded to one decimal place as well: 627.5 g.

If a calculation is done involving more than one operation, such as multiplying and adding, only the final answer should be rounded. Do not round the answers to any intermediate steps in the calculation. Base the rounding on the significant digits of the measurements used as if only multiplication or division had been done.

Measurements that are being added, subtracted, multiplied, or divided need to be expressed in the same units whenever possible. This should be done before beginning any calculation. In a problem such as 4.5 L + 0.7 mL, the liter unit must be converted to milliliters (or milliliters to liters) before the addition is done. Methods for converting measurement units will be described in a later section of this chapter.

PRACTICE PROBLEM SET 3.3

How many significant digits are in each of the following measurements?

1. 5.6 cm	11. 8.007 L	21. 1000. km
2. 4.8 mm	12. 3.00078 mL	22. 3000. g
3. 550 mL	13. 15 g	23. $10\overline{0}0$ km
4. 5600 mg	14. 23 m	24. $3\overline{0}00$ km
5. 0.005 mL	15. 15.0 g	25. $10\overline{0}0$ km
6. 0.002 g	16. 2.00 mL	26. $30\overline{0}0$ km
7. 6.420 mm	17. 0.000001 m	27. 2050 L
8. 12.020 L	18. 0.00000026 g	28. 5030 m
9. 1950.6 g	19. 1000 km	29. 0.0203600 mg
10. 5680.2 m	20. 3000 g	30. 0.00430500 mcg

Round off each of the following measurements to 3 significant figures.

31. 0.32591 m	35. 169,240 mcL	39. 800.00 g
32. 6259 g	36. 4.3×10^3 L	40. 10.095×10^{-5} L
33. 200 mg	37. 0.0029006 mcg	
34. 5 mL	38. 50,000 km	

Do the following problems, rounding each answer to the correct number of significant figures. Assume all the numbers represent measurements.

41. (136 m)(27 m)	44. (3.45 m)/(2.00 s)
42. (205 m)(23 m)	45. 3.45 cm + 22.2 cm − 0.0089 cm
43. (16.0 mL)/(5.8 min)	46. 7.4 L + 0.56 L − 0.0046 L

47. $\dfrac{(160\ \text{m})(3.7\ \text{m})}{8\ \text{m}}$

48. $\dfrac{(230\ \text{cm})(6.8\ \text{cm})}{4\ \text{cm}}$

49. $(5.62\ \text{cm})(4.63\ \text{cm}) + 5.67\ \text{cm}^2$

50. $(4.23\ \text{m})(1.07\ \text{m}) - 1.43\ \text{m}^2$

Decide whether each of the following numbers would be *exact* or *approximate*.

51. Second shift at the walk-in clinic gave 24 flu shots yesterday.
52. Each flu shot given at the clinic in Problem 51 contained 2.0 mL.
53. The thermostat at your house is set at 70°F.
54. There are 50 tongue depressors in a standard package.

Solve each of the following problems. Round answers appropriately.

55. You measure the lengths of the sides of a triangle to be 7.80 in., 5.69 in., and 4.675 in. What is the perimeter of the triangle?
56. If the average weight of a dime is 4.65 g, then how much do 25 of them weigh?
57. The formula for the area of a triangle is: $A = \frac{1}{2}bh$. The base length of a triangle is measured to be 28.85 cm and the height is 7.68 cm. What is the area of the triangle?
58. Three capsules are weighed on scales of differing sensitivities. The results are 17.6 mg, 17.78 mg, and 17.635 mg. Find the average weight of the three capsules.
59. If 12 injections of flu vaccine were given and each contained 2.25 mL, how many milliliters of vaccine were used altogether?
60. A patient has a roughly circular burn on his back with a diameter of 3.5 cm as measured by a nurse. What is the area of this burn? (The formula for the area of a circle is $A = \pi r^2$.)

SECTION 3.4   THE METRIC AND SI SYSTEMS

In the United States we have the misfortune of having to deal with several different systems of units whenever measurements are made. To work in areas related to medicine and health care, you will need to be familiar with at least four different systems of units. These are the metric system (SI), the U.S. Customary System—USCS (sometimes called the English system), the apothecary system, and the household units system. The values of units used in all of these systems have been set by international agreements and, in the United States, are standardized by the NIST (National Institute of Standards and Technology). The NIST is a branch of the U.S. Commerce Department and as such is an agency of the federal government. All of these systems will be discussed in this chapter.

The **SI unit system** (*Le Système International d'Unités*) is a decimal system of units for mass, length, time, and other physical quantities that is used worldwide under treaty agreements among nations. Most of the units will be familiar as **metric system** units. The SI consists of one primary unit for each quantitative property to be measured and a set of *prefixes* used with the primary units to create larger or smaller units. Table 3.2 lists the units of metric measurement that will be most important to you in your health career.

Table 3.2 Basic Units of Metric Measurement

Quantity Measured	Unit Name	Symbol
Length	Meter	m
Weight or Mass	Gram	g
Volume	Liter	L

When a prefix is placed on a base metric unit, a new unit of measure results that is equal to the product of the prefix factor and the base unit. Table 3.3 gives the names, values, and symbols for commonly used prefixes.

Table 3.3 Metric Prefixes

Prefix	Value	Symbol
Giga	$10^9 = 1,000,000,000$	G
Mega	$10^6 = 1,000,000$	M
Kilo	$10^3 = 1,000$	k
Hecto	$10^2 = 100$	H
Deka	$10^1 = 10$	da
no prefix used	$10^0 = 1$	—
Deci	$10^{-1} = 0.1$	d
Centi	$10^{-2} = 0.01$	c
Milli	$10^{-3} = 0.001$	m
Micro	$10^{-6} = 0.000001$	μ or mc
Nano	$10^{-9} = 0.000000001$	n

As a worker in allied health fields, you will most often use the prefixes kilo-, centi-, milli-, and micro-. The micro- prefix is often abbreviated with the Greek letter mu, μ, but in medical fields "mc" is commonly used to represent the micro- prefix. Therefore, microgram is abbreviated mcg instead of μg.

Another abbreviation that is often found in medical areas is cc. This abbreviation stands for "cubic centimeter" and is a volume unit. One cubic centimeter is equivalent to 1 milliliter: 1 mL = 1 cc. As noted in Chapter 1, in many hospitals mL is the preferred unit and the use of cc is discouraged.

Calculations in the medical field will frequently require that you convert one unit of measure to another. Units of measure can be converted only to other units that measure the same quantity. For example, units of volume (liters) cannot be converted into units of length (meters). However, all units of volume are compatible, so any unit of volume can be converted into another unit of volume. Table 3.4 shows the equivalents for the metric system of units that are used most often in medical areas.

Table 3.4 Common Metric Equivalents and Symbols

Equivalents for Liquid Volumes
1 mL (or ml, 1 milliliter) = 1 cc (or cm^3, one cubic centimeter)
1000 mL = 1 L (liter)
1000 cc = 1 L (liter)
Equivalents for Weights (Masses)
1 kg (kilogram) = 1000 g (grams)
1 g (gram) = 1000 mg (milligrams)
1 mg (milligram) = 1000 mcg (μg or micrograms)

Here we will cover the two most common methods of converting units of measure. The use of conversion factors, commonly called **dimensional** (or unit) **analysis**, is one common way of changing one unit of measure into another. A method that we will call "decimal bumping" uses the chart of prefixes to help move the decimal when a conversion is done in the metric system.

Conversion by Dimensional (or Unit) Analysis

Sometimes you may run across a situation in which several different units may be used to measure similar quantities in a problem, for example, liters and milliliters. In these cases, it will be necessary for you to convert the units so that they are the same or are compatible with other units in the problem. There are several methods by which to do the conversion. One is by use of a **conversion factor**, that is, the ratio of the unit you have to start with and the equivalent in the unit you want to change to. Tables of equivalents and conversion factors are found in the appendices at the end of this book.

EXAMPLE 9: Metric Volume Conversions Using Dimensional Analysis

Convert 0.375 liters (L) to milliliters (mL); 1 L = 1000 mL (see Table 3.3).

Solution

The conversion factor will be a ratio of these two values, either $\dfrac{1\ L}{1000\ mL}$ or $\dfrac{1000\ mL}{1\ L}$.

The unit to be canceled is liters (L), and to cancel it out, the same unit in the conversion factor needs to be in the denominator.

$$(0.375\ \cancel{L})\left(\frac{1000\ mL}{1\ \cancel{L}}\right) = 375\ mL$$

EXAMPLE 10: Metric Length Conversions Using Dimensional Analysis

Convert 70,000 m to kilometers.

Solution

The conversion factor to change meters to kilometers is 1 km = 1000 m.

$$(70{,}000\ \cancel{m})\left(\frac{1\ km}{1000\ \cancel{m}}\right) = 70\ km$$

EXAMPLE 11: Measuring Heights

A patient's height is measured to be 175 cm. What is this patient's height in meters (1 m = 100 cm)?

Solution

$$(175\ \cancel{cm})\left(\frac{1\ m}{100\ \cancel{cm}}\right) = 1.75\ m \quad \text{(remember to count significiant digits)}$$

EXAMPLE 12: Metric Weight Conversions Using Dimensional Analysis

Convert 2.5 m to millimeters (1 m = 1000 mm).

Solution

$$(2.5\ \cancel{m})\left(\frac{1000\ mm}{1\ \cancel{m}}\right) = 2500\ mm$$

The unit conversion method called *dimensional analysis* is used frequently. It may be used when converting units within a system as in these examples and is always used when converting between two entirely different systems of measurement.

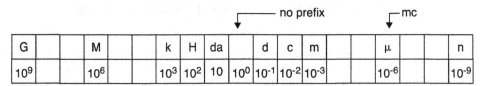

							no prefix					mc		
G		M		k	H	da		d	c	m		µ		n
10^9		10^6		10^3	10^2	10	10^0	10^{-1}	10^{-2}	10^{-3}		10^{-6}		10^{-9}

Figure 3.1 Decimal Bumping Chart

Conversions Done by Decimal Bumping

Metric prefixes are based on powers of 10. Thus the changing of prefixes on a given base unit involves multiplying or dividing by 10, 100, 1000, and so on. Figure 3.1 shows the commonly used metric unit prefixes. With this chart you may easily change metric unit sizes by simply counting blocks rather than trying to remember when to multiply or divide by 10, or 100, or 1000, and so on.

When you move one block on the chart you are either multiplying or dividing by 10; 2 blocks, 100; and so forth. If you choose any block on the chart as your starting point and move one or more blocks to the right, you are changing the unit to a smaller metric unit with the same base. If you move to the left, you are changing to a larger metric unit with the same base. The reason we are saying "the same base" is because the chart changes only the prefix on a given metric unit, not the base unit (meter, liter, or gram). You will see that no base measurement units are listed on the chart. The central block at 10^0 is the chart location for a metric base unit with *no prefix*. This method is quick and easy to use whenever you are doing simple conversions within the metric system.

EXAMPLE 13: Weight Conversions Using Decimal Bumping

6.78 mg = ? µg = ? mcg   (in medical usage, mcg will often be used in place of µg)

Solution

Consult Figure 3-1 to find the prefix that you have to start with, the m (milli) prefix. Also find the prefix that you wish to change to, the mc (micro) prefix.

Starting in the m prefix location, count boxes until you reach the mc box and note the direction. Here, the mc box is three boxes (places) to the right of the m box.

Now move the decimal point in the given number 3 places to the right and the unit is converted.

Thus, 6.78 mg = 6780 mcg.

Note: There is no reference made to which base unit is being used in the decimal bumping chart. So these conversions are also true: 6.78 mL = 6780 mcL and 6.78 mm = 6780 mcm.

From block to block on the chart, prefixes change by a value of 10^1 or 10^{-1} depending on the direction you move. You probably noticed that some blocks are blank. That is because there is no metric prefix for that particular power of 10. For example, there is no metric prefix equivalent to 10^4 or 10^5, only to the 10^3 and 10^6 powers. However, you must still count these empty blocks when changing prefixes.

EXAMPLE 14: Length Conversions Using Decimal Bumping

427 nm = ? mm

Solution

Find both the nano- and the milli- prefixes on the chart. Moving from nano- to milli- will move the decimal 6 places to the left. Add zeros as needed for placeholders. Thus, 427 nm = 0.000427 mm.

Chapter 3

In calculations where several measurements are involved, the same units should be used for all the measurements if at all possible. For example, if you are measuring lengths to find an area, measure all the lengths with the same ruler and use the same units (all inches, all centimeters, and so on). If this is not possible or has not been done, then you may end up converting one or more of the units to another before calculating.

EXAMPLE 15: Weight Conversions Using Decimal Bumping

$$\frac{(18.5 \text{ mg})(0.450 \text{ g})}{1.75 \text{ mg}} = ? \text{ mg}$$

Solution

Since the desired unit for the final answer is mg, all measurements in the problem itself should be converted to milligrams before solving.

$$0.450 \text{ g} = 450. \text{ mg} \quad (\text{“bump” the decimal 3 places to the right})$$

Substituting this into the problem,

$$\frac{(18.5 \text{ mg})(450. \text{ mg})}{1.75 \text{ mg}} = 4757.142857 \text{ mg}$$

Now, this product must be rounded to 3 significant figures since all the original measurements contain 3 significant figures. The correctly rounded answer is 4760 mg.

PRACTICE PROBLEM SET 3.4

Complete the following unit conversions.

1. 5698 mm = ? m
2. 23,000 mcg = ? mg
3. 565 L = ? kL
4. 298 g = ? kg
5. 7.4 g = ? mg
6. 3.69 L = ? mL

7. 6850 mcL = ? mL
8. 524 mcg = ? mg
9. 0.07 mg = ? g
10. 0.225 km = ? mm
11. 0.00076 L = ? mL
12. 0.00000088 g = ? ng

13. How many deciliters are in 300 mL?

14. A drug order for a patient reads, "give 250 mg" of an antibiotic, but the computer will only let the nurse enter grams of medication given. How many grams should she record?

15. 52 L = ? mg

16. 0.5 mm = ? g

17. Convert $\dfrac{4.5 \text{ g}}{1.0 \text{ L}}$ to mg/L.

18. Convert $\dfrac{88.0 \text{ km}}{1 \text{ hr}}$ to m/hr.

19. Convert $\dfrac{50.0 \text{ mL}}{1.0 \text{ min}}$ to L/min.

20. Convert $\dfrac{25.0 \text{ km}}{1.0 \text{ s}}$ to m/s.

Calculate as indicated and round to the correct number of significant figures based on the measurements in each problem.

21. 7.5 mL + 0.75 L = ? L

22. 4.6 g + 2300 mg = ? g

23. (4.2 mm)(6.75 mm) = ? mm^2

24. (5.78 m)(3.4 m) = ? m^2

25. 55.0 g + 9.76 dg + 5.67 mg = ?g

26. 4.5 mL + 0.0047 L – 3400 mcL = ? mL

27. $\dfrac{60 \text{ mL}}{5 \text{ min}} = ? \text{ mL/min}$

28. $\dfrac{3450 \text{ m}}{2.5 \text{ s}} = ? \text{ m/s}$

29. $\dfrac{0.09864 \text{ cm}^2}{3.67 \text{ cm}} = ? \text{ cm}$

30. $\dfrac{0.657889 \text{ m}^2}{2.457 \text{ m}} = ? \text{ m}$

31. A doctor orders 1 L of 5% dextrose water solution (D_5W) for his office. To fill this order, he ordered two cases. If standard case sizes are 1000 cc, 500 cc, and 250 cc, which size case did he order?

32. A doctor tells you to inject 1.75 cc of a vaccine into a patient. How many milliliters is this?

SECTION 3.5 HOUSEHOLD MEASUREMENT UNITS

The **household system** of measurement is commonly used in prescribing medications to be taken at home or for children's dosages. The SI (metric) system is strictly a decimal system. However, in the household system, and in the apothecary system discussed in the next section, fractions are commonly used to state the amounts of medications to be administered. Table 3.5 gives the equivalents for the most commonly used household units along with their abbreviations.

Table 3.5 Equivalents and Symbols for Household Units

Liquid Volume Equivalents
1 glass = 8 oz (ounces)
1 c (measuring cup) = 8 oz (ounces)
1 oz (ounce) = 2 T (tablespoons)
1 T (tablespoon) = 3 t (teaspoons)
1 t (teaspoon) = 60 gtt (drops)
Weight Equivalents
1 lb (pound) = 16 oz (ounces)

Conversions in this system will be done using the **dimensional analysis** method since the numbers do not have prefixes like the SI system. It should also be noted that these measurements are not extremely accurate when done by the patient at home using kitchen measuring cups and spoons. Generally, the doctor prescribing such a dosage is aware of this fact and has allowed for it in the amount prescribed so as not to either overdose or underdose the patient.

EXAMPLE 16: Volume Conversions Using Dimensional Analysis

A patient is to take 3 oz of a very strong laxative. How many tablespoons should the patient take?

$$3 \text{ oz} = ? \text{ T}$$

Solution

First look in the table of equivalents to discover that 1 oz = 2 T.

Now set up this information in fraction form so you can cancel the ounce unit in the original dosage. Then do the multiplication or division indicated.

$$(3 \text{ oz})\left(\frac{2 \text{ T}}{1 \text{ oz}} \right) = 6 \text{ T}$$

This patient should take 6 T in order to take a dosage equivalent to 3 oz.

EXAMPLE 17: Volume Conversions Using Dimensional Analysis

A doctor prescribes 15 gtt of an antispasmodic drug. How many teaspoons is this?

$$15 \text{ gtt} = ? \text{ t}$$

Solution

From the table of equivalents, 1 t = 60 gtt.

$$(15 \text{ g\hspace{-0.3em}t\hspace{-0.3em}t})\left(\frac{1 \text{ t}}{60 \text{ g\hspace{-0.3em}t\hspace{-0.3em}t}}\right) = \frac{15}{60} \text{ t} = \frac{1}{4} \text{ t}$$

So the patient should take one-fourth of a teaspoon of the medication.

Sometimes, the conversion of one unit to another may require the use of more than one conversion fraction. For example, to convert ounces into teaspoons using the information in our conversion table, you must first change ounces into tablespoons and then tablespoons into teaspoons. Look at Example 18 to see how this is done.

EXAMPLE 18: A Word Problem—Pediatric Dosage

Young's Rule for calculating pediatric dosages is

$$p = \frac{aA}{12 + a}$$

where a = the child's age in years
          A = the usual adult dose
          p = the pediatric dosage

If the recommended adult dosage of a certain medication is 2.00 oz, how many teaspoons would you give a 6-year-old child?

Solution

First substitute the known values into the formula:

$$p = \frac{(6)(2.00 \text{ oz})}{12 + 6} = \frac{12 \text{ oz}}{18} = 0.666666\ldots = \frac{2}{3} \text{ oz}$$

Now convert ounces to teaspoons: 1 oz = 2 T, and 1 T = 3 t.

$$\left(\frac{2 \text{ o\hspace{-0.3em}z}}{3}\right)\left(\frac{2 \text{ T}}{1 \text{ o\hspace{-0.3em}z}}\right)\left(\frac{3 \text{ t}}{1 \text{ T}}\right) = \frac{12 \text{ t}}{3} = 4 \text{ t}$$

The child should receive 4 t of the medication.

PRACTICE PROBLEM SET 3.5

Write each of the following measures using the proper numbers and unit abbreviations.

1. three tablespoons
2. four tablespoons
3. two and one-fourth cups
4. one and a quarter cups
5. five drops

6. two drops
7. one ounce
8. three ounces
9. four and one-half teaspoons
10. one and three-fourths teaspoons

Convert units as indicated

11. 1 T = ? oz	21. $\frac{1}{2}$ t = ? gtt	31. 30 gtt = ? T
12. 3 T = ? oz	22. $\frac{3}{4}$ t = ? gtt	32. 45 gtt = ? T
13. 20.0 oz = ? T	23. 15 gtt = ? t	33. 20 t = ? oz
14. 8.0 oz = ? T	24. 45 gtt = ? t	34. 4 t = ? oz
15. 4 t = ? T	25. $\frac{1}{4}$ glass = ? oz	35. $\frac{2}{3}$ t = ? oz
16. 12 t = ? T	26. $\frac{1}{8}$ glass = ? oz	36. $\frac{5}{8}$ t = ? oz
17. 2 T = ? t	27. 12 oz = ? glass	37. 48 oz = ? lb
18. $\frac{1}{2}$ T = ? t	28. 32 oz = ? glass	38. 128 oz = ? lb
19. 1 cup = ? T	29. $1\frac{1}{2}$ T = ? gtt	39. 2 lb = ? oz
20. $\frac{1}{2}$ cup = ? T	30. 4 T = ? gtt	40. $\frac{5}{8}$ lb = ? oz

41. Young's Rule for calculating pediatric dosages is

$$p = \frac{aA}{12 + a}$$

where a = the child's age in years
A = the usual adult dose
p = the pediatric dosage

If the recommended adult dosage of a certain medication is 3.75 oz, how many ounces would you give an 8-year-old child?

42. Using the formula in Problem 41, how much medication would you give a 5-year-old child if the usual adult dosage is 1.25 oz?

43. How many tablespoons of medication would you give the child in Problem 41?

44. How many teaspoons would you give the child in Problem 41?

45. Clark's Rule for determining pediatric dosages is

$$p = \frac{wA}{150}$$

where w = the child's weight in pounds
A = the usual adult dosage
p = the pediatric dosage

If a child weighs 22.0 lb and the usual adult dosage is 2.5 oz, how many teaspoons would you give the child?

46. Using the formula in Problem 45, what would the pediatric dosage, in teaspoons, be for a child with a weight of 50.0 lb if the adult dose is 6 oz?

47. How many drops would you give the child in Problem 45?

48. How many tablespoons would you give the child in Problem 45?

SECTION 3.6   THE APOTHECARY SYSTEM

The **apothecary system** is perhaps the oldest drug measurement system still in use today. It is not nearly as common as the metric or household systems, but is still used on drug labels and is used by some doctors in writing prescriptions. The units will be unfamiliar to you and some of the symbols used are strange. One unusual thing about this system is that the symbol for the unit *precedes* the numerical amount. You will also see *Roman numerals* used to specify amounts in the apothecary system as well as fractions. (See Chapter 1 for a review of Roman numerals.) In the apothecary system, a dosage of 5 grains would be written as gr 5 or gr v. Table 3.6 gives the equivalents and symbols for the most commonly used apothecary units.

Table 3.6 Equivalents and Symbols for the Apothecary System

Liquid Volume Equivalents
1 quart = qt 1 = 2 pints = pt 2 = pt ii
qt 1 = 32 fluid ounces = floz 32 = fl℥ 32 = fl℥ XXXII
pt 1 = 16 fluid ounces = floz 16 = fl℥ 16 = fl℥ xvi
fl℥ 1 = floz 1 = 8 fluid drams = fldr 8 = fl𝌆 8 = fl𝌆 viii
fldr 1 = fl𝌆 1 = 60 minims = min 60 = m 60 = m LX
Weights
oz 1 = ℥ 1 = 8 drams = 𝌆 8 = 𝌆 viii
1 dram = 𝌆 1 = 60 grains = gr 60 = gr LX

Some of the symbols used are not easy to write by hand. The symbol for dram is like a large number 3 but with a flat top: 𝌆. The symbol for ounce is like the symbol for dram but with a small letter z sitting up on the flat top of the dram symbol, like this: ℥. Also, using m for minim may seem confusing but in application problems it will be easy to distinguish from the same symbol used for the meter. Some persons use a script m for minims, like this: *m*. In this text, we will use min to stand for minims.

The minim was once said to equal 1 drop of water but has now been defined to be 0.06 mL of liquid volume. The grain was once equal to the weight of a plump grain of wheat but has now been standardized at about 60 mg.

EXAMPLE 19: Converting Volumes by Dimensional Analysis

If a patient was to receive 4 fluid drams (fl𝌆 4) of an antacid, how many fluid ounces (fl℥) would this be equivalent to?

$$fl𝌆\ 4 = ?\ fl℥$$

Solution

From the table of equivalents, fl℥ 1 = fl𝌆 8 (floz 1 = fldr 8).

$$(\cancel{fldr}\ 4)\left(\frac{floz\ 1}{\cancel{fldr}\ 8}\right) = floz\ \frac{4}{8} = floz\ \frac{1}{2}$$

So, 4 fluid drams is equivalent to one-half of a fluid ounce.

EXAMPLE 20: Converting Volumes by Dimensional Analysis

A doctor has ordered that a patient be given fl𝌆 xvi of an antacid. How many fluid ounces would the patient be given?

$$fl𝌆\ xvi = ?\ fl℥ \quad \text{(translation: 16 fluid drams = ? fluid ounces)}$$

Solution

From the table of equivalents: 1 fluid ounce = 8 fluid drams (fl℥ 1 = fl𝌆 8, or floz 1 = fldr 8).

$$(\cancel{fldr}\ 16)\left(\frac{floz\ 1}{\cancel{fldr}\ 8}\right) = floz\ \frac{16}{8} = floz\ 2 = fl℥\ 2$$

The patient should be given 2 floz (fl℥ 2) of the antacid.

Look back at Examples 19 and 20. Note that the symbols were "translated" into words in most cases. If the apothecary system is new to you, this will help you sort out a problem involving these units. You can always write your final answer with the symbols, but you can work it out using words or more familiar abbreviations like floz for "fluid ounce" instead of fl℥.

You may find it necessary to use more than one conversion factor in order to end up with the unit you need. Look at Example 21 to see this type of conversion.

EXAMPLE 21: Converting Volumes by Unit Analysis

qt $\frac{1}{2}$ = fl℥ ? (translation: one-half quart = how many fluid drams?)

Solution

To do this conversion using the table of apothecary equivalents will require that you first convert quarts to ounces (qt 1 = floz 32) and then convert ounces to fluid drams (floz 1 = fldr 8).

$$\left(qt\, \frac{1}{2} \right) \left(\frac{floz\ 32}{qt\ 1} \right) \left(\frac{fldr\ 8}{floz\ 1} \right) = fldr\, \frac{256}{2} = fldr\ 128 = \quad fl℥\ 128$$

EXAMPLE 22: Converting Weights by Unit Analysis

℈ 3 = gr ? (translation: 3 drams equals how many grains?)

Solution

On the table of apothecary equivalents you will find that 1 dram equals 60 grains (℈ 1 = gr 60).

$$(dram\ 3) \left(\frac{gr\ 60}{dram\ 1} \right) = gr\, \frac{180}{1} = gr\ 180$$

PRACTICE PROBLEM SET 3.6

Write each of the following measures using the proper numbers and unit abbreviations. Use both Hindu-Arabic numbers, fractions, and Roman numerals whenever possible.

1. five and one-half grains
2. six and one-half grains
3. five minims
4. twenty-three minims
5. four drams
6. seven and one-half drams
7. four fluid drams
8. eighteen drams
9. fourteen fluid ounces
10. five and one-half fluid ounces
11. one-fifteenth of a grain
12. one-eighth of a grain
13. three and one-half quarts
14. two and one-fourth quarts
15. seven pints
16. thirty-two pints
17. five and twenty-five-hundredths fluid ounces
18. one-thousandth of a fluid ounce
19. seventy-five drams
20. forty-two drams

Convert units as indicated.

21. fl℥ iss = fl℥ ?
22. fl℥ ss = fl℥ ?
23. pt xiv = fl℥ ?
24. pt iv = fl℥ ?

25. pt v = fl ʒ ?
26. pt ixss = fl ʒ ?
27. gr 210 = ʒ ?
28. gr XL = ʒ ?
29. min xv = fl ʒ ?
30. min 50 = fl ʒ ?
31. qt xv = fl ʒ ?
32. qt 2 = fl ʒ ?

33. fl ʒ 12 = fl ℥ ?
34. fl ʒ XL = fl ℥ ?
35. ℥ $\frac{1}{4}$ = gr ?
36. ʒ $2\frac{3}{4}$ = gr ?
37. qt $\frac{1}{4}$ = pt ?
38. qt $6\frac{3}{4}$ = pt ?
39. pt $\frac{1}{8}$ = min ?
40. pt $\frac{7}{8}$ = min ?

SECTION 3.7 CONVERTING BETWEEN MEASUREMENT SYSTEMS

It is often necessary to convert between the various systems of measurement. Although a prescription may be written using the apothecary system, most dosages or labels on medicines and drugs use the metric units. Most of the conversions are done by the unit analysis method, as shown in the previous three sections of this chapter.

In order to do conversions between the metric, apothecary, and household systems, a table of equivalent values or conversion factors is needed. In Table 3.7 you will find some **conversion factors** that will be useful in this effort. The table is limited to the units in each measurement system that are most often used in allied health areas.

Table 3.7 Approximate Equivalents Between SI, Apothecary, and Household Units

Metric	Apothecary	Household
Liquid Volumes	**Liquid Volumes**	**Liquid Volumes**
30 or 32 mL (30 mL is used most)	fl ℥ 1 = fl ʒ 8	2 T
4 or 5 mL (5 mL is used most)	fl ʒ 1 = min 60	1 t = 60 gtt
	min 1	1 gtt
15 mL	fl ʒ 4	1 T
1 mL = 1 cc	min 15 or 16	15 or 16 gtt
Weights	**Weights**	**Weights**
60 mg	gr 1	
1 g	gr 15	
1 kg	gr 15,000 = oz 35.2	2.2 lb
0.45 kg	oz 16	1 lb
Lengths	**Lengths**	**Lengths**
2.54 cm	None	1 in.

EXAMPLE 23: Converting Weight Measurements

$$gr\ 10 = ?\ mg$$

Solution

These units are measures of weight, so locate the equivalent needed in Table 3.7. Then set up the conversion fraction so 'gr' will cancel, leaving the answer in mg. In Table 3.7, gr 1 = 60 mg.

$$(\cancel{gr}\ 10)\left(\frac{60\ mg}{\cancel{gr}\ 1}\right) = 600\ mg$$

EXAMPLE 24: Converting Weight Measurements

The label on a certain medication indicates that the vial contains 1.50 g. How many grains of drug are in a vial?

Solution

Table 3.7 tells us that 1 g = gr 15. Set up the conversion fraction so that 'g' will cancel, leaving the answer in 'gr'.

$$(1.50 \text{ g})\left(\frac{\text{gr } 15}{1 \text{ g}}\right) = \text{gr } 22.5$$

EXAMPLE 25: Converting Volume Measurements

You are directed to give 8 t of a liquid medication to a patient. How many milliliters is this?

Solution

From Table 3.7, 1 t = 5 mL. Set up the conversion fraction so that 't' will cancel, leaving the answer in 'mL'.

$$(8 \text{ t})\left(\frac{5 \text{ mL}}{1 \text{ t}}\right) = 40 \text{ mL}$$

Please note that had you chosen to use 1 t = 4 mL, the result would have been only 32 mL, not 40 mL. This shows you that some of the equivalents between the various systems are approximate at best.

EXAMPLE 26: Converting Weight Measurements

A patient weighs 100 lb 8 oz. How many kilograms does this equal?

Solution

From Table 3.7, 1 kg = 2.2 lb.
However, you must first convert 100 lb 8 oz to just pounds.
From Table 3.7, 1 lb = 16 oz.

$$(8 \text{ oz})\left(\frac{1 \text{ lb}}{16 \text{ oz}}\right) = \frac{8}{16} \text{ lb} = \frac{1}{2} \text{ lb}$$

But, since fractions are not used in the metric system, this is 0.5 lb. This gives the patient's weight as 100.5 lb. Now convert the weight to kilograms.

$$(100.5 \text{ lb})\left(\frac{1 \text{ kg}}{2.2 \text{ lb}}\right) = \frac{100.5}{2.2} \text{ kg} = 45.681818\ldots \text{ kg}$$

Since our weight measurement has 4 significant digits, we round to 45.68 kg.

PRACTICE PROBLEM SET 3.7

1. gr $\frac{3}{4}$ = ? mg
2. gr $\frac{1}{2}$ = ? mcg
3. 40.0 mL = floz ?
4. 25.0 mL = fl℥ ?
5. 2 T = ? mL
6. 4.5 T = ? mL

7. 10 mL = ? t
8. 12 mL = ? t
9. fl℥ ss = ? mL
10. floz iv = ? mL
11. 8.75 mcg = gr?
12. 5.0 mcg = gr ?

13. min 8 = ? gtt
14. min 14 = ? gtt
15. fl℥ xxii = ? mL
16. fl℥ xiv = ? mL
17. 5.0 t = ? mL
18. 8.5 t = ? mL

19. $10 \text{ t} = \text{fl} \bar{3}$?

20. $10 \text{ T} = \text{fl} \bar{3}$?

21. $0.100 \text{ L} = \text{fl} \bar{3}$?

22. $100.0 \text{ mL} = \text{fl} \bar{3}$?

23. $\text{fl} \bar{3} \text{ iiss} = \text{fl} \bar{3}$?

24. $\text{fl} \bar{3} \text{ viiss} = \text{min}$?

25. $\text{qt ss} = ? \text{ gtt}$

26. $\text{pt iss} = ? \text{ gtt}$

27. $45 \text{ gtt} = \text{fl} \bar{3}$?

28. $250 \text{ gtt} = \text{fl} \bar{3}$?

29. $0.25 \text{ lb} = \text{gr}$?

30. $\text{gr } 6\bar{0}00 = ? \text{ lb}$

31. $1200. \text{ gtt} = ? \text{ cups}$

32. $4 \text{ cups} = \text{min}$?

33. $\text{fl} \bar{3} \text{ } 2 = ? \text{ cc}$

34. $\text{fl} \bar{3} \text{ } 3 = ? \text{ cc}$

35. $4.5 \text{ cc} = \text{min}$?

36. $\text{min } 8 = ? \text{ cc}$

37. $200 \text{ lb} = ? \text{ kg}$

38. $125 \text{ lb} = ? \text{ kg}$

39. $0.50 \text{ g} = \text{gr}$?

40. $2.5 \text{ g} = \text{gr}$?

SECTION 3.8   TEMPERATURE SCALES

Thermometers are rulers developed for measuring the relative amount of heat in the location of the thermometer. Temperature scales are like the markings of a ruler and were originally developed using two base-line physical phenomena: the freezing point of pure water and the boiling point of pure water. There are several temperature scales in general use in the United States: the Fahrenheit, Celsius, and Kelvin scales. Other scales are in use in specialized areas, but these three are widely used in allied health applications.

The Fahrenheit Temperature Scale

The **Fahrenheit temperature scale** was set up by a German physicist named Daniel Gabriel Fahrenheit (1686–1736). He was also the inventor of the mercury-in-glass thermometer that is still in common use today. Mr. Fahrenheit's scale has 180 steps between the freezing point and boiling point of water. A step is a *degree* and temperatures are expressed in "degrees Fahrenheit" (°F). On the Fahrenheit temperature scale, the freezing temperature of water is 32°F and the boiling temperature of water is 212°F.

One of the most common temperature measurements made in allied health careers is, of course, a patient's body temperature. Many times a digital thermometer will be used for this purpose, and it is a simple matter to read and record the temperature in any scale that the thermometer may be set for. However, glass thermometers are still very common and some practice and skill are needed to accurately read such thermometers. Figure 3.2 shows you an oral thermometer and its scale markings.

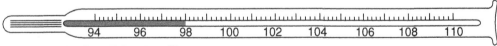

Figure 3.2 An Oral, Fahrenheit Thermometer

EXAMPLE 27: Reading Glass Thermometers

Read the temperature indicated by each of the following thermometers.

a.

Solution

As you can see, the colored liquid is up to the mark that is halfway between the 98 and 100 markings on the scale. This is the location of the 99-degree mark. The patient's temperature is 99°F.

b.

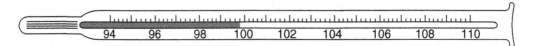

Solution

As you can see, the colored liquid is four tick marks past the 99°F location. Each tick mark is equivalent to two-tenths of a degree. The patient's temperature is 99.8°F.

The Celsius Temperature Scale

The **Celsius temperature scale**, which was called the *centigrade scale* at one time, was named after Anders C. Celsius (1701–1744). This temperature scale has 100 steps (degrees) between the freezing and boiling points of water. This means that a step (degree) on the Celsius scale is larger than a degree on the Fahrenheit scale. On the Celsius temperature scale, the freezing temperature of water is 0°C and the boiling temperature of water is 100°C. The Celsius "degree" is about twice as large as the Fahrenheit "degree" (1°C = 1.8°F).

Both the Fahrenheit and Celsius temperature scales measure very low temperatures as *negative* numbers. In some areas of application, like those medical areas dealing with the gas laws (inhalation therapy, and so on), these negative temperatures can result in incorrect calculations. To overcome this potential problem, *absolute temperature scales* are used. Theoretically, the lowest possible temperature is *absolute zero*. This temperature is estimated to be –273°C on the Celsius scale and –459°F on the Fahrenheit scale.

The Kelvin Temperature Scale

This scale was named in honor of Lord Kelvin (William Thomson, 1824–1907). On the **Kelvin temperature scale**, *absolute zero* is the zero temperature location. In theory, no temperature lower than absolute zero is possible. This means that the Kelvin temperature scale will have no negative temperatures on it.

An unusual thing about the Kelvin scale is that the units are called *Kelvins* rather than *degrees*. Absolute zero on the Kelvin scale is 0 K (zero Kelvins). The Kelvin and Celsius scales have the same-size units so that a step of 1°C is the same size step as 1 K. The freezing temperature of water on this scale is 273.15 K and the boiling temperature is 373 K (three hundred seventy-three Kelvins).

Conversions Between the Kelvin, Celsius, and Fahrenheit Scales

The conversion of a temperature measured on one of these scales to the equivalent temperature on one of the other scales is done by formula, as follows:

Temperature Conversion Formulas		
$T_C = \dfrac{T_F - 32}{1.8}$	$T_F = 1.8T_C + 32$	$T_K = T_C + 273$

EXAMPLE 28: Converting Fahrenheit to Celsius

Change 70.0°F to the equivalent number of degrees Celsius.

Solution

First, choose the formula that starts with the temperature scale that you wish to switch to. In this case the proper formula is

$$T_C = \frac{T_F - 32}{1.8}$$

Substituting for T_F,

$$T_C = \frac{90.0 - 32}{1.8}$$
$$T_C = \frac{38°}{1.8}$$
$$T_C = 21.111\ldots°$$

Thus, 70.0°F = 21.1°F (remember to round based on significant digits).

EXAMPLE 29: Converting Celsius to Fahrenheit

Change 20.0°C to degrees Fahrenheit.

Solution

Here you should choose $\qquad T_F = 1.8T_C + 32$.

Now substitute the value of T_C:

$$T_F = 1.8(20.0) + 32$$
$$T_F = 36 + 32$$
$$T_F = 68°$$

So, 20.0°C = 68.0°F (remember to round based on significant digits).

EXAMPLE 30: Converting Celsius to Kelvin

Convert 8.00°C to the equivalent temperature Kelvin.

Solution

The proper formula is $T_K = T_C + 273$.

Substitute for T_C:

$$T_K = 8.00 + 273$$
$$T_K = 281$$

Thus, 8.00°C = 281 K (remember, no degree symbol).

EXAMPLE 31: Converting Fahrenheit to Celsius

Convert 20.0°F to the equivalent Celsius temperature.

Solution

$$T_C = \frac{T_F - 32}{1.8}$$

$$T_C = \frac{20.0 - 32}{1.8}$$

$$T_C = \frac{-12}{1.8}$$

$T_C = -6.666\ldots$ °F $= -6.67$°F (remember to round based on significant digits).

EXAMPLE 32: Converting Celsius to Fahrenheit

Convert –88.0°C to the equivalent number of degrees Fahrenheit.

Solution

$$T_F = 1.8T_C + 32$$
$$T_F = 1.8(-88.0) + 32$$
$$T_F = -158.4 + 32$$

$T_F = -126.4$°C $= -126$°C (remember to round based on significant digits).

PRACTICE PROBLEM SET 3.8

Convert each of the following temperatures as indicated.

1. 89.0°F = ? °C
2. 350°F = ? °C
3. 115°C = ? K
4. 60°C = ? K
5. 25.0°C = ? °F
6. 42.0°C = ? °F
7. 4.00°F = ? °C

8. 0.50°F = ? °C
9. –40.0°F = ? °C
10. –15.0°F = ? °C
11. 4.00 K = ? °C
12. 400.0 K = ? °C
13. –15.0°C = ? °F
14. –32.0°C = ? °F

15. 800.0°C = ? °F
16. 1500.0°C = ? °F
17. 98.6°F = ? °C = ? K
18. 32.0°F = ? °C = ? K
19. 200.0 K = ? °C = ? °F
20. 500.0 K = ? °C = ? °F

What temperature do each of the following thermometers indicate?

21.

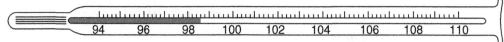

22.

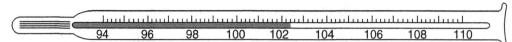

23.

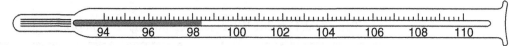

24.

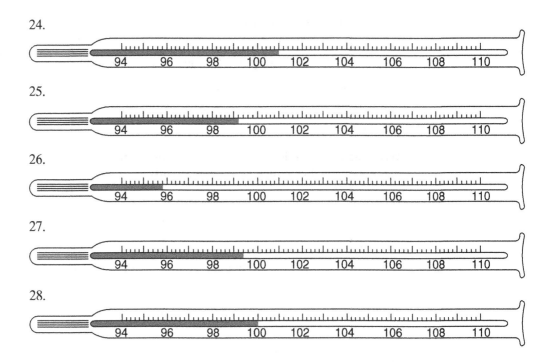

25.

26.

27.

28.

Chapter Summary

In this chapter you were introduced to the very important area of measurements. Measurements will be part of your everyday concerns in virtually any allied health profession. Being familiar with the primary unit systems and how to convert from one unit to another will be a very useful to you. Also, the fact that measurements you may make are only as good as your instrumentation allows is important for you to understand. You must learn to adjust calculated results to reflect your instrumentation's precision and accuracy.

Important Terms and Formulas

$a \times 10^n$

accuracy

apothecary system

approximate numbers

Celsius temperatures

conversion factors

dimensional analysis

exact numbers

Fahrenheit temperatures

household units

Kelvin temperatures

length

mass

measurements

metric system

military time

precision

scientific notation

SI unit system

significant digits

time

unit analysis

volume

weight

Formulas Used

$$T_C = \frac{T_F - 32}{1.8} \qquad T_F = 1.8T_C + 32 \qquad T_K = T_C + 273$$

Write each of the following numbers in scientific notation.

1. 0.00567
2. 550,000
3. 100

4. 0.000000007
5. 4.6

Write each of the following *measurements* in scientific notation, being careful to maintain the proper significant digit count in your answer.

6. 8900 L
7. 0.000006 g
8. 450.0 mL

9. 6.0 m
10. 0.005600 mg

Remove each of the following numbers from scientific notation.

11. 6.79×10^{-8}
12. 2.843×10^{-3}
13. 9.23×10^{4}

14. 2.9×10^{0}
15. 8×10^{-1}

How many significant digits are in each of the following measurements?

16. 0.02360 mg
17. 562.0 m
18. 3.00260 L

19. 4.50×10^{4} g
20. 6.5×10^{-8} mL

Write out the names of each of the following units.

21. mcg
22. ʒ
23. flʒ
24. min
25. mL

26. gr
27. °
28. nL
29. t
30. gtt

31. What is the difference between an exact number and an approximate number?
32. What is the difference between the accuracy of a measurement and its precision?
33. Are the measurements 45 mL and 45.0 mL the same? Why or why not?
34. Why do you need to learn several different systems of measurement?
35. What do the significant digits in a measurement tell you?

Convert each of the following units as indicated.

36. flʒ $\frac{1}{6}$ = min ?
37. oz $\frac{1}{2}$ = flʒ ?
38. $\frac{1}{4}$t = ? gtt
39. 2 cups = ? oz
40. 0.75 L = ? cc
41. 1.45 L = ? mL
42. 76 mcg = ? mg
43. ʒ 96 = ʒ ?
44. flʒ 3 = min ?

45. min 4 = gtt ?
46. 8 T = ? t
47. 0.76 kg = ? g
48. 1000 mg = gr ?
49. 8 t = ? mL
50. $\frac{1}{2}$T = ? gtt
51. 8 lb 4 oz = ? kg
52. flʒ 2 = ? t
53. flʒ 2 = ? gtt

54. gr XLIV = ? g
55. fl℥ xvss = ? mL
56. 65.0°C = ? °F

57. −78.0°C = ? K
58. 108°F = ? °C
59. −8.00°F = ? °C

60. Which of these volumes is the largest: 4.56×10^3 nL, 4.56 mcL, or 0.00456 mL?

61. Three samples are weighed on an electronic scale with the following weights obtained: 0.53698 g, 0.55567 g, and 0.52514 g. Write each of these weights in scientific notation.

62. What is the difference between the largest and smallest weight in Problem 61? Express your answer in scientific notation.

63. If 15 injections of flu vaccine were given and each contained 1.25 mL, how many milliliters of vaccine were used altogether?

64. A doctor orders 1 L of 10% dextrose water solution ($D_{10}W$) for his office. To fill this order, he ordered four cases. If standard case sizes are 1000 cc, 500 cc, and 250 cc, which size cases did he order?

65. Clark's Rule for determining pediatric dosages is

$$p = \frac{wA}{150}$$

where w = the child's weight in pounds

A = the usual adult dosage

p = the pediatric dosage

If a child weighs 35.0 lb and the usual adult dosage is 2.00 oz, how many teaspoons would you give the child?

66. How many drops would you give the child in Problem 65?

Chapter Test

Write each of the following in scientific notation.

1. 765,000,000
2. 0.00000067
3. 9.45

Remove each of the following from scientific notation.

4. 6.098×10^0
5. 7.93×10^{-5}
6. 3.497×10^8

Round off each of the following measurements to 3 significant digits.

7. 56873 mg
8. 0.00678 L
9. 50.00999 m

Do each of the following calculations using the measurements given and round off your answer properly.

10. $(4.56 \text{ m})(3.7 \text{ m}) = ? \text{ m}^2$
11. If 1 penny weighs 3.56 g, how much do 10 such pennies weigh?
12. 23.45 mL + 67.8 mL + 6.7899 mL

Convert units as indicated.

13. gr xviiss = ? mg

14. 6.78 mL = ? L

15. $1\frac{3}{4}$ T = ? gtt

16. 0.2 mg = ? mcg

17. 0.45 L = fl℥ ?

18. min 15 = ? gtt

19. gr 4 = ? g

20. $4\frac{1}{2}$ t = ? gtt

21. 37°C = ? °F

22. −60°C = ? K

23. −10°F = ? °C

24. 0.12 mg = gr ?

25. fl℥ 20 = fl℥ ?

26. A patient has a roughly circular burn on her back with a diameter of 2.15 cm as measured by a nurse. What is the area of this burn? (The formula for the area of a circle is $A = \pi r^2$.)

27. A doctor tells you to inject 1.25 cc of a vaccine into a patient. How many milliliters is this?

28. Clark's Rule for determining pediatric dosages is

$$p = \frac{wA}{150}$$

where w = the child's weight in pounds

A = the usual adult dosage

p = the pediatric dosage

What would the pediatric dosage, in teaspoons, be for a child with a weight of 45.0 lb if the adult dose is 4 oz?

29. How many tablespoons would you give the child in Problem 28?

30. How many fluid drams would you give the child in Problem 28?

MEDICATION LABELS, PRESCRIPTIONS, AND SYRINGE CALCULATIONS

Objectives for Chapter 4

After completing this chapter the student should be able to:

1. Extract important information regarding medication types or forms, dosage rates, dosage recommendations, medication storage information, expiration dates, and other patient-related information from medical labels and product inserts.

2. Read and properly interpret prescriptions for medications and medical orders regarding dosage, type or form of medication, method of administration, and directions referring to patient care as written by physicians.

3. Do all necessary calculations involving syringes and the administration of medications with them.

SECTION 4.1   READING MEDICATION LABELS AND INSERTS

One of the many critical functions that may be performed by allied health professionals is the administration of drugs to patients. Drugs are prescribed for patients to help the body fight off infections or for other therapeutic purposes. Drugs can save the life of a patient or threaten that life if improperly chosen or improperly administered. All medical professionals included in the chain of drug administration (from the person who prescribes a drug, to the pharmacist who fills the prescription, to the person who then administers the drug) are equally responsible for the patient's safety. All of these persons need to be careful to *assure that the right drug is given in the right amount to the right patient in the right way.*

In this section, you will be looking at labels for various medications and learning what to look for and what all the various information there tells you. In Chapter 5, you will calculate dosages based on label information. Some labels are easy to read and some are so small that you might need to use a magnifying glass to read them. However, it is imperative that you do read them and carefully compare the information on the label with the medication prescribed. Do not ever assume that since a pharmacist sent it to you to administer that the medication is correct. You need to check it out for yourself. Remember that you are responsible to the patient as much as the doctor or pharmacist.

Not all medication labels are the same in format but they do all have certain information in common. In Figure 4.1 you will see a medication label with many of its parts pointed out. There is a list below the label that shows you what is being pointed out. Following this list is a more detailed discussion of each item on the label.

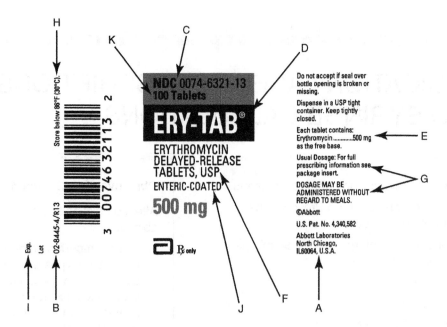

A. Manufacturer

B. Manufacturer's lot number

C. National Drug Code number (NDC)

D. Trade name and generic name of the drug

E. Amount of drug per dose

F. United States Pharmacopedia (USP)

G. Dosage recommendations

H. Storage instructions

I. Expiration date

J. Form of the drug in this container

K. Total amount of drug in this container

As you can see, there are a lot of things to look at on this label and this list does not point out everything on the label. Some of the items are more important than others, and the order of the list is not intended to indicate the order of importance of the items listed. Now we will look at the label in Figure 4-1 in some detail.

A. The *manufacturer* of this drug is Abbott Laboratories.

B. The *manufacturer's lot number* is 02-8445-4/R13 and likely encodes the facility that made the drug and the date on which this particular bottle was filled. This kind of information allows the manufacturer to track a particular batch of a drug in the event that some defect should be found and that batch needs to be removed from use.

C. The *National Drug Code number* (NDC) for this drug is NDC 0074-6321-13. This is an identifying number for this drug assigned by the Drug Enforcement Agency (DEA), an agency of the federal government of the United States.

D. The **trade name** of this drug is Ery-Tab. The trade name of a drug is indicated by the symbol ® following the name. The **generic name** of this drug is erythromycin. Many different drug companies may be manufacturing the same drug but each may give it their own trade name for sale in the marketplace. For example, perhaps the best known trade name for acetominophen is Tylenol®, yet every drug store chain and mass marketer has its own trade name for the same drug.

BE CAUTIOUS ABOUT DRUG NAMES! Many drugs that are entirely different have very similar-sounding names. You cannot afford to choose the wrong drug from a supply cabinet or other source and then administer it to a patient. This could have possibly disastrous effects on the patient and on your career. For example, Celexa® is not the same as Celebrex®, fluconasole is not fluorouracil, and glyguride is not glipizide. Just be careful to compare the prescribed drug name with the label name before administering a dose to a patient. CHECK NAMES LETTER-FOR-LETTER.

E. The *amount of drug* per dose for this drug is 500 mg of erythromycin per tablet in the container.

F. The **United States Pharmacopedia (USP)** designation means that this drug was manufactured in a way that conforms to the standards set by the United States Pharmacopedia, which sets the formulations for all drugs available in the United States.

G. There are several *dosage recommendations* or brief guidelines given here. Some labels may not give any directions on the label itself and will, as this label does, direct the user to refer to a more *detailed printed insert* enclosed with the drug.

H. The storage instructions indicate that this drug should be stored at temperatures below 86°F/30°C. If a drug is not completely used at once, it is important to follow the storage instructions carefully. If a drug requires refrigeration, then leaving it out at room temperature may severely impact its effectiveness or alter its effect on the patient.

I. The *expiration date* shown on a drug label is also very important to note. After the expiration date the drug may have lost its original potency or it may react differently when a patient takes it. **NEVER** give an expired drug to a patient.

J. The *form of the drug* in this container is tablet form. The tablets are called "delayed release" and are said to be "enteric coated"on the label. This means that the tablets should not be crushed or divided in any way as that would defeat the delayed release of this drug into the system with possible bad consequences for the patient. Drugs are dispensed in many forms, including tablet, caplet, capsule, powder, gel, cream, and liquid, just to name a few.

K. The *total amount* of drug originally in this container is one hundred (100) tablets.

In many cases some information will be found on a drug label in several places. For example, the NDC is on the label in Figure 4-1 in two places, and the generic name and amount of drug per tablet are on the label in three places. Other information may also appear on the label as well. The label that we are looking at now has several warnings on it as well as the color of the tablets and the symbol that is embossed on the tablets by Abbott Laboratories as they are manufactured.

EXAMPLE 1: Reading a Prozac® Label

Read the following label and find the information available there in the categories A–K as shown in Figure 4-1 and in the following list.

A. Manufacturer: Manufactured by Eli Lilly and Company.

B. Manufacturer's lot number: No control number shown.

C. National Drug Code number: NDC 0777-5120-58.

D. Trade name and generic name: The trade name is Prozac® and the generic name is fluoxetine hydrochloride.

E. Amount of drug per dose: 20 mg in each 5 mL.

F. United States Pharmacopedia code: No apparent USP code seen.

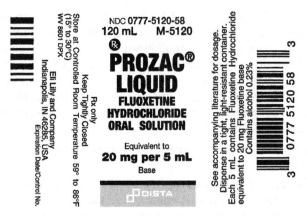

G. Dosage recommendations: "See accompanying literature" means that this information is on a printed insert.

H. Storage instructions: Store at a temperature between 59°F and 86°F (15°C and 30°C).

I. Expiration date: No expiration date is shown.

J. Form of drug in this container: This is a liquid solution for oral administration.

K. Total amount of drug in this container: The container holds 120 mL of the solution.

EXAMPLE 2: Reading a Provera® Label

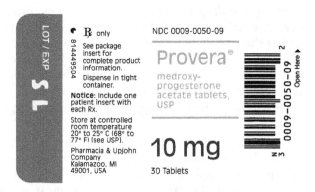

Read the label above and furnish the following information:

Trade name / generic name: _____

Form of medication: _____

Strength: _____

Amount in this container: _____

Recommended dosage: _____

Expiration date: _____

Special storage instructions: _____

NDC: _____

Manufactured according to USP standards?: _____

Here are the answers:

Trade name / generic name: <u>Provera® / medroxy-progesterone</u>

Form of medication: <u>tablets</u>

Strength: <u>10 mg/tab</u>

Amount in this container: <u>30 tablets</u>

Recommended dosage: <u>see package insert</u>

Expiration date: <u>none shown</u>

Special storage instructions: <u>store at regulated room temperature 20°–25°C</u>
<u>(68°–77°F)</u>

NDC: <u>0009-0050-09</u>

Manufactured according to USP standards?: <u>yes</u>

Inserts in Drug Packages

If more detailed instructions are needed in order to safely administer a medication to a patient or to be sure that proper storage procedures are being followed, refer to the *insert* that most manufacturers include with each container of a drug. This insert will contain all of the label information but in much more detail. It will also include chemical descriptions of the drug, list all known drug interactions, and list all known drug reactions or side effects and any necessary warnings or precautions.

PRACTICE PROBLEM SET 4.1

Read each of the following labels carefully and supply the following information for each one: (a) the manufacturer's name, (b) the brand name of the drug, (c) the generic name of the drug, (d) the administration route that should be used with the drug, (e) the total amount of medication (mL, number of capsules, etc.) in an unopened container, and (f) the amount of drug per tablet, mL, etc.

1.

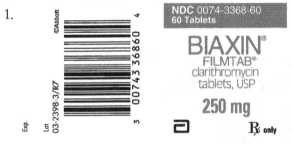

Source: Label ©Abbott Laboratories. Used with permission.

2.

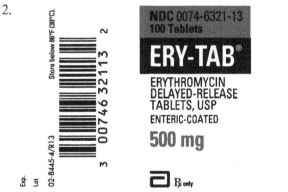

Source: Label © Abbott Laboratories. Used with permission.

3.

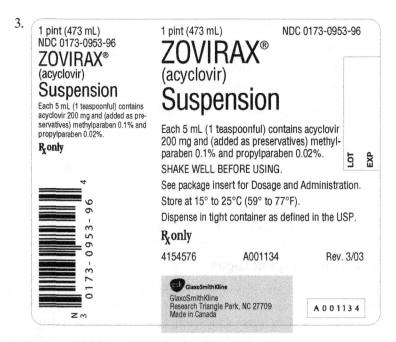

Source: Reproduced with permission of GlaxoSmithKline.

4.

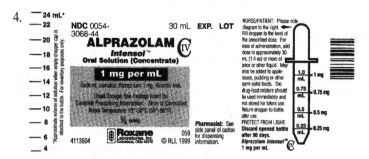

Source: Label © Roxane Laboratories. Used with permission.

5.

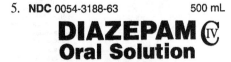

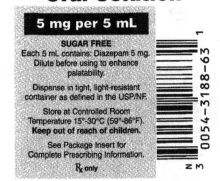

LOT
EXP.

4116001//04   © RLI, 2004

Source: Label © Roxane Laboratories.
Used with permission.

6.

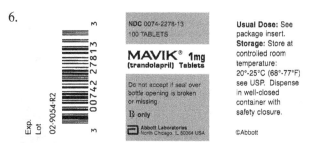

NDC 0074-2278-13
100 TABLETS

MAVIK® **1mg**
(trandolapril) **Tablets**

Do not accept if seal over
bottle opening is broken
or missing.

℞ only

Abbott Laboratories
North Chicago, IL 60064 USA

Usual Dose: See
package insert.
Storage: Store at
controlled room
temperature:
20°-25°C (68°-77°F)
see USP. Dispense
in well-closed
container with
safety closure.

©Abbott

Source: Label © Abbott Laboratories. Used with permission.

7.

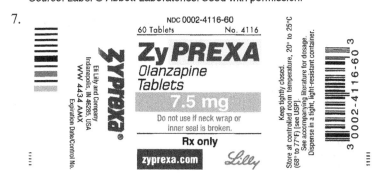

NDC 0002-4116-60

60 Tablets   No. 4116

Zy PREXA
Olanzapine
Tablets

7.5 mg

Do not use if neck wrap or
inner seal is broken.

Rx only

zyprexa.com   *Lilly*

Eli Lilly and Company
Indianapolis, IN 46285, USA
VW 4434 AMX

Expiration Date/Control No.

Keep tightly closed.
Store at controlled room temperature, 20° to 25°C
(68° to 77°F) [see USP].
See accompanying literature for dosage.
Dispense in a tight, light-resistant container.

Source: Copyright Eli Lilly & Co. All rights reserved. Used with permission.

8.

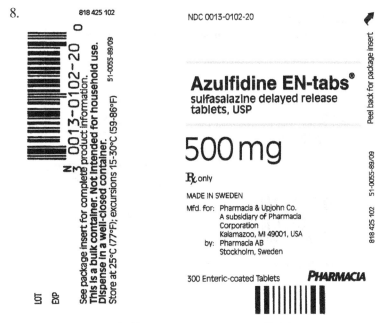

818 425 102

NDC 0013-0102-20

Azulfidine EN-tabs®
sulfasalazine delayed release
tablets, USP

500 mg

℞ only

MADE IN SWEDEN

Mfd. for: Pharmacia & Upjohn Co.
A subsidiary of Pharmacia
Corporation
Kalamazoo, MI 49001, USA
by: Pharmacia AB
Stockholm, Sweden

300 Enteric-coated Tablets   **PHARMACIA**

See package insert for complete product information.
This is a bulk container. Not intended for household use.
Dispense in a well-closed container.
Store at 25°C (77°F); excursions 15-30°C (59-86°F)

51-0055-89/09

LOT EXP

Peel back for package insert

Source: Reproduced with permission of Pfizer, Inc. All rights reserved.

9.

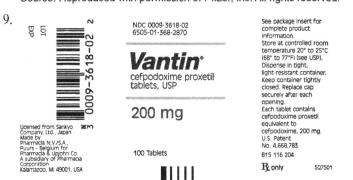

EXP LOT

NDC 0009-3618-02
6505-01-368-2870

Vantin®
cefpodoxime proxetil
tablets, USP

200 mg

100 Tablets

Licensed from Sankyo
Company, Ltd., Japan
Made by
Pharmacia N.V./S.A.,
Puurs - Belgium for
Pharmacia & Upjohn Co.
A subsidiary of Pharmacia
Corporation
Kalamazoo, MI 49001, USA

See package insert for
complete product
information.
Store at controlled room
temperature 20° to 25°C
(68° to 77°F) [see USP].
Dispense in tight,
light-resistant container.
Keep container tightly
closed. Replace cap
securely after each
opening.
Each tablet contains
cefpodoxime proxetil
equivalent to
cefpodoxime, 200 mg.
U.S. Patent
No. 4,668,783
815 116 204

℞ only   5Q7501

Source: Reproduced with permission of Pfizer, Inc. All rights reserved.

Medication Labels, Prescriptions, and Syringe Calculations

10.

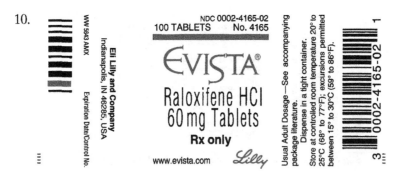

NDC 0002-4165-02
100 TABLETS   No. 4165

EVISTA®
Raloxifene HCl
60 mg Tablets
Rx only
www.evista.com   *Lilly*

WW 5643 AMX

Eli Lilly and Company
Indianapolis, IN 46285, USA

Expiration Date/Control No.

Usual Adult Dosage—See accompanying package literature.
Dispense in a tight container.
Store at controlled room temperature 20° to 25°C (68° to 77°F); excursions permitted between 15° to 30°C (59° to 86°F).

3 00002-4165-02 1

11.

NDC 0009-7224-01   5 ml

Lymphocyte Immune
Globulin, Anti-Thymocyte
Globulin (Equine)
Atgam®

250 mg protein
(50 mg per mL)

Rx only

For I.V. use only. For suggested dose, refer to package insert.
U.S. License No. 1216.
ATTENTION—May contain particles; this is normal. Use 0.2μ to 1.0μ in-line filter. See insert.   816 661 002
Pharmacia & Upjohn Company
Kalamazoo, MI 49001, USA

12.

NDC 0009-5190-03

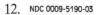

Detrol LA

tolterodine tartrate
extended release capsules

2 mg

500 Capsules

N
3 0009-5190-03 8

Rx only
See package insert for complete product information.
Store at 25°C (77°F); excursions permitted to 15°-30°C (59°-86°F) (see USP Controlled Room Temperature). Protect from light.
U.S. Patent No. 5,382,600

Manufactured for: Pharmacia & Upjohn Company • A subsidiary of Pharmacia Corporation • Kalamazoo, MI 49001, USA
By: International Processing Corporation Winchester, Kentucky 40391, USA

818270001

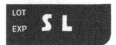

LOT
EXP   **S L**

13.

See package insert for complete product information.
Dispense in a well-closed container.
Store at 25°C (77°F); excursions 15-30°C (59-86°F)
MADE IN SWEDEN
Mfd. for: Pharmacia & Upjohn Co.
A subsidiary of Pharmacia Corporation
Kalamazoo, MI 49001, USA
by: Pharmacia AB
Stockholm, Sweden

819 022 000   51-0052-89/08

PHARMACIA

NDC 0013-0101-01

Azulfidine®

sulfasalazine tablets, USP

500 mg

100 Tablets   Rx only

THIS PACKAGE FOR HOUSEHOLDS
WITHOUT YOUNG CHILDREN

N
3 0013-0101-01 2

Peel back for package insert

14. ℞ only

Usual Dosage: Two capsules in a single daily administration. For additional prescribing information read package insert.

Dispense in a tight container as defined in the USP.

Keep tightly closed.

Store at 25°C (77°F); excursions permitted to 15°-30°C (59°-86°F) [see USP Controlled Room Temperature].

Each capsule contains: rifabutin, USP 150 mg.

LOT   EXP

NDC 0013-5301-17

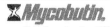
rifabutin capsules, USP

150 mg

N3 0013-5301-17 2

MADE IN ITALY

Manufactured for:
Pharmacia & Upjohn Company
A subsidiary of Pharmacia Corporation
Kalamazoo, MI 49001, USA

by: Pharmacia Italia S.p.A.
Ascoli Piceno, Italy

819 076 000   100002067 00

100 Capsules   **PHARMACIA**

15. FOR ORAL USE ONLY.
STORAGE
Before Reconstitution:
Store below 86°F (30°C).
After Reconstitution:
Store suspension between 41°F (5°C) and 86°F (30°C). Protect from freezing.
DOSAGE AND USE
See accompanying prescribing information.
MIXING DIRECTIONS:
Tap bottle lightly to loosen powder. Add 24 mL of distilled water or Purified Water (USP) to the bottle. Shake well.
SHAKE WELL BEFORE EACH USE.
DISCARD UNUSED PORTION AFTER 2 WEEKS.
This package contains **1400 mg** fluconazole in a natural orange-flavored mixture.*

NDC 0049-3450-19
35 mL when reconstituted

DIFLUCAN®
(Fluconazole for Oral Suspension)

ORANGE FLAVORED

40 mg/mL
when reconstituted

Pfizer Roerig
Division of Pfizer Inc, NY, NY 10017

3 N 0049-3450-19 2

* When reconstituted as directed, each teaspoonful (5 mL) contains 200 mg of fluconazole.

Rx only

05-4800-32-3

1223
MADE IN USA

16. FOR ORAL USE ONLY.
STORAGE
Before Reconstitution:
Store below 86°F (30°C).
After Reconstitution:
Store suspension between 41°F (5°C) and 86°F (30°C). Protect from freezing.
SHAKE WELL BEFORE EACH USE.
DISCARD UNUSED PORTION AFTER 2 WEEKS.
MIXING DIRECTIONS
Tap bottle lightly to loosen powder. Add 24 mL of distilled water or Purified Water (USP) to the bottle. Shake well.
DOSAGE AND USE
See accompanying prescribing information.
This package contains **350 mg** fluconazole in a natural orange-flavored mixture.*

NDC 0049-3440-19
35 mL when reconstituted

DIFLUCAN®
(Fluconazole for Oral Suspension)

ORANGE FLAVORED

10 mg/mL
when reconstituted

Pfizer Roerig
Division of Pfizer Inc, NY, NY 10017

3 N 0049-3440-19 3

* When reconstituted as directed, each teaspoonful (5 mL) contains 50 mg of fluconazole.

Rx only

05-4799-32-3

1222
MADE IN USA

17. FOR ORAL USE ONLY.
Store dry powder below 30°C (86°F).
PROTECT FROM FREEZING.
DOSAGE AND USE
See accompanying prescribing information.
MIXING DIRECTIONS:
Tap bottle to loosen powder.
Add 15 mL of water to the bottle.
After mixing, store suspension at 5° to 30°C (41° to 86°F).
Oversized bottle provides extra space for shaking.
After mixing, use within 10 days.
Discard after full dosing is completed.
SHAKE WELL BEFORE USING.
Contains 1200 mg azithromycin.

NDC 0069-3140-19
1200 mg (30 mL when mixed)

Zithromax®
(azithromycin for oral suspension)

CHERRY FLAVORED

200 mg* per 5 mL

Pfizer Pfizer Labs
Division of Pfizer Inc, NY, NY 10017

www.zithromax.com

N3 0069-3140-19 0

* When constituted as directed, each teaspoonful (5 mL) contains azithromycin dihydrate equivalent to 200 mg of azithromycin.

Rx only

05-5015-32-2

6424
MADE IN USA

18. Store at or below 86°F (30°C).

Dispense in tight containers (USP).

DOSAGE AND USE
See accompanying prescribing information.

*Each tablet contains azithromycin dihydrate equivalent to 600 mg of azithromycin.

NDC 0069-3080-30
30 Tablets   Rx only

Zithromax®
(azithromycin) 600

600 mg*

Pfizer Pfizer Labs
Division of Pfizer Inc, NY, NY 10017

N3 0069-3080-30 4

05-5185-31-2

6440
MADE IN USA

19.

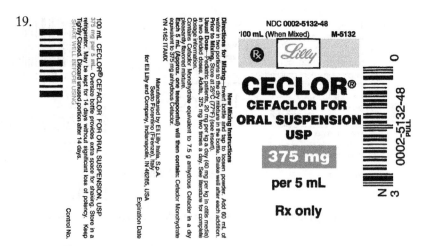

20.

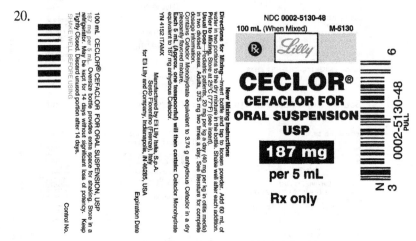

SECTION 4.2 ABBREVIATIONS USED ON PRESCRIPTIONS AND MEDICAL ORDERS

The number of abbreviations used in the medical professions is large and can be confusing. The letters used for an abbreviation may often seem to have nothing to do with the words. The reason for this is that many of the abbreviations are based on medical terms that have their roots in Latin or Greek rather than the English that we speak. You may also see Roman numerals used on prescriptions and medical orders.

Constant efforts are being made to standardize medical abbreviations. The idea is to improve the communication between various caregivers. One such group, *The Joint Commission on Accreditation of Health Care Organizations* (JACHO), has made a list of what they call "dangerous" abbreviations, symbols, and acronyms that are not to be used by any health care group that the organization accredits. The current list is given in Table 4-1 You may still see these abbreviations used out of habit, but they will slowly disappear from common use.

It is likely that other unclear or easily confused abbreviations will be eliminated from use in the future. Various Web sites, such as JACHO.org and drugintel.com, keep up with ongoing changes. Some states and individual health care providers have specified additional prohibited abbreviations and units that they no longer use. Many physicians and other health providers are using computer programs to write prescriptions, and these

Table 4.1 Abbreviations Prohibited by JACHO

Abbreviation or Symbol	Potential Problem	Use Instead
U (unit)	mistaken for the numbers 0 or 4 or cc	write "unit"
IU (International Unit)	mistaken for IV (intravenous) or the number 10	write "International Unit"
Q.D., QD, q.d., qd (daily) Q.O.D., QOD, q.o.d., qod (every other day)	mistaken for each other	write "daily" write "every other day"
trailing zero (X.0 mg)	decimal point is missed	write "X mg" unless the trailing zero is required to show the level of precision
lack of leading zero (.X mg)	decimal point is missed	write "0.X mg"
MS	can mean morphine sulfate or magnesium sulfate	write "morphine sulfate" or "magnesium sulfate"
MSO_4 and $MgSO_4$	confused with one another	write "morphine sulfate" or "magnesium sulfate"

automatically translate the abbreviations and symbols into the word meanings. JACHO has listed additional abbreviations and symbols that will possibly be eliminated in the near future. See Table 4.2.

Even with these abbreviations eliminated, the list of approved abbreviations is still very long. We will not attempt to be exhaustive here, but will attempt to categorize abbreviations into groups with similar meanings, such as drug administration routes, amounts, or other categories (Tables 4.3 through 4.6).

Taken together, ID, IM, IV, and subQ are known as **parenteral** administration routes. They are injections and infusions. There are several other injections routes, including intra-arterial (IA, into an artery), intracardial (IC, into the heart), intraosseous (IO, into bone), and intraspinal (IS, into the spine). These were not included in Table 4.3, as only qualified physicians may use these administration routes.

In writing and reading prescriptions and medical orders, care *must* be taken. Often, a cursory reading of or sloppy writing on a medical order will lead to problems for an innocent patient. Write clearly and proofread what you have written. Read carefully and in detail.

Table 4.2 Additional Abbreviations and Symbols for Possible Future Elimination

Abbreviation or Symbol	Potential Problem	Use Instead
> (greater than) < (less than)	misinterpreted as the number "7" or the lettter "L" and confused with one another	write "greater than;" write "less than"
abbreviations for drug names	misinterpreted due to similar abbreviations for multiple drugs	write drug names in full
apothecary units	unfamiliar to many practitioners and confused with metric units	use metric units
@	mistaken for the number "2"	write "at"
cc	mistaken for U (units) when poorly written	write "mL" or "milliliters"
μg	mistaken for mg (milligrams) resulting in a 1000-fold overdose	write "mcg" or "micrograms"

Table 4.3 Routes of Drug Administration

Abbreviation	Meaning
a.d.	right ear (dexter ear)
a.s.	left ear (sinister ear)
a.u.	both ears
buc. or buccal	inside the cheek
IM	intramuscular, into the muscle
inj.	injection
IV	into a vein
IVP	intravenous push
IVPB	intravenous piggy back
ID	beneath the skin
o.d.	right eye (dexter eye)
o.l. or o.s.	left eye (sinister eye)
o.u. or o_2	both eyes
p.o.	by mouth
R or p.r.	rectal
subL or SL	sublingual, under the tongue
Sub-Q or subQ	into the subcutaneous tissue
top	topically (on the skin)
V or p.v. or vag	vaginal (in the vagina)

Table 4.4 Abbreviations Referring to Time or Frequency of Administration

Abbreviation	Meaning
a.c.	before meals
ad	up to
ad lib	at your pleasure or freely
a.m.	morning
ATC	around the clock
b.i.d.	twice a day
d.	day
disc or D.C.	discontinue
e.m.p.	as directed
h or hr	hour
HS or hs	at bed time (hour of sleep)
noct	night
p.c.	after meals

Table 4.4 Abbreviations Referring to Time or Frequency of Administration (*contd.*)

Abbreviation	Meaning
p.m.	afternoon
p.r.n.	as needed
qh	every hour
q2h, q3h, q4h	every 2, 3, or 4 hours
qid	four times a day
s.o.s.	if there is need
stat	immediately
tid	three times a day
T.I.W.	three times a week

Table 4.5 Abbreviations Related to Amounts

Abbreviation	Meaning
aa	of each
amp	ampule or ampoule
c.	with
cc	cubic centimeter
cap.	capsule
dil.	dilute
div.	divide
g. or GM or g	gram
gr.	grain
gtt.	drop
HS	half strength
mcg or μg	microgram
mg	milligram
mL or ml	milliliter
NMT	not more than
O	pint
qs	a sufficient quantity
qs ad	a sufficient quantity to make
ss	one-half
tsp	teaspoon
T	tablespoon
x	times
w/	with
w/o or s.	without

Table 4.6 Other Commonly Used Medical Abbreviations

Abbreviation	Meaning
aq.	water
ASA	aspirin
BM	bowel movement
BP	blood pressure
BS	blood sugar
BSA	body surface area
CHF	congestive heart failure
comp.	compound
disp.	dispense
DW	distilled water
D5W	dextrose 5% in water
elix.	elixir
et	and
ex aq.	in water
fl or fld.	fluid
H	hypodermic
HA	headache
HBP	high blood pressure
HT	hypertension
M.	mix
N&V	nausea and vomiting
NMT	not more than
non rep. or N.R.	do not repeat
NPO	nothing by mouth
N.S. or NS	normal saline
oint.	ointment
pulv.	powder
R.L. or R/L	Ringer's lactate
SOB	shortness of breath
sol.	solution
sup.	suppository
susp.	suspension
syr.	syrup
tab.	tablet
TPN	total parenteral nutrition
tr.	tincture
ung.	ointment

Table 4.6 Other Commonly Used Medical Abbreviations (*contd.*)

Abbreviation	Meaning
URI	upper respiratory infection
USP	United States Pharmacopedia
UTI	urinary tract infection
VS	vital signs
WBC	white blood cell count

PRACTICE PROBLEM SET 4.2

The following exercises list either an abbreviation on the meaning of an abbreviation. Fill in the blank with either the abbreviation, if a meaning is given, or a meaning, if an abbreviation is given.

#	Abbreviation	Meaning
1	p.o.	
2	IM	
3		rectal
4		sublingual
5	a.c.	
6	p.c.	
7		as needed
8		if there is need
9	mcg	
10	NMT	
11		tincture
12		tablet
13	BSA	
14	ASA	
15		one-half
16		without
17	b.i.d.	
18	IVPB	
19		into a vein
20		on the skin
21	p.v.	
22	ATC	
23	ad lib	
24	stat	
25	q4h	

26. As a group, ID, IV, IM, and sub-Q are known as _____ administrations.

READING AND INTERPRETING PRESCRIPTIONS AND MEDICAL ORDERS

As with the previous sections of this chapter, our goal in this section is not to teach you how to administer drugs. Our goal is to teach you how to read and interpret medical orders and prescriptions. In the first two sections of this chapter, you were shown how to read drug labels and given some information about abbreviations that will be written on prescriptions. Here you will use the information learned to "translate" a drug or medication order into the words and actions necessary to properly administer the medication required.

IMPORTANT:
If you are unsure of what a medical order or prescription says, *ask, never assume!*

THE FIVE "RIGHTS" FOR GIVING MEDICATIONS:
If you are giving a medication to a patient be sure that you give

the right drug

in the right dose

by the right route

at the right time

to the right patient.

A **medical order** (medication order) is a drug order written in a hospital, nursing home, or other such medical facility for an inpatient. A **prescription** (Figure 4-2) is a drug order written in an office or clinic or for a patient being discharged. In most states, only licensed physicians may write medical orders or prescriptions. Some states do allow nurse practitioners, physician assistants, and other certified persons to write such orders.

Not all medical orders and prescriptions follow the same format but they must all contain certain essential information. There are eleven items to note on the prescription in Figure 4.2. We will look at each of these separately.

1. *The patient's full name* (John Vernon Doe) must appear on the prescription. Other information necessary to identify the person for whom the medication is intended may be included as well. In this case, the patient's address and age are also given.

2. *The date* (01/15/2007) on which the prescription was written must be included. Generally, pharmacies will not fill "old" prescriptions.

3. *The drug name* (Acetaminophen) must be given. It may be the generic or manufacturer's name.

Figure 4.2 A Sample Prescription

Phone: (336) 555-5555	DEA# 0000000000

Ima Doctor, M. D.
5555 Physicians Way
Saxapahaw, NC 27249

Patient's Name: John Vernon Doe   Age: 34 Date: 01/15/2007

Address: 2525 East Main Street, Saxapahaw, NC 27249

R$_x$: Acetaminophen 500 mg caplets #30

po q8h X10d. for pain

Refill: 0   X   Generic and/or equivalent allowed

Physician's Signature: Ima Doctor, M.D.

4. *The dosage amount* (500 mg in caplet form) must be given.

5. *The administration route* (po, by mouth) must be given.

6. *The frequency* (q8h, every eight hours) with which the patient is to take the medication.

7. *The duration* (X 10d, enough for days) is the number of days that the patient is to take the medication.

8. *The quantity or amount* (#30, q8h = 3 per day for 10 days = 30 caplets) that the pharmacist is to dispense.

9. *A checkoff blank or box allowing a generic substitute* to be dispensed by the pharmacist in place of a brand-name drug. If a brand name is given and the prescription does not indicate that a generic may be substituted, the pharmacist will dispense the more expensive brand-name drug. Some drugs that are new on the market may not have a generic equivalent available until after some time on the market.

10. *The physician's signature* (Ima Doctor, M.D.) must be on the prescription.

11. *The physician's DEA number* (United States Drug Enforcement Agency registration number) must be on the prescription if the drug prescribed is a controlled substance such as a narcotic.

EXAMPLE 3: Translating a Prescription

A physician writes a prescription as follows: give cephalexin 0.5 g p.o. t.i.d. X10d.

a. Translate the prescription into words.

b. Assuming only 250-mg capsules are available, calculate one dose.

c. How many capsules are needed altogether to fill this prescription?

Solution

a. Give cephalexin (generic name), one-half gram per dose, by mouth, three times a day for ten days.

b. $0.5 \text{ g} = 500 \text{ mg}, \dfrac{500 \text{ mg per dose}}{250 \text{ mg per capsule}} = 2$ capsules for one dose

c. $\left(\dfrac{2 \text{ cap}}{\text{dose}}\right)\left(\dfrac{3 \text{ dose}}{\text{day}}\right) = \dfrac{6 \text{ cap}}{\text{day}}$

$\left(\dfrac{6 \text{ cap}}{\text{day}}\right)(10 \text{ days}) = 60$ capsules are needed to fill the prescription.

EXAMPLE 4: Translating a Prescription

A physician writes a medical order as follows: nitroglyercin gr 1/400 subL prn.

a. Translate the prescription into words.

b. Assuming only 0.3-mg tablets are available, calculate one dose.

c. How many tablets are needed altogether to fill this order?

Solution

a. Give 1/400 grain of nitroglycerin, under the tongue, as needed.

b. $\left(\text{gr}\dfrac{1}{400}\right)\left(\dfrac{60 \text{ mg}}{\text{gr } 1}\right)\left(\dfrac{1 \text{ tablet}}{0.3 \text{ mg}}\right) = \dfrac{1}{2}$ tablet

c. This part cannot be calculated since the physician specified "as needed."

A CAUTION about "prn" orders:

Find out the maximum number of safe dosages per day that may be given to a patient and the number of days that this maximum dosage may be continued. You want to be sure that a patient is not overmedicated by taking too much medication "as needed."

PRACTICE PROBLEM SET 4.3

For each of the following drug orders give (a) the route of administration in words; (b) the number of tablets, capsules, milliliters, etc. necessary for one dose; (c) the number of tablets, capsules, milliliters, etc. per day; and (d) the total number of tablets, capsules, milliliters, etc. necessary altogether. Each problem will give the dosage available per tablet or capsule. Remember, it may not be possible to calculate all of the answers for every problem.

1. Ordered: aspirin gr VI po q4h X 5 d. for pain. Dosage available: 325-mg tablets.
2. Ordered: 300 mcg nitroglycerin subL stat. Dosage available: 0.3-mg scored tablets.
3. Ordered: Celebrex 0.2 g p.o. qd. X 15 d. for pain. Dosage available: 100-mg tablets.
4. Ordered: Heparin 15000 U subQ bid X 4 d. Dosage available: 5-mL multiuse vial supplying 10,000 U per mL.
5. Ordered: Morphine sulfate gr 1/4 IM stat. Dosage available: 15-mg/mL vials.
6. Ordered: Percocet tablet q4h X 7 d.
7. Ordered: Ampicillin 500 mg p.o. qid X 5 d. Dosage available: 250-mg capsules.
8. Ordered: Codeine sulfate gr ss p.o. q4h until further notice. Dosage available: 30-mg tablets.
9. Ordered: Digoxin elix. 20 mcg stat po. Dosage available: 60-mL container labeled 50 mcg/mL.
10. Ordered: Clonidine 0.4 mg p.o. bid X 3 d. Dosage available: 0.1-mg tablets.
11. Ordered: acetaminophen 650 mg p.o. q4h X 5 d. Dosage available: 650-mg tablets.
12. Ordered: Penicillin G 2 million U IM qid X 7 d. Dosage available: 1 million units/vial.
13. Ordered: Meperidine hydrochloride 20 mg IM q4h X 3 d. for pain. Dosage available: 1-mL single-use vials labeled 25 mg/mL.
14. Ordered: Atropine sulfate 200 mcg subQ stat. Dosage available: 20-mL multiuse vial labeled 0.4 mg/mL.
15. Ordered: Tigan 200 mg IM q8h X 4d for nausea. Dosage available: 3-mL single-use vials labeled 100 mg/mL.
16. Ordered: Phenobarbital gr 1/4 p.o. t.i.d. X 3 d. Dosage available: 120-mL elixir labeled 3 mg/mL.
17. Ordered: Lasix 40 mg p.o. q12h X 4d Dosage available: 40-mg scored tablets.
18. Ordered: Dexamethasone 3 mg p.o. q12h X 10 d. Dosage available: 1.5-mg tablets.
19. Ordered: Loratidine 5 mg qd. X 5 d. Dosage available: 1 mg/mL syrup.
20. Ordered: Darvon 1 g p.o. q4h. Dosage available: 100 mg tablets.

SECTION 4.4   SYRINGE CALCULATIONS

A **hypodermic syringe** is a medical instrument that is used to administer sterile liquid medications through the skin. Syringes are used in all of the *parenteral* administration routes discussed in Section 4.2 of this chapter. Figure 4-3 shows the parts of a syringe.

In addition to standard syringes, there are specialized syringes, such as *insulin syringes*, which are marked in USP units; *tuberculin syringes*, which have slim barrels and hold only 1 cc when full; and syringes that are prefilled with exact amounts of medication. The most commonly used syringes are pictured in Figure 4-4.

The syringes labeled A, B, and C are large-capacity syringes that are used to add medications to IV infusions. Syringe A is a 20-cc (mL) syringe calibrated in whole cc's (mL's) (1.0 cc or 1.0 mL per mark). Syringe B is a 10-cc (mL) syringe calibrated in fifths of a cc

Figure 4.3 Syringe Parts and Calibration Marks

Source: From *Medical Dosage Calculations,* 8th ed., by Olsen, Giangrasso, and Shrimpton; published by Prentice Hall Health, ISBN# 0-13-113479-5.

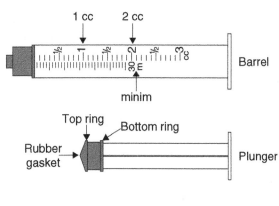

Figure 4.4 Commonly Used Syringes

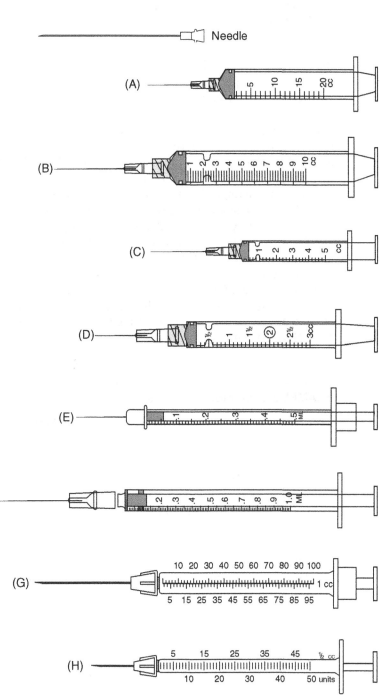

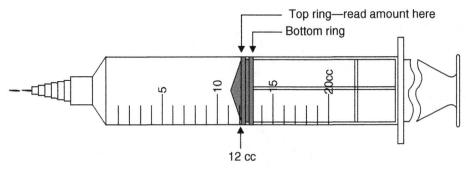

Figure 4.5 Filling a Syringe

Source: From *Medical Dosage Calculations,* 8th ed., by Olsen, Giangrasso, and Shrimpton; published by Prentice Hall Health, ISBN# 0-13-113479-5.

(0.2 cc or 0.2 mL per mark). Syringe C is a 5-cc (mL) syringe calibrated in tenths of a cc (0.1 cc or 0.1 mL per mark).

Syringes D through H are used in parenteral injections. Syringe D is a 3-cc (mL) syringe calibrated in tenths of a cc (0.1 cc or 0.1 mL). Syringe E is a $\frac{1}{2}$-cc syringe. It is numbered in tenths of a cc and each mark is one-hundredth of a cc (0.01 cc or 0.01 mL per mark). Syringe F is a tuberculin syringe with a 1-cc (mL) capacity and is calibrated in hundredths of a cc (0.01 cc or 0.01 mL). Syringe G is a U-100 insulin syringe and is to be used for injecting insulin only. It has a capacity of 1.0 cc (mL) and is calibrated in units of 100 units/mL. Syringe H is a U-100 Lo-Dose insulin syringe with a capacity of $\frac{1}{2}$ cc (mL). It is calibrated in units. There are also 30-units Lo-Dose syringes available. Like syringe G, Lo-Dose insulin syringes should only be used for injections of insulin.

Syringes come in many capacities and are marked in milliliters, mL, or cubic centimeters, cc, minums, m, or units (1 unit = 0.01 cc = 0.01 mL). Often, two scales will be printed on the same syringe. Commons sizes are 1 cc or 1 mL (remember: 1 cc = 1 mL), 3 cc, 5 cc, . . . , up to 100 cc. When filling a syringe, you should draw the liquid into the syringe so that the top ring of the rubber gasket on the plunger aligns with the bottom of the desired amount marked on the barrel of the syringe. Figure 4-5 shows a 20-cc (20-mL) syringe filled to the 12-cc (12-mL) mark.

EXAMPLE 5: Syringe Markings

How much does each line on the syringe pictured here represent? What amount of liquid is in the syringe?

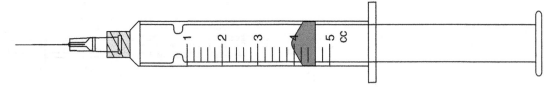

Solution

This is a 5-cc syringe. If you count marks starting at, say, the 2-cc mark and ending at the 3-cc mark, there are 5 divisions:

$$\frac{1 \text{ cc}}{5 \text{ marks}} = 0.2 \text{ cc per mark}$$

The syringe contains 4.2 cc.

If you examine the different types of syringes closely, it is easy to see that they are not all calibrated the same as the one in Example 5. Common calibrations are whole cc's (1 cc per mark), fifths of a cc (0.2 cc per mark), tenths of a cc (0.1 cc per mark), and hundredths of a cc (0.01 cc per mark). If you calculate the amount of a drug that needs to be injected, you need to round your answer so that it corresponds to the calibration marks of the syringe to be used to administer the injection.

EXAMPLE 6: Rounding Based on Syringe Calibration Marks

A dosage amount is calculated to be 1.45 mL. If you were to use a standard 3-cc syringe as shown in Figure 4-4, how should the dosage be rounded, if at all?

Solution

If you read the marking on the 3-cc syringe carefully, you will see that it is calibrated in tenths of a cc (0.1 cc per mark). This means that your dosage amount needs to be rounded to the nearest tenth of a cc. (Remember: 1 cc = 1 mL.) Thus, 1.45 mL should be rounded to 1.5 mL (1.5 cc).

EXAMPLE 7: Rounding Based on Syringe Calibration Marks

A nurse has chosen a tuberculin syringe to give an injection. Her calculations yield a dosage of 0.738 mL. To what place should she round her answer?

Tuberculin syringes are calibrated in hundredths of a mL (0.01 mL), so round to the nearest hundredth: 0.738 mL = 0.74 mL.

Just as there are different-size syringes for different purposes, there are also different size **needles** to choose from. Which size needle to use is determined by a number of factors, such as the administration route, the site of administration, the size and age of a patient, the viscosity ("thickness" or "stickiness") of the medication itself, and other factors. As this is only an introductory look at syringes, we will not go into a great deal of detail about choosing the proper needle size in this book.

The diameter of the hollow metal tube that is the needle is called its *gauge*. Gauges run from 14, which is a large-diameter needle, to 27, which is a small-diameter needle. Lengths of needles are usually in the range of $\frac{3}{8}$ in. up to 2 in. In general, the longer the needle, the larger the gauge.

PRACTICE PROBLEM SET 4.4

Refer back to Figure 4.4 to answer these questions.

True or False:
1. You may use a tuberculin syringe to give 1.1 mL of medication.
2. 100 U of insulin may be measured in a tuberculin syringe.
3. The larger the diameter of a needle, the higher its gauge number.
4. Longer needles have higher gauge numbers.
5. A 3-cc syringe may be used to give precisely 1.55 mL of medication.

Indicate which type and size of syringe should be used to make each of the following injections, and give the properly rounded amount that should be administered.

6. A dosage calculation yields 11.225 mL of a medication to be administered through an IV drip of D5W.
7. A nurse needs to inject 0.825 mL, subQ.

8. A nurse needs to inject 5.64 mL into a 1-L bag of RL.
9. An injection is to be given IM and the calculated amount is 1.6333 . . . mL.
10. An injection is to be given IM and the calculated amount is 2.575 mL.

In each of the following problems, a doctor has prescribed an injection and the available drug concentration and amounts are given. You are to decide which type of syringe would be appropriate to use, round the prescribed dosage accordingly, and give both the type of syringe and actual amount that will be administered.

11. Give 200 mg IM of a drug that is 165 mg/mL.
12. Give 200,000 U IM of a drug that is 400,000 U/mL.
13. Add 450 mg to a 100-mL IVPB. The drug concentration is 40 mg/mL.
14. Give 500,000 U of penicillin from a supply that is 300,000 U/mL.
15. Give 30 mg IM from a supply that is 25 mg/mL.

Chapter Summary

In this chapter you have been given a brief overview of several areas related to the administration of medications. All of these areas are very important to the patients that you may serve in any number of allied health professions. Please understand that this is not a comprehensive treatment and more study and training on your part will be necessary before you can truly apply any of this information in a true clinical situation.

Important Terms

generic name

hypodermic syringe

medical order

parenteral

prescription

trade name

USP (United States Phermacopedia)

Important Cautions and Warnings

1. BE CAUTIOUS ABOUT DRUG NAMES

2. NEVER GIVE AN EXPIRED DRUG TO A PATIENT

3. DO NOT BREAK TABLETS INTO HALVES OR QUARTERS UNLESS THEY ARE SCORED FOR THAT PURPOSE

4. READ ALL MEDICAL ORDERS OR PRESCRIPTIONS VERY CAREFULLY

The Five RIGHTS for Giving Medications:

1. the Right Drug
2. in the Right Dose
3. by the Right Route
4. at the Right Time
5. to the Right Patient

Chapter Review Problems

Read each of the following labels carefully and supply the required information for each one: (a) the manufacturer's name, (b) the brand name of the drug, (c) the generic name of the drug, (d) the administration route that should be used with the drug, (e) the total amount of medication (mL, number of capsules, etc.) in an unopened container, and (f) the amount of drug per tablet, mL, etc.

1.

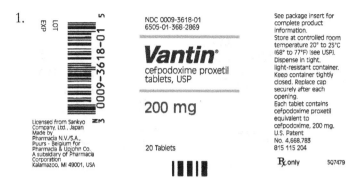

NDC 0009-3618-01
6505-01-368-2869

Vantin®

cefpodoxime proxetil
tablets, USP

200 mg

20 Tablets

LOT
EXP

Licensed from Sankyo
Company, Ltd., Japan
Made by
Pharmacia N.V./S.A.,
Puurs - Belgium for
Pharmacia & Upjohn Co.
A subsidiary of Pharmacia
Corporation
Kalamazoo, MI 49001, USA

See package insert for
complete product
information.
Store at controlled room
temperature 20° to 25°C
(68° to 77°F) [see USP].
Dispense in tight,
light-resistant container.
Keep container tightly
closed. Replace cap
securely after each
opening.
Each tablet contains
cefpodoxime proxetil
equivalent to
cefpodoxime, 200 mg.
U.S. Patent
No. 4,668,783
815 115 204

℞ only   5Q7479

2.

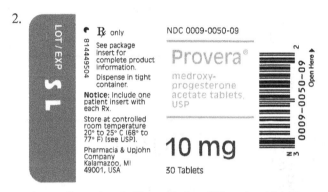

℞ only
See package
insert for
complete product
information.
Dispense in tight
container.
Notice: Include one
patient insert with
each Rx.

Store at controlled
room temperature
20° to 25° C (68° to
77° F) [see USP].

Pharmacia & Upjohn
Company
Kalamazoo, MI
49001, USA

LOT / EXP

81444950-4

NDC 0009-0050-09

Provera®

medroxy-
progesterone
acetate tablets,
USP

10 mg

30 Tablets

3.

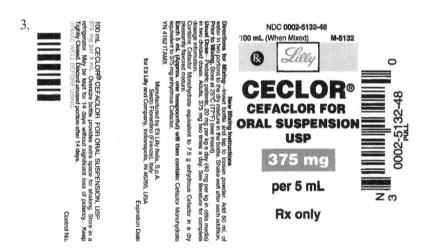

NDC 0002-5132-48
100 mL (When Mixed)   M-5132

℞   *Lilly*

CECLOR®
CEFACLOR FOR
ORAL SUSPENSION
USP

375 mg

per 5 mL

Rx only

4.

℞ only

See package insert for
complete product
information.

Store at 25°C (77°F);
excursions permitted
to 15°-30°C (59°-86°F)
[see USP Controlled
Room Temperature].

Protect from light.

U.S. Patent No. 5,382,600

NDC 0009-5190-02

Detrol®LA

tolterodine tartrate
extended release
capsules

2 mg

90 Capsules   **PHARMACIA**

Manufactured for
Pharmacia & Upjohn
Company
A subsidiary of
Pharmacia Corporation
Kalamazoo, MI
49001, USA

By
International Processing
Corporation
Winchester, Kentucky
40391, USA

818261001

LOT
EXP   **S L**

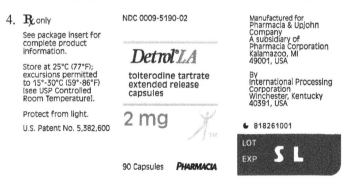

Medication Labels, Prescriptions, and Syringe Calculations

5.

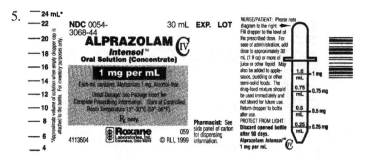

Source: Label © Roxane Laboratories. Used with permission.

6.

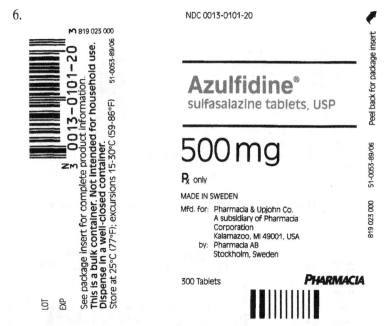

Source: Reproduced with permission of Pfizer, Inc. All rights reserved.

The following exercises list either an abbreviation or the meaning of an abbreviation. Fill in the blank with either the abbreviation, if a meaning is given, or a meaning, if an abbreviation is given.

#	Abbreviation	Meaning
7		by mouth
8		nothing by mouth
9	cap.	
10	susp.	
11	t.i.w.	
12		every 8 hours
13		if needed
14	p.v.	

For each of the following drug orders, give (a) the route of administration in words, (b) the number of tablets, capsules, milliliters, etc. necessary for one dose, (c) the number of tablets, capsules, milliliters, etc. per day, and (d) the total number of tablets, capsules, milliliters, etc. necessary altogether. Each problem will give the dosage available per tablet or capsule. Remember, it may not be possible to calculate all of the answers for every problem.

15. Ordered: aspirin gr IV po q4h X 3 d. for pain. Dosage available: 81-mg chewable tablets.

16. Ordered: 400 mcg nitroglycerin subL stat. Dosage available: 0.4-mg scored tablets.

17. Ordered: Keflex 25 mg p.o. q6h X 10 d. Dosage available: 125 mg/5-mL powder for oral suspension.

18. Ordered: Heparin 20000 U subQ bid X 2 d. Dosage available: 5-mL multiuse vial supplying 10,000 U per mL.

19. Ordered: Morphine sulfate gr 1/2 IM stat. Dosage available: 15-mg/mL vials.

Indicate which type and size of syringe should be used to make each of the following injections, and give the properly rounded amount that should be administered.

20. A dosage calculation yields 11.375 mL of a medication to be administered through an IV drip of D5W.

21. A nurse needs to inject 0.500 mL, subQ.

22. A nurse needs to inject 4.25 mL into a 1-L bag of RL.

23. An injection is to be given IM and the calculated amount is 1.3333. . . mL.

Chapter Test

Read each of the following labels carefully and supply the required information for each one: (a) the manufacturer's name, (b) the brand name of the drug, (c) the generic name of the drug, (d) the administration route that should be used with the drug, (e) the total amount of medication (mL, number of capsules, etc.) in an unopened container, and (f) the amount of drug per tablet, mL, etc.

1.
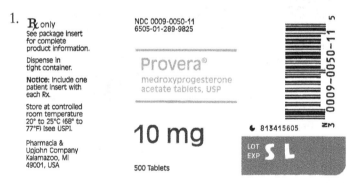

Source: Reproduced with permission of Pfizer, Inc. All rights reserved.

2.
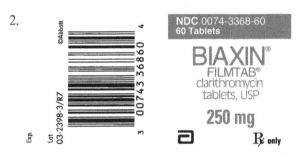

Source: Label © Abbott Laboratories. Used with permission.

3.

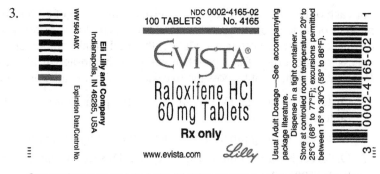

4.

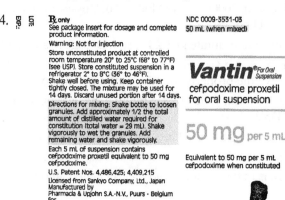

Rx only
See package insert for dosage and complete product information.

Warning: Not for injection

Store unconstituted product at controlled room temperature 20° to 25°C (68° to 77°F) (see USP). Store constituted suspension in a refrigerator 2° to 8°C (36° to 46°F). Shake well before using. Keep container tightly closed. The mixture may be used for 14 days. Discard unused portion after 14 days.

Directions for mixing: Shake bottle to loosen granules. Add approximately 1/2 the total amount of distilled water required for constitution (total water = 29 mL). Shake vigorously to wet the granules. Add remaining water and shake vigorously.

Each 5 mL of suspension contains cefpodoxime proxetil equivalent to 50 mg cefpodoxime.

U.S. Patent Nos. 4,486,425; 4,409,215
Licensed from Sankyo Company, Ltd., Japan
Manufactured by
Pharmacia & Upjohn S.A.-N.V., Puurs - Belgium
for
Pharmacia & Upjohn Company
Kalamazoo, MI 49001, USA
817 152 101
5Q5355

NDC 0009-3531-03
50 mL (when mixed)

Vantin For Oral Suspension
cefpodoxime proxetil
for oral suspension

50 mg per 5 mL

Equivalent to 50 mg per 5 mL cefpodoxime when constituted

Pharmacia
&Upjohn

5.

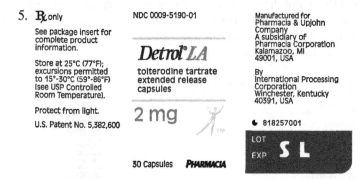

Rx only

See package insert for complete product information.

Store at 25°C (77°F); excursions permitted to 15°-30°C (59°-86°F) (see USP Controlled Room Temperature).

Protect from light.

U.S. Patent No. 5,382,600

NDC 0009-5190-01

Detrol LA
tolterodine tartrate
extended release
capsules

2 mg

30 Capsules **PHARMACIA**

Manufactured for
Pharmacia & Upjohn
Company
A subsidiary of
Pharmacia Corporation
Kalamazoo, MI
49001, USA

By
International Processing
Corporation
Winchester, Kentucky
40391, USA

818257001

LOT
EXP **S L**

The following exercises list either an abbreviation or the meaning of an abbreviation. Fill in the blank with either the abbreviation, if a meaning is given, or a meaning, if an abbreviation is given.

#	Abbreviation	Meaning
6	aq.	
7	IVPB	
8	subQ	
9	ss	
10		drop
11		beneath the skin
12		before meals
13		Immediately

For each of the following drug orders give (a) the route of administration in words, (b) the number of tablets, capsules, milliliters, etc. necessary for one dose, (c) the number of tablets, capsules, milliliters, etc. per day, and (d) the total number of tablets, capsules, milliliters, etc. necessary altogether. Each problem will give the dosage available per tablet or capsule. Remember, it may not be possible to calculate all of the answers for every problem.

14. Ordered: Ampicillin 500 mg p.o. qid X 10 d. Dosage available: 250-mg capsules.

15. Ordered: Codeine sulfate gr 1 p.o. q4h until further notice. Dosage available: 30-mg tablets.

16. Ordered: Digoxin elix. 150 mcg stat p.o. Dosage available: 60-mL container labeled 50 mcg/mL.

17. Ordered: Clonidine 0.2 mg p.o. bid X 3 d. Dosage available: 0.1-mg tablets.

Indicate which type and size of syringe should be used to make each of the following injections, and give the properly rounded amount that should be administered.

18. Give 250 mg IM of a drug that is 165 mg/mL.

19. Give 100,000 U IM of a drug that is 400,000 U/mL.

20. Add 300 mg to a 100-mL IVPB. The drug concentration is 40 mg/mL.

21. Give 250,000 U of penicillin from a supply that is 300,000 U/mL.

22. Give 20 mg IM from a supply that is 25 mg/mL.

5

MODELING HEALTH APPLICATIONS WITH RATIOS AND PROPORTIONS

Objectives for Chapter 5

After completing this chapter the student should:

1. Have a basic knowledge of the uses of ratios and proportions in several common areas of allied health careers.

2. Be able to understand and manipulate formulas that are in the form of proportions.

3. Have a deeper knowledge of how to approach word problems and similar problems in the world of work.

4. Understand the basic terminology used in the health areas discussed.

SECTION 5.1   INTRODUCTION

In Chapter 2 you reviewed ratios and methods for solving proportions. Recall that a **ratio** is an amount of one thing relative to another—a comparison of two values. The label on the drug Ceclor states it contains 375 mg per 5 mL. This is a ratio of the amount of drug present per amount of solution. **Proportions** are equal ratios and allow us to adjust amounts or volumes without changing the prescribed ratio. For example, if a patient requires 375 mg of Ceclor, he should be given 5 mL. However, if he requires 750 mg of the drug, he should be given twice as much, or 10 mL. Adjustments such as these can be easily done with proportions using the **cross-multiplication property**.

Cross-Multiplication Property

To solve a proportion, we use the property of proportions that states

The cross products of any true proportion are equal.

If $\dfrac{a}{b} = \dfrac{c}{d}$, then $ad = bc$, where $b \neq 0$ and $d \neq 0$.

In this section of the book, you will apply these techniques to the solution of a variety of problems in the allied health field. This is not intended to be an exhaustive presentation of all possible areas of use, but simply an introduction to real-world applications of ratios and proportion in the health care profession.

This chapter is written so that each section is independent of the others and, at your instructor's choice, you can omit whole sections without getting lost or missing explanations of any mathematical techniques. For example, you can cover Sections 5.2 and 5.5 only and not get confused or need any information from the other sections of the chapter in order to successfully complete your work.

SECTION 5.2 RATIOS AND PROPORTIONS IN DOSAGE CALCULATIONS

In giving medications to patients, it is often left to the nurse, certified medical assistant, or other properly trained personnel to get the medication and administer the amount prescribed by the physician. This is an important task and care needs to be taken to ensure that proper dosages are given. Either overmedication or undermedication may have severe consequences for the patient. In other, more specific courses you will learn how to administer medications and the terminology that is used there. As you have seen in Chapter 4, abbreviations are often used. For example, in addition to giving medications by mouth (orally or p.o.), you may also give medications IM (intramuscularly), IV (intravenously), or SC (subcutaneously). The method used varies with the medication to be given. You may see some of these abbreviations in problems here, but they are not an important part of the calculations required in this section.

When a physician orders a medication to be given in his office, he will generally prescribe the amount of a particular drug for the nurse or assistant to give. The nurse will then go to the medical storage area to get the medication and measure out enough to match the dosage prescribed.

Look at Example 1 to see a situation that will require us to use a proportion to determine how much of a stock medication should be given.

EXAMPLE 1: Using a Proportion to Calculate a Dosage Amount

A physician orders you, the nurse, to give 300,000 units of penicillin IM to a particular patient. You go to the medical storage area and find a supply of penicillin. The label on the stock supply reads 400,000 units per mL. What amount, in mL, should you give the patient?

Solution

The stock supply label is really a ratio that compares the amount of penicillin per volume of liquid in the container, in this case:

$$\frac{400,000 \text{ units pencillin}}{1 \text{ mL}}$$

If we set up a second ratio comparing the dosage we wish to give with the amount that we should give the patient, we have the following ratio:

$$\frac{300,000 \text{ units pencillin}}{x}$$

Now we can set up a proportion using these two ratios and solve for the volume of the stock supply of penicillin that we need to give the patient using the cross-multiplication property:

$$\frac{400,000 \text{ units pencillin}}{1 \text{ mL}} = \frac{300,000 \text{ units pencillin}}{x} \qquad \text{Set up a proportion.}$$

$$(400,000 \text{ units})(x) = (300,000 \text{ units})(1 \text{ mL}). \qquad \text{Cross-multiply.}$$

$$\frac{400,000 \text{ units}(x)}{400,000 \text{ units}} = \frac{300,000 \text{ units}(1 \text{ mL})}{400,000 \text{ units}} \qquad \begin{array}{l}\text{Use the Division} \\ \text{Property of Equality.}\end{array}$$

$$x = 0.75 \text{ mL} \qquad \text{Simplify.}$$

This indicates that if you carefully measure out 0.75 mL of the stock solution, it will contain 300,000 units of penicillin.

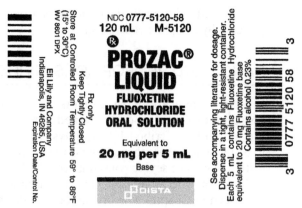

Figure 5.1 Label for Prozac Liquid

Using our knowledge of proportions, we can create a formula to help us calculate correct dosages using stock medications. The parts of the dosage formula that are called "stock" are amounts read from the label of the medication that is on the shelf. For example, look at the drug label for Prozac Liquid shown in Figure 5.1. The ratio stated on the label, 20 mg per 5 mL, represents the given ratio, or "stock" amount, for this medication. The numerator of the second ratio is the prescribed amount of medication that the doctor wants to have administered to the patient. The denominator of the second ratio is the volume or weight of the stock that should be measured and administered to the patient in order to ensure the prescribed amount of medication is given. Remember that the units in both the numerator and denominator should be alike when setting up a proportion.

A Basic Dosage Calculation Formula

$$\frac{\text{Amount of "drug" in the stock}}{\text{Per volume or weight}} = \frac{\text{Amount of "drug" prescribed}}{\text{Volume or weight of stock needed}}$$

Look at the use of this formula in the next few examples.

EXAMPLE 2: Using the Basic Dosage Formula

You are asked to administer 250 mg of Ceclor® orally to a patient with a urinary tract infection. In the drug cabinet you find a 150-mL bottle of Ceclor® labeled 125 mg/5 mL Suspension. How much of the stock supply should you measure out and give to the patient? Give your answer in milliliters and in teaspoons.

Solution

The labeled medication states that there are 125 mg of medication in every 5 mL of suspension (solution). Set up the two ratios using our formula in order to determine the number of milliliters of the suspension that should be administered in order for the patient to receive 250 mg of medication.

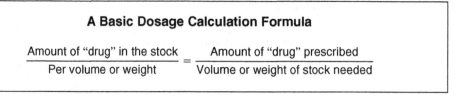

$$\frac{125\,mg}{5\,mL} = \frac{250\,mg}{x}$$ Substitute the values that are known.

$$(125\,mg)(x) = (5\,mL)\,(250\,mg)$$ Cross-multiply.

$$x = \frac{(5\,mL)(250\,\cancel{mg})}{125\,\cancel{mg}}$$ Use the Division Property of Equality.

$$x = 10\ mL$$ Simplify.

The patient should be given 10 mL of Ceclor®. We know from our earlier work with conversions that t = 5 mL. Therefore, this patient should be given 2 t of medication.

EXAMPLE 3: Calculating Dosages from Medication Labels

You are asked to administer 200 mg of fluconazole orally to a patient. In the drug cabinet you find a stock solution of fluconazole with the label pictured here. How much of the stock supply should you measure out and give to the patient?

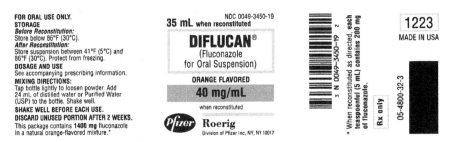

Solution

Carefully read the label. You can see that it indicates that there are 40 mg of fluconazole in each milliliter of the contents of this supply.

$$\frac{\text{Amount of "drug" in the stock}}{\text{Per volume or weight}} = \frac{\text{Amount of "drug" prescribed}}{\text{Volume or weight of stock needed}}$$

$$\frac{40\ mg}{1\,mL} = \frac{200\ mg}{x}$$ Substitute the values that are known.

$$(40\ mg)(x) = (200\ mg)(1\ mL)$$ Cross-multiply.

$$x = \frac{(200\,\cancel{mg}\,)(1\ mL)}{40\,\cancel{mg}}$$ Use the Division Property of Equality.

$$x = 5\ mL$$ Simplify.

Thus, to give the prescribed 200 mg of fluconazole, you should administer 5 mL (or 1 t) of the stock solution. (Recall that 5 mL = 1 t.)

EXAMPLE 4: Tablet Dosages

A physician has ordered that a patient be given 1.5 g of sulfasalazine. The hospital pharmacy has the medication in tablet form as shown on the following label. How many tablets should the patient be given?

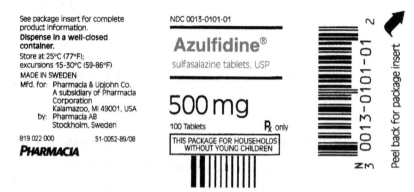

Solution

Carefully read the label. You will notice that the ordered amount and the available tablets are given in two different units. Using the decimal bumping procedure from Chapter 3, convert 1.5 g to milligrams by moving the decimal point 3 places to the right. 1.5 g = 1500 mg. Now set up the two ratios, cross-multiply, and solve as follows:

$$\frac{\text{Amount of ``drug'' in the stock}}{\text{Per volume or weight}} = \frac{\text{Amount of ``drug'' prescribed}}{\text{Volume or weight of stock needed}}$$

$$\frac{500 \text{ mg}}{1 \text{ tab}} = \frac{1500 \text{ mg}}{x} \qquad \text{Substitute the values that are known.}$$

$$(500 \text{ mg})(x) = (1 \text{ tab})(1500 \text{ mg}) \qquad \text{Cross-multiply.}$$

$$x = \frac{(1 \text{ tab})(1500 \text{ mg})}{500 \text{ mg}}. \qquad \text{Use the Division Property of Equality.}$$

$$x = 3 \text{ tablets} \qquad \text{Simplify.}$$

Some Basic Rules Regarding Tablets

Unless a **tablet** is scored properly, do not break it into halves or quarters. Tablets that are unscored may be broken, but you should never assume that you can do this without first referring to the literature that accompanies the medicine, checking with the pharmacy, or seeing it clearly stated on the product label. Many tablet labels have a warning that states: "Do not break or crush." However, even if the label does not say this, do not break the pills unless the literature says that you may do so.

Some tablets are coated (**enteric**) so that they will survive stomach acids for a time and be absorbed through the intestines. Other tablets are formulated to dissolve slowly (timed-release, slow-release, or sustained-release tablets) and thus be absorbed over a long time period. If one of these types of tablets is broken or crushed and then taken by a patient, it may be ineffective or even dangerous for the patient.

In general, the fewer the number of tablets that can be given to obtain the correct dosage, the better it will be for the patient. One reason for this is that many patients have trouble swallowing tablets and other oral medications. For example, one 100-mg tablet is better than two 50-mg tablets if the higher-dosage tablet is available from the pharmacy.

Dosages Based on Body Weight

Body weight is an important factor in dosages of medication for both adults and children. Some medication labels specify the amount of medication to be administered per pound or per kilogram of weight. That is one reason that you are always required to be weighed when you visit the doctor! Individual dosages may be calculated in mg or mcg per lb or kg, per day. Then, the total daily dosage may be divided into several doses to be administered throughout the day. For example, if the order says q.6.h, that indicates 4 doses per day; or if it says t.i.d., that indicates 3 doses per day. Because body weight is extremely important for infant dosages, measurements are usually done in kilograms (kg). Adult weights may be recorded as pounds (lb) or kilograms (kg) and can be converted as necessary.

Ratios and proportions can be used to calculate medication based on body weight. Look at the following example of calculating the correct dosage of medication for a child.

EXAMPLE 5: Calculating Dosages Based on Body Weight

A doctor prescribed ampicillin for a child who weighs 9.1 kg. The label on the box recommends a dosage of 100 mg/kg/day.

    a. Calculate the correct daily amount of ampicillin that the child should receive.

    b. If the label states that there are 250 mg of ampicillin per 5 mL of liquid, how many milliliters should this child be given daily?

Solution

    a. Using a ratio, we know that the recommended dosage is

$$\frac{100 \text{ mg}}{1 \text{ kg}}$$

$$\frac{100 \text{ mg}}{1 \text{ kg}} = \frac{x}{9.1 \text{ kg}}$$ Set up a proportion using the child's weight to determine the correct dosage.

$$(100 \text{ mg})(9.1 \text{ kg}) = x(1 \text{ kg})$$ Cross-multiply.

$$\frac{(100 \text{ mg})(9.1 \text{ kg})}{1 \text{ kg}} = x$$ Use the Division Property of Equality.

$$910 \text{ mg} = x$$ Simplify.

Thus, this child should receive 910 mg of ampicillin daily.

    b. To determine the number of milliliters of stock medication that should be administered, we will use another proportion. The dosage strength stated on the label is

$$\frac{250 \text{ mg}}{5 \text{ mL}}$$

$$\frac{250 \text{ mg}}{5 \text{ mL}} = \frac{910 \text{ mg}}{x}$$ Using the dosage amount just calculated, set up a proportion to find our answer.

$$(250 \text{ mg})x = (910 \text{ mg})(5 \text{ mL})$$ Cross-multiply.

$$x = \frac{(910 \text{ mg})(5 \text{ mL})}{250 \text{ mg}}$$ Use the Division Property of Equality.

$$x = 18.2 \text{ mL}$$ Simplify.

Therefore, this 9.1-kg child should be given approximately 18 mL of the stock medication daily in order to receive the correct dosage of 910 mg of ampicillin daily. If divided into 3 doses per day, the child would be given 6 mL per dose.

EXAMPLE 6: Calculating a Safe Dosage Range

A child weighs 18.5 kg and is prescribed medication with a dosage of 125 mg q8h. The label on the box recommends a daily dosage of 10–20 mg/kg/day, and the strength of the medication is listed as 125 mg per 5 mL. Is the prescribed dosage safe for this child?

Solution

First calculate the minimum and maximum dosages for a child weighing 18.5 kg. We will use the dimensional analysis method instead of proportions for this example.

Minimum: **Maximum:**

$$18.5 \text{ kg} \times \frac{10 \text{ mg}}{\text{kg}} = 185 \text{ mg/day} \qquad 18.5 \text{ kg} \times \frac{20 \text{ mg}}{\text{kg}} = 370 \text{ mg/day}$$

The order for 125 mg q8h results in a daily dosage of 125 mg × 3 times a day = 375 mg/day. Although this is slightly over the maximum recommended daily dosage, the difference of 5 mg between the ordered dosage and recommended dosage is small. The doctor has probably ordered it due to the 125 mg/5 mL strength of the drug. This results in an easy dosage of 5 mL (or 1 t) 3 times a day.

Note that discrepancies in drug dosages are much more critical if the required dosages are small amounts. For example, the difference between 2 mg and 5 mg is probably much more significant that the difference between 122 mg and 125 mg. It is also true that very young patients and geriatric patients are more easily affected by discrepancies in dosages. Other factors that may be critical include weight, especially low body weight, and the medical condition of the patient. If you are in doubt about the accuracy of a dosage that has been ordered, you should call the physician to verify the order, especially for a high-risk patient.

PRACTICE PROBLEM SET 5.2

Find the appropriate label for the medication prescribed in Problems 1–30, and use the information on the label to answer the questions.

1. A doctor orders that a child be given 75 mg q12h of cefpodoxime proxetil. How many milliliters should be given in each dose?
2. You are to give a patient 10 mg of liquid Prozac. How many milliliters should you give the patient?

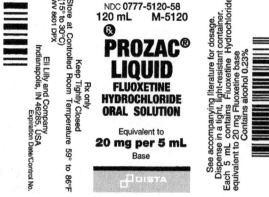

Source: Reproduced with permission of Pfizer, Inc. All rights reserved.

Source: Copyright Eli Lilly & Co. All rights reserved. Used with permission.

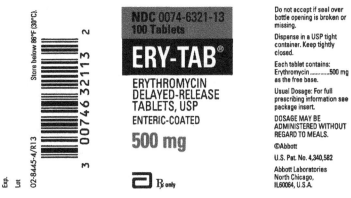

Source: Label © Abbott Laboratories. Used with permission.

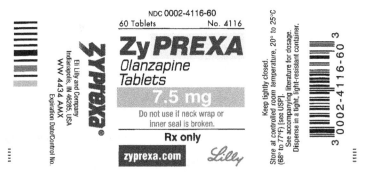

Source: Copyright Eli Lilly & Co. All rights reserved. Used with permission.

3. A physician orders 1500 mg of erythromycin for a patient. How many tablets should be given if the following label represents the only available supply of this drug? Should these tablets be split or crushed? Why or why not?

4. How many tablets of ZyPrexa® should you give in order to fill an order for 15 mg?

5. How many grams of medication are in three Zithromax tablets?

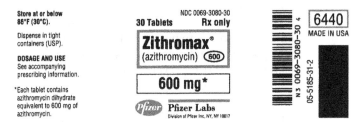

Source: Reproduced with permission of Pfizer, Inc. All rights reserved.

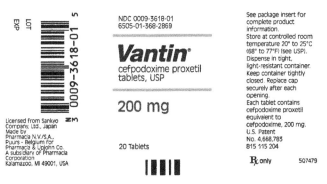

Source: Reproduced with permission of Pfizer, Inc. All rights reserved.

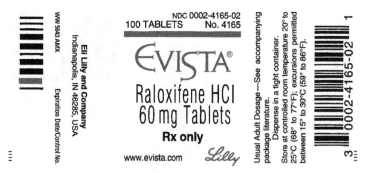

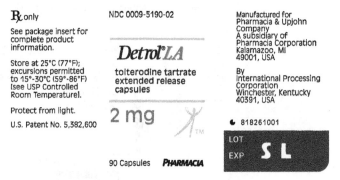

6. How many grams of medication are in four Vantin tablets?
7. How many raloxifene HCL tablets need to be given so that the patient gets a dose of 0.06 g?
8. How many capsules of Detrol LA® should be taken if the order is for 1 daily dose of 4 mg?
9. The prescribed dosage of medroxyprogesterone is 10 mg daily for 5 days. How many tablets should the patient take per day?
10. A patient is prescribed a daily dose of 0.4 g of Vantin® for acute maxillary sinusitis. If this daily dose is to be divided into 2 doses (1 every 12 hours), how many tablets will the patient take during one day? How many will he take for each individual dose?
11. An order for 0.4 g acyclovir per dose is prescribed for a patient with shingles. How many milliliters of this medication should the patient take per dose?
12. A patient is prescribed a dose of 0.5 mg of alprazolam, 3 times daily. How many milliliters per day should he take? How many milliliters per dose?

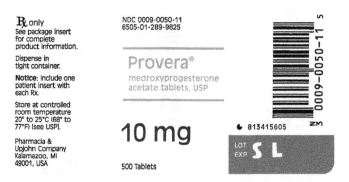

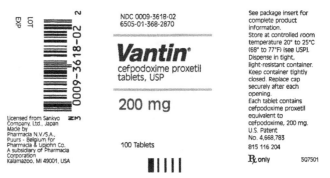

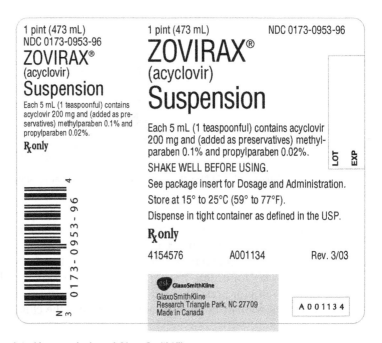

13. How many caplets of tolterodine tartrate should a patient take if a dosage of 2 mg is prescribed?
14. How many tablets of Mavik® are necessary for a dosage of 2 mg?
15. How many milliliters of diazepam will be needed daily for a patient who has been prescribed a dose of 10 mg, 3 times a day?
16. If a pediatric patient is given a dose of 2.5 mL of Prozac®, how many milligrams of medication were given in that dose?

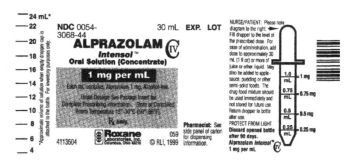

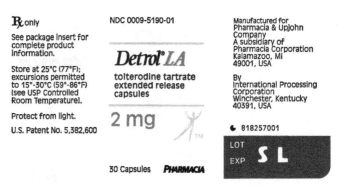

Source: Reproduced with permission of Pfizer, Inc. All rights reserved.

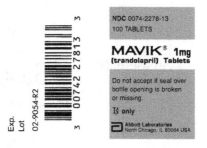

Source: Label © Abbott Laboratories. Used with permission.

17. A 50-lb child is prescribed Zithromax for pneumonia with an intial dose of 200 mg on day 1 followed by 100 mg once a day for days 2–5. How many milliliters of medication will be needed for the initial dose and then for the last 4 doses?
18. A doctor orders 150 mg fluconazole for a patient. How many milliliters are needed?
19. A doctor prescribes a dose of 1 t of Ceclor® twice daily for a child with otitis media. How many milligrams of medication is the child receiving in each dose?

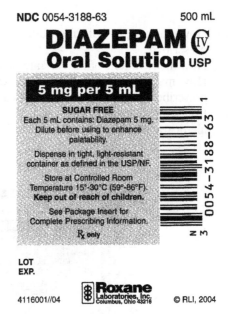

Source: Label © Roxane Laboratories. Used with permission.

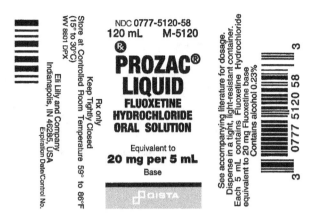

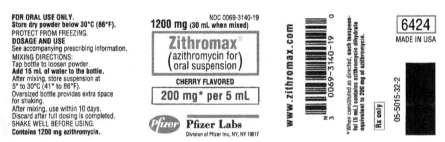

20. A doctor prescribes a dose of $\frac{1}{2}$ teaspoon of Ceclor® twice daily for a small child with pharyngitis. How many milligrams of medication is the child receiving in each dose?

21. How many tablets are needed to give a dose of 10 mg of olanzapine? Assume that you may split the tablets if necessary.

22. How many tablets are needed to give a dose of 0.5 g of clarithromycin?

23. If you were to give 1 t of cefpodoxime proxetil to a patient, what is the dose in milligrams?

24. To give a dose of 400 mg of azithromycin, how many teaspoons would you give?

25. If you inject 10 mL of lymphocyte immune globulin into a patient's IV, what dose of medication will she receive?

26. For chickenpox, an adult patient is prescribed 800 mg of acyclovir 4 times daily for 5 days. How many teaspoons of medication should be taken for a single dose?

27. If 3 mL of diazepam is given to a patient, how many milligrams of medication did the patient receive?

28. A woman is prescribed a 60-mg daily dose of Evista® for osteoporosis. How many tablets should she take per day?

29. If you inject 15 cc of lymphocyte immune globulin into a patient's IV, what dose in milligrams are you giving the patient?

30. If you were told to give 1200 mg of Zithromax®, how many milliliters would you give? How many tablespoons is this?

FOR ORAL USE ONLY.

STORAGE
Before Reconstitution:
Store below 86°F (30°C).
After Reconstitution:
Store suspension between 41°F (5°C) and
86°F (30°C). Protect from freezing.

SHAKE WELL BEFORE EACH USE.

DISCARD UNUSED PORTION AFTER 2 WEEKS.

MIXING DIRECTIONS
Tap bottle lightly to loosen powder. Add 24 mL
of distilled water or Purified Water (USP) to the
bottle. Shake well.

DOSAGE AND USE
See accompanying prescribing information.
This package contains **350 mg** fluconazole in a
natural orange-flavored mixture.*

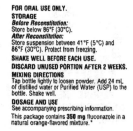

NDC 0049-3440-19
35 mL when reconstituted

DIFLUCAN®
(Fluconazole
for Oral Suspension)

ORANGE FLAVORED

10 mg/mL
when reconstituted

Pfizer **Roerig**
Division of Pfizer Inc, NY, NY 10017

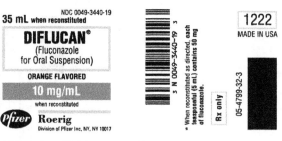

1222
MADE IN USA

* When reconstituted as directed, each
teaspoonful (5 mL) contains 50 mg
of fluconazole.

Rx only

05-4799-32-3

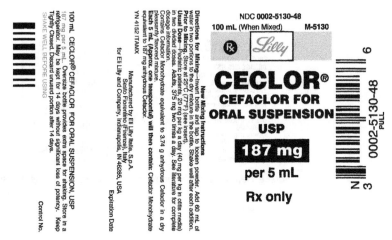

NDC 0002-5130-48
100 mL (When Mixed)   M-5130

℞   *Lilly*

CECLOR®
CEFACLOR FOR
ORAL SUSPENSION
USP

187 mg

per 5 mL

Rx only

0002-5130-48

100 mL CECLOR® CEFACLOR FOR ORAL SUSPENSION, USP
187 mg per 5 mL. Oversize bottle provides extra space for shaking. Store in a refrigerator. May be kept for 14 days without significant loss of potency. Keep Tightly Closed. Discard unused portion after 14 days.
SHAKE WELL BEFORE USING

Control No.

New Mixing Instructions
Directions for Mixing—Invert bottle and tap to loosen powder. Add 60 mL of water in two portions to the dry mixture in the bottle. Shake well after each addition.
Prior to Mixing Store at 25°C (77°F) (see insert).
Usual Dose—Pediatric patients, 20 mg per kg a day (40 mg per kg in otitis media) in two divided doses. Adults, 375 mg two times a day. See literature for complete dosage information.
Contains Cefaclor Monohydrate equivalent to 3.74 g anhydrous Cefaclor in a dry pleasantly flavored mixture.
Each 5 mL (Approx. one teaspoonful) will then contain Cefaclor Monohydrate equivalent to 187 mg anhydrous Cefaclor.

Manufactured by Eli Lilly Italia, S.p.A.
Sesto Fiorentino (Firenze), Italy
for Eli Lilly and Company, Indianapolis, IN 46285, USA

Expiration Date

YN 4152 1TAMX

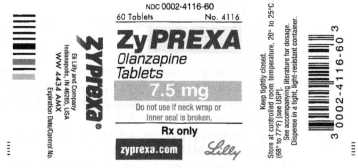

NDC 0002-4116-60
60 Tablets   No. 4116

Zy PREXA
Olanzapine
Tablets

7.5 mg

Do not use if neck wrap or
inner seal is broken.

Rx only

zyprexa.com   *Lilly*

Zyprexa®

Eli Lilly and Company
Indianapolis, IN 46285, USA
WW 4434 AMX

Expiration Date/Control No.

Keep tightly closed.
Store at controlled room temperature, 20° to 25°C
(68° to 77°F) [see USP].
See accompanying literature for dosage.
Dispense in a tight, light-resistant container.

0002-4116-60

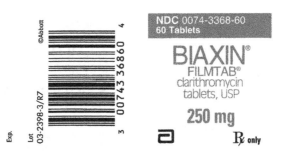

NDC 0074-3368-60
60 Tablets

BIAXIN®
FILMTAB®
clarithromycin
tablets, USP

250 mg

℞ only

©Abbott

Lot 03-2398-3/R7

Exp.

6505-01-354-8582
Store tablets at 15° to 30°C (59° to 86°F).
Do not accept if seal over bottle opening
is broken or missing.
Dispense in a USP tight,
light-resistant container.
Each tablet contains:
250 mg clarithromycin.
Usual Adult Dose: One or two tablets
every twelve hours.
See enclosure for full prescribing
information.
Filmtab – Film-sealed tablets, Abbott.
Mfd. by Abbott Pharmaceuticals PR Ltd.
Barceloneta, PR 00617
For Abbott Labs, N. Chicago, IL 60064 USA

Source: Label © Abbott Laboratories. Used with permission.

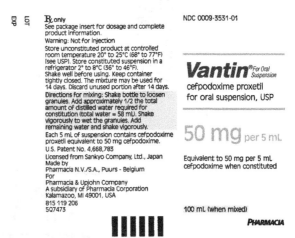

LOT
EXP

℞ only
See package insert for dosage and complete
product information.
Warning: Not for injection
Store unconstituted product at controlled
room temperature 20° to 25°C (68° to 77°F)
[see USP]. Store constituted suspension in a
refrigerator 2° to 8°C (36° to 46°F).
Shake well before using. Keep container
tightly closed. The mixture may be used for
14 days. Discard unused portion after 14 days.
Directions for mixing: Shake bottle to loosen
granules. Add approximately 1/2 the total
amount of distilled water required for
constitution (total water = 58 mL). Shake
vigorously to wet the granules. Add
remaining water and shake vigorously.
Each 5 mL of suspension contains cefpodoxime
proxetil equivalent to 50 mg cefpodoxime.
U.S. Patent No. 4,668,783
Licensed from Sankyo Company, Ltd., Japan
Made by
Pharmacia N.V./S.A., Puurs - Belgium
For
Pharmacia & Upjohn Company
A subsidiary of Pharmacia Corporation
Kalamazoo, MI 49001, USA
815 119 206
5Q7473

NDC 0009-3531-01

Vantin® For Oral
Suspension
cefpodoxime proxetil
for oral suspension, USP

50 mg per 5 mL

Equivalent to 50 mg per 5 mL
cefpodoxime when constituted

100 mL (when mixed)

PHARMACIA

Source: Reproduced with permission of Pfizer, Inc. All rights reserved.

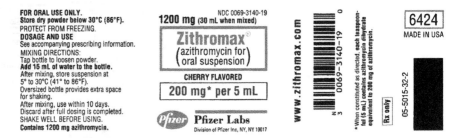

FOR ORAL USE ONLY.
Store dry powder below 30°C (86°F).
PROTECT FROM FREEZING.
DOSAGE AND USE
See accompanying prescribing information.
MIXING DIRECTIONS:
Tap bottle to loosen powder.
Add 15 mL of water to the bottle.
After mixing, store suspension at
5° to 30°C (41° to 86°F).
Oversized bottle provides extra space
for shaking.
After mixing, use within 10 days.
Discard after full dosing is completed.
SHAKE WELL BEFORE USING.
Contains 1200 mg azithromycin.

NDC 0069-3140-19
1200 mg (30 mL when mixed)

Zithromax®
(azithromycin for
oral suspension)

CHERRY FLAVORED

200 mg* per 5 mL

Pfizer **Pfizer Labs**
Division of Pfizer Inc, NY, NY 10017

www.zithromax.com

0069-3140-19

*When constituted as directed, each teaspoon-
ful (5 mL) contains azithromycin dihydrate
equivalent to 200 mg of azithromycin.

Rx only

05-5015-32-2

6424
MADE IN USA

Source: Reproduced with permission of Pfizer, Inc. All rights reserved.

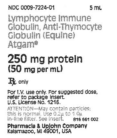

NDC 0009-7224-01   5 mL

Lymphocyte Immune
Globulin, Anti-Thymocyte
Globulin (Equine)
Atgam®

250 mg protein
(50 mg per mL)

℞ only

For I.V. use only. For suggested dose,
refer to package insert.
U.S. License No. 1216.
ATTENTION—May contain particles;
this is normal. Use 0.2μ to 1.0μ
in-line filter. See insert.   816 661 002
Pharmacia & Upjohn Company
Kalamazoo, MI 49001, USA

Source: Reproduced with permission of Pfizer, Inc. All rights reserved.

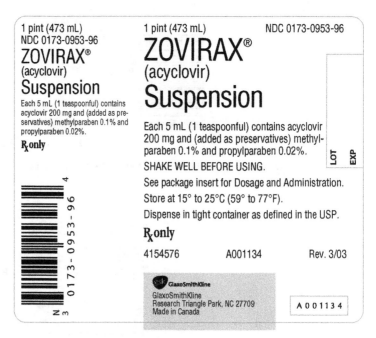

1 pint (473 mL)
NDC 0173-0953-96
ZOVIRAX®
(acyclovir)
Suspension

Each 5 mL (1 teaspoonful) contains
acyclovir 200 mg and (added as preservatives) methylparaben 0.1% and
propylparaben 0.02%.

R_x only

1 pint (473 mL)   NDC 0173-0953-96
ZOVIRAX®
(acyclovir)
Suspension

Each 5 mL (1 teaspoonful) contains acyclovir
200 mg and (added as preservatives) methylparaben 0.1% and propylparaben 0.02%.

SHAKE WELL BEFORE USING.

See package insert for Dosage and Administration.

Store at 15° to 25°C (59° to 77°F).

Dispense in tight container as defined in the USP.

R_x only

4154576   A001134   Rev. 3/03

GlaxoSmithKline
GlaxoSmithKline
Research Triangle Park, NC 27709
Made in Canada

A 0 0 1 1 3 4

Source: Reproduced by permission of GlaxoSmithKline.

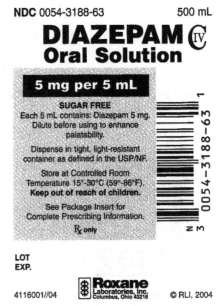

NDC 0054-3188-63   500 mL

DIAZEPAM ℂIV
Oral Solution

5 mg per 5 mL

SUGAR FREE
Each 5 mL contains: Diazepam 5 mg.
Dilute before using to enhance
palatability.

Dispense in tight, light-resistant
container as defined in the USP/NF.

Store at Controlled Room
Temperature 15°-30°C (59°-86°F).
Keep out of reach of children.

See Package Insert for
Complete Prescribing Information.

R_x only

LOT
EXP.

4116001//04   **Roxane**
Laboratories, Inc.
Columbus, Ohio 43216   © RLI, 2004

Source: Label © Roxane Laboratories. Used with permission.

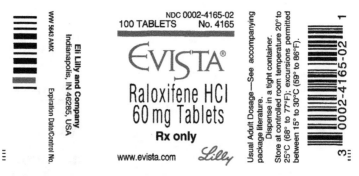

WW 5643 AMX
Eli Lilly and Company
Indianapolis, IN 46285, USA

Expiration Date/Control No.

NDC 0002-4165-02
100 TABLETS   No. 4165

EVISTA®

Raloxifene HCl
60 mg Tablets

Rx only

www.evista.com   *Lilly*

Usual Adult Dosage—See accompanying
package literature.
Dispense in a tight container.
Store at controlled room temperature 20° to
25°C (68° to 77°F); excursions permitted
between 15° to 30°C (59° to 86°F).

Source: Copyright Eli Lilly & Co. All rights reserved. Used with permission.

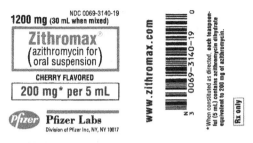

31. Polymox® is a brand of amoxicillin whose label recommends the child dosage to be 20 to 40 mg/kg/day. The label also states that this stock solution contains 125 mg of medication per 5 mL of solution. Calculate the minimum daily dosage of medication for a child who weighs 10.5 kg. How many milliliters of the stock solution will be administered to achieve this daily dosage?

32. Use the information in the previous problem and calculate the maximum daily dosage of amoxicillin and the number of milliliters of this medication to be administered to a child weighing 10.5 kg.

33. Kefzol® is given to children to treat infections. For severe infections, a dosage of 45 mg/lb/day is recommended. If a child weighs 60 lb, how much daily medication should he receive for a severe infection? If the label recommends 4 doses per day, how much medication will be contained in each dose?

34. The initial dose of Zithromax® in oral suspension for the treatment of a child with acute otitis media is 10 mg/kg as a single dose. If a child weighs 12.5 kg, how much medication should be given as the intial dose? On days 2 through 5, the child should received 5 mg/kg. How much medication will the child receive on each day after the initial dose?

35. The doctor has ordered 125 mg Amoxil® oral suspension to be given 3 times a day for an infant weighing 6.2 kg. If the label states that the usual child dosage is 20 to 40 mg/kg/day, calculate the per dose dosage range. Is the amount prescribed a correct dosage?

36. A physician has ordered 5 mL (1 t) tid ceflacor for a pediatric patient weighing 18.2 kg. The strength on the bottle is 187 mg/5 mL and the recommended dosage is 20–40 mg/kg/day. Is the amount prescribed a correct dosage?

37. The initial dose of morphine should be 2 to 10 mg/70 kg of body weight. A dose of 12 mg of morphine is ordered for a 90-kg patient. Is the amount prescribed a correct dosage?

38. The recommended intital dose of Azulfidine EN-tabs® for a child 6 years of age and older is 40 to 60 mg/kg of body weight in each 24-hour period, divided into 3 to 6 doses. The order for a 22.5-kg child is 200 mg 4 times a day. Is the amount prescribed a correct dosage?

SECTION 5.3   RATIOS, PROPORTIONS, FORMULAS, AND DIMENSIONAL ANALYSIS IN MULTISTEP DOSAGE CALCULATIONS

In Section 5.2, you learned the proportion method for calculating the correct dosages of medication to administer. The formula method of calculating dosage amounts is a derivative of the proportion method. The proportion method teaches you a method that you can always use if you understand the relationships among the quantities. However, some people prefer formulas and have no difficulty in memorizing them and using them correctly. Look at the proportion for dosage calculation from Section 5.2:

$$\frac{\text{Amount of "drug" in the stock}}{\text{Per volume or weight}} = \frac{\text{Amount of "drug" prescribed}}{\text{Volume or weight of stock needed}}$$

Let's assign variables to each of the numerators and denominators in order to create a formula. Let H = amount of "drug" in stock or on hand, Q = volume or weight of drug on hand, D = amount of "drug" prescribed, and A = volume or weight of stock needed to administer.

Using these variables in our proportion, we have

$$\frac{H}{Q} = \frac{D}{A}$$

If we cross multiply we have

$$HA = DQ$$

and solving for A (amount to administer),

$$A = \frac{DQ}{H} = D \times \frac{Q}{H}$$

This formula is useful since you can replace the variables with the given values for each problem and calculate the answer quickly. However, since this is a derivative of the original proportion, if you forget the formula, you can easily re-create it by using the proportion method.

EXAMPLE 7: Calculating Dosages Using a Formula

The label on a concentrated drug solution states that there are 75 mg of medication in 5 mL. If the order calls for 225 mg of medication, how many milliliters should be administered?

Solution

$$\text{Formula: } A = D \times \frac{Q}{H}$$

Recall that

H = amount of "drug" in stock or on hand = 75 mg

Q = volume or weight of drug on hand = 5 mL

D = amount of "drug" prescribed = 225 mg

A = volume or weight of stock needed to administer = unknown

Substitute the given values into the formula and solve.

$$A = 225 \text{ mg} \times \frac{5 \text{ mL}}{75 \text{ mg}} = 15 \text{ mL}$$

Therefore, 15 mL of the stock medication should be administered.

In the last section, most of the problems that you worked were one-step problems. However, in many instances, more than one step may be required to calculate the proper dosage. For example, if your patient's weight is measured in pounds and the medication dosage is only defined for weight in kilograms, a conversion from pounds to kilograms must be done before the correct dosage can be calculated. These multistep problems can be done using the ratio and proportion method, the formula method, or dimensional analysis. Dimensional analysis was introduced in Chapter 3 as a method of converting measurements to different units. In these next examples, we will look at some multistep dosage calculations and demonstrate different solution methods.

EXAMPLE 8: Metric to Apothecary to Capsule Conversions

The doctor orders 900 mg of aspirin for a patient. The available medication is gr 5 caplets. How many caplets of this medication should the patient be given?

Solution

Proportion Method

Our first job is to determine the apothecary equivalent in grains for a 900-mg dose of aspirin. We will set up a proportion using the equivalent $\dfrac{\text{gr } 1}{60 \text{ mg}}$.

$$\frac{\text{gr } 1}{60 \text{ mg}} = \frac{x}{900 \text{ mg}} \qquad \text{Set up the proportion.}$$

$$(\text{gr } 1)(900 \text{ mg}) = x \, (60 \text{ mg}) \qquad \text{Cross-multiply.}$$

$$\frac{(\text{gr } 1)(900 \text{ mg})}{60 \text{ mg}} = x \qquad \text{Use the Division Property of Equality.}$$

$$\text{gr } 15 = x \qquad \text{Simplify.}$$

Now that we have determined the equivalent dosage in the apothecary system, we can use this result to determine the number of caplets to dispense using another proportion.

$$\frac{1 \text{ caplet}}{\text{gr } 5} = \frac{x}{\text{gr } 15} \qquad \text{Set up the proportion.}$$

$$(1 \text{ caplet})(\text{gr } 15) = x \, (\text{gr } 5) \qquad \text{Cross-multiply.}$$

$$\frac{(1 \text{ caplet})(\text{gr } 15)}{\text{gr } 5} = x \qquad \text{Use the Division Property of Equality.}$$

$$3 \text{ caplets} = x \qquad \text{Simplify.}$$

Therefore, the patient should be given 3 caplets in order to receive the prescribed amount of 900 mg.

Dimensional Analysis Method

The requirement of the problem is to convert 900 mg to grains and then grains to caplets. We can set up a series of conversion fractions that can be multiplied together in one calculation to accomplish these steps. For this conversion, we include the following equivalents: 60 mg = gr 1 and gr 5 = 1 caplet.

$$900 \text{ mg} \times \frac{\text{gr } 1}{60 \text{ mg}} \times \frac{1 \text{ caplet}}{\text{gr } 5} = \frac{900 \text{ caplets}}{300} = 3 \text{ caplets}$$

By using the equivalents in fraction form, the conversions are completed in one series of calculations using dimensional analysis.

In most doctor's offices, patients are weighed in pounds. However, many medications have recommended dosages, especially for children, based on weights in kilograms. Therefore, there must first be a conversion of the weight in pounds to kilograms before the correct dosage amount can be calculated. Look at the next example involving a dosage calculation dependent on a weight conversion.

EXAMPLE 9: Weight Conversions for Dosage Calculations

A child has a mild upper respiratory tract infection and her doctor orders erythromycin drops 125 mg p.o. q6h. The label on the bottle reads, "Usual dose for Children: 30–50 mg/kg/day; 100 mg per 2.5 mL (dropperful)." Calculate the recommended daily dosage range if the child weighs 32 lb. Determine if the ordered amount is within the recommended range. If so, calculate the correct dose in milliliters that should be administered to the child.

Solution

Proportion Method

First use a proportion to convert the child's weight to kilograms since the label indicates that the dosage is based on weight in kilograms. We will use the fact that 1 kg = 2.2 lb for part of our proportion.

$$\frac{2.2\ \text{lb}}{1\ \text{kg}} = \frac{32\ \text{lb}}{x} \qquad \text{Set up the proportion.}$$

$$(2.2\ \text{lb})x = (32\ \text{lb})(1\ \text{kg}) \qquad \text{Cross-multiply.}$$

$$x = \frac{(32\ \cancel{\text{lb}})(1\ \text{kg})}{2.2\ \cancel{\text{lb}}} \qquad \text{Use the Division Property of Equality.}$$

$$x = 14.5\ \text{kg} \qquad \text{Simplify.}$$

Using the dosage on the label, the minimum amount of medication is 30 mg/kg/day and the maximum is 50 mg/kg/day. We will use these ratios to calculate the safe range of daily medication. Again we will set up proportions.

Minimum Dosage: **Maximum Dosage:**

$$\frac{30\ \text{mg}}{1\ \text{kg}} = \frac{x}{14.5\ \text{kg}} \qquad\qquad \frac{50\ \text{mg}}{1\ \text{kg}} = \frac{x}{14.5\ \text{kg}}$$

$$(30\ \text{mg})(14.5\ \text{kg}) = (1\ \text{kg})(x) \qquad (50\ \text{mg})(14.5\ \text{kg}) = (1\ \text{kg})(x)$$

$$\frac{(30\ \text{mg})(14.5\ \cancel{\text{kg}})}{1\ \cancel{\text{kg}}} = x \qquad\qquad \frac{(50\ \text{mg})(14.5\ \cancel{\text{kg}})}{1\ \cancel{\text{kg}}} = x$$

$$435\ \text{mg} = x \qquad\qquad\qquad 725\ \text{mg} = x$$

The recommended dosage for this patient ranges from 435 mg daily to 725 mg daily. The ordered amount is 125 mg p.o. q6h, which is 125 mg 4 times a day, resulting in a daily dosage of 500 mg. This is within the recommended range.

To determine the amount to administer in order to ensure that this dosage is received, set up another proportion using the information on the label (100 mg per 2.5 mL).

$$\frac{100\ \text{mg}}{2.5\ \text{mL}} = \frac{125\ \text{mg}}{x} \qquad\qquad\qquad\qquad \text{Set up the proportion.}$$

$$(x)(100\ \text{mg}) = (125\ \text{mg})(2.5\ \text{mL}) \qquad\qquad \text{Cross-multiply.}$$

$$x = \frac{(125\ \cancel{\text{mg}})(2.5\ \text{mL})}{100\ \cancel{\text{mg}}} = 3.125\ \text{mL} \qquad \text{Use the Division Property of Equality and simplify.}$$

Therefore, approximately 3 mL of this medication should be given every 6 hours.

Dimensional Analysis

If we calculate the minimum and maximum daily dosages using dimensional analysis, we will convert the weight from pounds to kilograms, and use the lower-range ratio to calculate the minimum amount of medication in one calculation. We will do a similar setup for the maximum amount.

$$\text{Minimum Amount: } 32 \text{ lb} \times \frac{1 \text{ kg}}{2.2 \text{ lb}} \times \frac{30 \text{ mg}}{1 \text{ kg}} = 436.4 \text{ mg}$$

$$\text{Maximum Amount: } 32 \text{ lb} \times \frac{1 \text{ kg}}{2.2 \text{ lb}} \times \frac{50 \text{ mg}}{1 \text{ kg}} = 727.3 \text{ mg}$$

The slight difference in answers occurs because a rounded answer was used in the second calculation of the proportion method.

Body surface area (BSA) is another factor that may be used in calculating dosages for a number of drugs. For example, dosages of certain medications for patients undergoing cancer chemotherapy or patients with severe burns are calculated using body surface area. Body surface area is given in square meters (m^2) using the patient's weight and height. A formula with these variables can be used for the calculation but many people use a graph called a nomogram, consisting of weight and height variables, to find the BSA. A nomogram for calculating BSA is found in the appendix of this book.

There are two formulas used for calculating BSA, depending on the information given. One uses kilogram (kg) and centimeter (cm) measurements, and the other uses pound (lb) and inch (in.) measurements. They are both given here.

Calculating Body Surface Area

Metric Units:	U.S. Customary Units:
$\text{BSA} = \sqrt{\dfrac{\text{Weight in kg} \times \text{Height in cm}}{3600}}$	$\text{BSA} = \sqrt{\dfrac{\text{Weight in lb} \times \text{Height in in.}}{3131}}$

Note: BSA is measured in m^2.

EXAMPLE 10: Calculating Dosages Using Body Surface Area

A physician orders 40 mg/m^2 of prednisone for a patient who weights 160 lb and is 5 ft 8 in. How many mg of this drug should be administered?

Solution

The units of height and weight are U.S. Customary units, so we will convert the height to inches and substitute these values into the formula to find the BSA.

$$5 \text{ ft } 8 \text{ in.} = 5 \text{ ft} \times 12\frac{\text{in.}}{\text{ft}} = 60 \text{ in.} + 8 \text{ in.} = 68 \text{ in.}$$

$$\text{BSA} = \sqrt{\frac{\text{Weight in lb} \times \text{Height in in.}}{3131}} \qquad \text{U.S. Customary Units Formula}$$

$$= \sqrt{\frac{160 \text{ lb} \times 68 \text{ in.}}{3131}} \qquad \text{Substitute the given values.}$$

$$\text{BSA} = \sqrt{\frac{10880}{3131}} = \sqrt{3.474928} = 1.86 \text{ m}^2 \qquad \begin{array}{l}\text{Simplify the fraction and} \\ \text{take its square root.}\end{array}$$

Now use a proportion to complete the problem.

$$\frac{40 \text{ mg}}{1 \text{ m}^2} = \frac{x}{1.86 \text{ m}^2} \qquad \text{Set up the proportion.}$$

$$(40 \text{ mg})(1.86 \text{ m}^2) = (1 \text{ m}^2)(x) \qquad \text{Cross-multiply.}$$

$$\frac{(40 \text{ mg})(1.86 \text{ m}^2)}{1 \text{ m}^2} = x \qquad \text{Use the Division Property of Equality.}$$

$$74.4 \text{ mg} = x \qquad \text{Simplify.}$$

Therefore, 74.4 mg of prednisone should be administered to this patient.

In the last example, you can also set up an easy multiplication problem to find the dosage after finding the BSA by doing the following calculation:

$$1.86 \text{ m}^2 \times \frac{40 \text{ mg}}{\text{m}^2} = 74.4 \text{ mg}$$

Use the approach that seems easiest and most logical to you for all of these problems.

EXAMPLE 11: Using Metric Units to Calculate BSA and Determine Dosages

A child weighs 7.7 kg and is 40 cm tall. The recommended dosage of a medication that has been prescribed for this child is 5 mg per m². Calculate this child's BSA and then the correct amount of medication to administer.

Solution

$$\text{BSA} = \sqrt{\frac{\text{Weight in kg} \times \text{Height in cm}}{3600}} \qquad \text{Metric Units Formula}$$

$$\text{BSA} = \sqrt{\frac{7.7 \text{ kg} \times 40 \text{ cm}}{3600}} \qquad \text{Substitute the given values.}$$

$$\text{BSA} = \sqrt{\frac{308}{3600}} = \sqrt{0.085555} = 0.29 \text{ m}^2 \qquad \begin{array}{l}\text{Simplify the fraction and} \\ \text{take its square root.}\end{array}$$

To calculate the correct dosage,

$$0.29 \text{ m}^2 \times \frac{5 \text{ mg}}{\text{m}^2} = 1.45 \text{ mg}$$

The correct dosage of medication for this child is 1.45 mg.

The formulas for calculating BSA require computations using a calculator. The use of a diagram called a **nomogram** is another way to estimate a patient's BSA rather easily using a straight line to connect given values in order to find the unknown value. To use a nomogram, find the patient's height and weight. The height can be in either centimeters or inches, and the weight in pounds or kilograms because the nomogram has scales for both. Place a straightedge extending from the patient's height in the left column to a patient's weight in the right column. Then read the value at the place where the straightedge interests the Surface Area (SA) column. The scale is logarithmic so read it carefully. This is the patient's estimated body surface area in m². Use this method for the patient in Example 10 to see if you can arrive at the same BSA as was calculated by using the formula.

PRACTICE PROBLEM SET 5.3

1. A patient's order is 35 mg of codeine phosphate by subcutaneous injection. Available in stock is 50 mg in 1 mL of liquid for SC Injection. How many milliliters will you administer?

2. A doctor orders 250 mg of amoxicillin trihydrate orally for your patient. The stock solution that is available is 125 mg in 5 mL of syrup. How many milliliters of stock solution will you administer?

3. A patient is to be given 30 mg of frusemide intravenously and 10 mg in 1 mL of liquid for IV injection is available. How many milliliters should you administer?

4. A doctor orders 10 mg of haloperidol decanoate to be given to a patient by intramuscular injection and 50 mg/mL of liquid for IM injection is available. How many milliliters will you administer?

5. A client is ordered 1000 milligrams of sodium valproate orally by his physician. The stock solution available contains 200 mg in 5 mL of syrup. How many milliliters should you administer to the patient?

6. A geriatric patient is ordered a daily dose of 75 mg of thioridazine orally by her doctor. It is to be divided into 3 doses. The stock solution available is labeled 25 mg in 5 mL of suspension. How many milliliters should the patient take for each dose? How many teaspoons is this?

To solve Problems 7–10, find the appropriate label for the medication prescribed in the problem, and use the information on the label to answer the questions. The labels follow Problem 11.

7. A patient is ordered 0.25 g of cefpodoxime proxetil. How many milliliters should be given to the patient? How many teaspoons is this?

8. A patient is ordered 0.6 g of azithromycin. How many milliliters should be given to the patient? How many teaspoons is this?

9. In order to give gr $\frac{1}{6}$ medroxyprogesterone to a patient, how many tabs should be given?

10. In order to give gr 5 rifabutin to a patient, how many capsules should be given?

11. A doctor orders tetracycline elixir qid for a child weighing 60 lb at a dosage of 8 mg/kg/day in equally divided doses. How many mg would 1 dose contain? The tetracycline in stock is labeled 50 mg per 5 mL. How many milliliters should be administered?

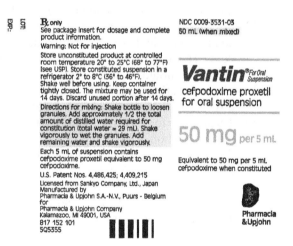

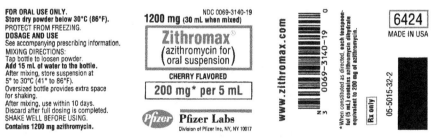

Modeling Health Applications with Ratios and Proportions

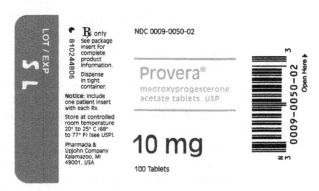

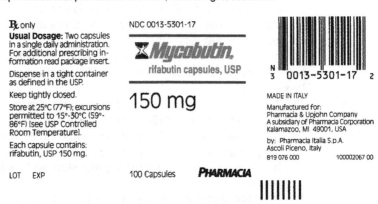

12. A doctor orders quinidine for an adult patient weighing 108 lb at a dosage of 25 mg/kg/day q6h. How many milligrams should each dose contain? The stock of quinidine is supplied as 300-mg tablets. How many tablets should be given?

13. The doctor orders ampicillin IVPB for a child weighing 55 lb at a dosage of 20 mg/kg/day in 4 equally divided doses. How many milligrams should be given per dose? The ampicillin is supplied as 250 mg in 1.5 mL after reconstitution. How many milliliters should be administered?

14. The medication order is 4.5 g q4h p.o. The patient weighs 253 lb. The recommended dose is 40–50 mg/kg/day. Is the ordered dose safe?

15. The order is for erythromycin 2500 mg p.o. q6h for a 187-lb patient. The safe range for this medication is 30–50 mg/kg/day. Is the ordered dose safe?

16. The pediatrician prescribes Cefadyl 5 mg qid IM for a child weighing 20 kg. The label lists the recommended dosage as 1–3 mg/kg/day. Is the ordered dose safe?

17. The recommended pediatric dose of Ancef® is 80–160 mg/kg/day. The doctor ordered 200 mg Ancef IV q4h for a child weighing 12 kg. Is the ordered dose safe?

18. The doctor orders garamycin 35 mg IM q6h for a child weighing 44 lb. According to the label, the recommended dose is 6–7.5 mg/kg/day in 4 equally divided doses. Garamycin is supplied as 80 mg/mL. Is the order within the safe range? How many milliliters should be administered?

19. A child with a fever is ordered Tylenol® suspension $\frac{1}{2}$ tsp p.o. q4h prn. The child weighs 33 lb. The label states that the recommended dose is 25–35 mg/kg/day q4h prn. The medication is supplied as 325 mg per 10 mL. Is the ordered dose in the safe range? If so, how many milliliters should be administered?

20. A 2-year-old child weighs 30 lb and the doctor has ordered Tolectin 100 mg p.o. qid. The medication on hand is in 200-mg scored tablets. The recommended dosage for children 2 years and older is 15 to 30 mg/kg/day. Is the ordered dose in the safe range? If so, how many tablets should be given?

21. Calculate the BSA of a patient who is 86 cm tall and weighs 12.8 kg. Verify your results using the nomogram in Appendix B.

22. Calculate the BSA of a patient who is 112 cm tall and weighs 21.5 kg. Verify your results using the nomogram in Appendix B.
23. Calculate the BSA of a patient who is 5 ft 8 in. tall and weighs 210 lb. Verify your results using the nomogram in Appendix B.
24. Calculate the BSA of a patient who is 6 ft 1 in. tall and weighs 275 lb. Verify your results using the nomogram in Appendix B.
25. The BSA of the patient is 2.13 m^2. The physician ordered indinavir 375 mg/m^2. How many capsules would you administer if the label reads 0.25 g/capsule?
26. The BSA of the patient is 1.69 m^2. The physician ordered 30 mg/m^2 of Nembutal. How many capsules are needed if the label reads 50 mg/capsule?
27. The doctor orders thyroid 16.25 mg/m^2. If each tablet contains 32.5 mg, how many tablets would you administer to a patient who is 164 cm tall and weighs 94 kg?
28. The recommended dosage of a particular medication is 175 mcg/m^2. If the patient is 152 cm tall and weighs 50 kg, how much medication should be administered?
29. The doctor orders CeeNU for a child whose height is 38 in. and whose weight is 45 lb. The first recommended dose is a single oral dose of 130 mg/m^2. Find the recommended first dose of this medication for this patient.
30. The recommended dosage of a medication is 0.4 mg/m^2. The patient is 5 ft 6 in. tall and weighs 170 lb. Find the recommended dosage for this patient.

SECTION 5.4   RATIOS AND PROPORTIONS IN X-RAY APPLICATIONS

In making and interpreting the results of x-rays, it is important to understand the relationships between three quantities that are factors in every x-ray. These quantities are the **exposure time**, the level of the **electrical current** that is used for an exposure, and the **distance** between the x-ray machine and the x-ray film on which the exposure will be recorded. Using various combinations of time, current, and distance, many different x-ray pictures may be taken for different purposes.

The time of an exposure, t, is usually short and will be measured in seconds and fractions of a second. X-rays do cause damage to living tissue, so exposure must be limited for health reasons. The level of electric current is measured in milliamperes, mA, and determines the penetrating power of the x-rays produced by the machine. Distances may be measured in any convenient unit, but inches (in.), and centimeters, (cm) are most commonly used. Figure 5.2 shows the various distances that may need to be carefully measured especially if measurements of bone lengths, thickness, or other measurements are to be made on the resulting x-ray film itself.

We will now examine the various relationships that are possible between the three variables time, current, and distance. To make this a little easier, we will look at pairs of variables. First we will assume that the time for an exposure has been set and will look at the relationship between current and distance. Then we will set the current to one value and see what the relationship between time and distance is. Lastly, we will set a distance and investigate the relationship between time and current.

Current-to-Distance Relationship (Time Held Constant)

If the exposure time, in seconds, is set at a constant value, the type of exposure will then be determined by the current level (in milliamperes, mA) and the distance (in inches or centimeters) between the focal point of the x-ray machine and the x-ray film (this is the focus-to-film distance as shown in Figure 5.2). The ratio of the original current setting to the square of the original FFD is equal to the ratio of the new current setting that we wish to use to the square of the new FFD needed in order to keep the new x-ray exposure the same as the original in intensity. The current, mA, is directly proportional to the square of the focus-to-film distance, FFD.

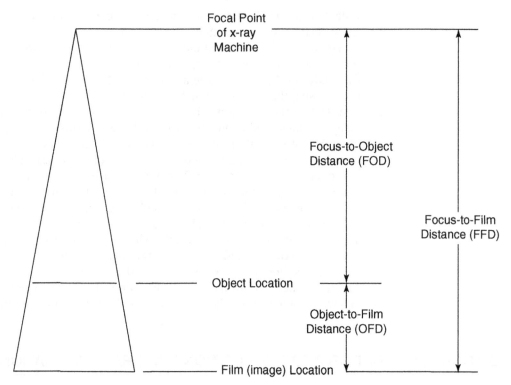

Figure 5.2 Distances to Measure

Current-to-Distance Proportion

$$\frac{\text{Original mA}}{(\text{Original FFD})^2} = \frac{\text{New mA}}{(\text{New FFD})^2}$$

EXAMPLE 12: Exposure Calculation with Time Held Constant

A patient's wrist was x-rayed at a distance of 30 in. with the current level set at 7.5 mA. If a second x-ray is to be taken at a distance of 20 in., at what level should we set the current in order to give the patient's wrist the same exposure as in the first x-ray?

Solution

$$\frac{\text{Original mA}}{(\text{Original FFD})^2} = \frac{\text{New mA}}{(\text{New FFD})^2} \qquad \text{Start with the basic formula.}$$

$$\frac{7.5 \text{ mA}}{(30 \text{ in.})^2} = \frac{x}{(20 \text{ in.})^2} \qquad \text{Substitute known values.}$$

$$\frac{7.5 \text{ mA}}{900 \text{ in.}^2} = \frac{x}{400 \text{ in.}^2} \qquad \text{Simplify the exponents.}$$

$$(x)(900 \text{ in.}^2) = (7.5 \text{ mA})(400 \text{ in.}^2) \qquad \text{Cross-multiply.}$$

$$900x = 3000 \text{ mA} \qquad \text{Simplify.}$$

$$\frac{900x}{900} = \frac{3000}{900} \text{ mA} \qquad \text{Use the Division Property of Equality.}$$

$$x = 3.333\ldots \text{ mA} \qquad \text{Simplify.}$$

So the new current setting should be 3.3 mA in order to keep the overall exposure the same intensity as the original x-ray. Remember, the current is directly proportional to the square of the focus-to-film distance. Thus a decrease in distance should result in a decrease in the current used.

Time-to-Distance Relationship (Current Held Constant)

If the current, in milliamperes (mA), is set at a constant value, the type of exposure that results depends upon the time that the x-ray machine is on and the distance between the focus of the x-ray machine and the x-ray film. In Figure 5.2, the distance from the focus point to the film location is shown. The ratio of the original exposure time to the square of the original FFD used is equal to the ratio of the new exposure time that we wish to use to the square of the new FFD needed in order keep the new x-ray exposure the same as the original in intensity. The exposure time is directly proportional to the square of the focus-to-film distance.

Time-to-Distance Proportion

$$\frac{\text{Original } t}{(\text{Original FFD})^2} = \frac{\text{New } t}{(\text{New FFD})^2}$$

EXAMPLE 11: Exposure Calculation with Current Held Constant

An x-ray of a patient's arm was made with a focus-to-film distance (FFD) of 18 in. with an exposure time of 0.3 s. If a new x-ray is to be taken at a distance of 30 in., what time of exposure should be used if the technician wishes to keep the same exposure on the new film?

Solution

$$\frac{\text{Original } t}{(\text{Original FFD})^2} = \frac{\text{New } t}{(\text{New FFD})^2} \qquad \text{Start with the basic formula.}$$

$$\frac{0.3 \text{ s}}{(18 \text{ in.})^2} = \frac{x}{(30 \text{ in.})^2} \qquad \text{Substitute known values.}$$

$$\frac{0.3 \text{ s}}{324 \text{ in.}^2} = \frac{x}{900 \text{ in.}^2} \qquad \text{Simplify the exponents.}$$

$$(0.3 \text{ s})(900 \text{ in.}^2) = (x)(324 \text{ in.}^2) \qquad \text{Cross multiply.}$$

$$324x = 270 \text{ s} \qquad \text{Simplify.}$$

$$\frac{324x}{324} = \frac{270}{324} \text{ s} \qquad \text{Use the Division Property of Equality.}$$

$$x = 0.8333\ldots \text{ s} \qquad \text{Simplify.}$$

Thus the new exposure time required in order to keep the new exposure the same as the original exposure on the film is 0.83 s. The increase in exposure time is required because as the FFD increases, the number of x-rays reaching each square inch of film each second is decreased. This is due to something called the *inverse square law*, which may be studied in detail in any good physics book.

It is important to note here that changing any of the various distances shown in Figure 5.2 will also change the relative size of the image that is shown on the developed x-ray film. Just like a photographic camera, the size of the image on the film is a factor of the distances between the camera lens, the film, and the object being photographed.

Current-to-Time Relationship (Distance Held Constant)

If the distances are set at a constant value, the type of exposure that results will then depend upon the level of the current, in milliamperes (mA), and the time of the exposure. The following formula is used for this relationship. Assuming that the FFD is held constant, the current in milliamperes varies inversely with the time of the exposure. This means that if the current setting is *increased*, then the time of the exposure must be *decreased* in order to keep the exposure the same intensity.

Current-to-Time Proportion

$$\frac{\text{Original mA}}{\text{New } t} = \frac{\text{New mA}}{\text{Original } t}$$

EXAMPLE 14: Exposure Calculation with Distance Held Constant

An x-ray was done with the current set at 30 mA and an exposure time of 3 s. If the current setting is changed to 150 mA, what should the time of this new exposure be?

Solution

$$\frac{\text{Original mA}}{\text{New } t} = \frac{\text{New mA}}{\text{Original } t} \qquad \text{Start with the basic formula.}$$

$$\frac{30 \text{ mA}}{x} = \frac{150 \text{ mA}}{3 \text{ s}} \qquad \text{Substitute the known values.}$$

$$(x)(150 \text{ mA}) = (3 \text{ s})(30 \text{ mA}) \qquad \text{Cross multiply.}$$

$$150x = 90 \text{ s} \qquad \text{Simplify.}$$

$$\frac{150x}{150} = \frac{90}{150} \text{ s} \qquad \text{Use the Division Property of Equality.}$$

$$x = 0.6 \text{ s} \qquad \text{Simplify.}$$

So the new exposure time needed is 0.6 s. In an inverse relationship, the values go in different directions. Here the current setting was increased, and the time of the exposure decreased as a result.

Image Magnification

In general, the images on x-ray films are magnified when compared with the size of the actual object being x-rayed. Depending upon the various distances involved, the magnification may be very small or it may be significant. In some medical procedures having the actual size of the object being x-rayed is important. When x-raying bones under muscle tissue or in images of unborn children, it is not possible to make a direct measurement of the size needed. There are two commonly used methods of making measurements on the x-ray film and then mathematically calculating the actual size of the bone or other structure x-rayed.

One method involves knowing the focus-to-film distance (FFD), the focus-to-object distance (FOD), and the object-to-film distance (OFD). Please refer to Figure 5.2 to see where these distances are. In the following proportion, the word *image* refers to the x-ray itself, and the word *object* refers to the actual item being x-rayed.

Image Magnification Proportion Using Measured Distances

$$\frac{\text{Image length}}{\text{Object length}} = \frac{\text{Focus-to-film distance}}{\text{Focus-to-object distance}}$$

$$\frac{\text{Image length}}{\text{Object length}} = \frac{\text{FFD}}{\text{FOD}}$$

Note: FOD = FFD − OFD

EXAMPLE 15: Calculating a Distance from an X-ray Image

A radiographic technician made an x-ray image of the head of an unborn child. The technician noted that the focus-to-film distance (FFD) was 80 cm and the object-to-film distance (OFD) was 16 cm. The biparietal diameter of the unborn child's head was measured on the x-ray film and found to be 9.85 cm. (The biparietal diameter of a skull is the shortest diameter and is measured approximately from temple to temple.) What is the *actual* biparietal diameter of the child's head?

Solution

First, list the given information:

FFD = 80 cm, OFD = 16 cm, image length = 9.85 cm
FOD = FFD − OFD
FOD = 80 cm − 16 cm = 64 cm

$$\frac{\text{Image length}}{\text{Object length}} = \frac{\text{FFD}}{\text{FOD}} \qquad \text{Start with the basic formula.}$$

$$\frac{9.85 \text{ cm}}{x} = \frac{80 \text{ cm}}{64 \text{ cm}} \qquad \text{Substitute known values.}$$

$$(x)(80 \text{ cm}) = (9.85 \text{ cm})(64 \text{ cm}) \qquad \text{Cross multiply.}$$

$$80x = 630.4 \text{ cm} \qquad \text{Simplify.}$$

$$\frac{80x}{80} = \frac{630.4}{80} \text{ cm} \qquad \text{Use the Division Property of Equality.}$$

$$x = 7.88 \text{ cm} \qquad \text{Simplify.}$$

Thus the actual biparietal diameter of the unborn child's head is 7.88 cm.

A second method of determining the actual size of an object pictured on an x-ray is to place a measuring rod of known length at the same distance from the focus as the object being x-rayed. This method is really more reliable than the method previously shown. With this method, no distances need to be measured by the x-ray technician.

Image Magnification Proportion Using a Measuring Rod

$$\frac{\text{Measuring rod's image length}}{\text{Measuring rod's actual length}} = \frac{\text{Image length}}{\text{Object's length}}$$

EXAMPLE 16: Calculating a Distance Based on the Length of a Measuring Rod

On an x-ray of an unborn child, the biparietal diameter of the skull is measured to be 12.2 cm. On the same x-ray, a 10-cm-long measuring rod is 13.0 cm long. What is the actual biparietal diameter of the child's skull?

Solution

$$\frac{\text{Measuring rod's image length}}{\text{Measuring rod's actual length}} = \frac{\text{Image length}}{\text{Object's length}}$$

$$\frac{13.0 \text{ cm}}{10.0 \text{ cm}} = \frac{12.2 \text{ cm}}{x} \qquad \text{Substitute the known values.}$$

$$(x)(13.0 \text{ cm}) = (10.0 \text{ cm})(12.2 \text{ cm}) \qquad \text{Cross-multiply.}$$

$$13.0x = 122 \text{ cm} \qquad \text{Simplify.}$$

$$\frac{13.0x}{13.0} = \frac{122}{13.0} \text{ cm} \qquad \text{Use the Division Property of Equality.}$$

$$x = 9.4 \text{ cm} \qquad \text{Simplify.}$$

So the actual biparietal diameter of the unborn child is 9.4 cm.

PRACTICE PROBLEM SET 5.4

Identify each of the following variables and give the units in which they are measured:

1. mA
2. t
3. FFD
4. FOD
5. OFD
6. s
7. In a given examination, the current employed by a technician was 8.00 mA, and an FFD of 40.0 in. was used. If a new exposure is to be made at a distance of 30.0 in., what current should be used in order for the second exposure to have the same intensity as the first?
8. A technician took an x-ray with the current set at 7.50 mA and an FFD of 24.0 in. If a new exposure is to be made at a distance of 36.0 in., what current should be used in order for the second exposure to have the same intensity as the first?
9. An x-ray of a patient is taken with an FFD of 16.0 in. with an exposure time of 0.100 s. If another exposure is to be taken with an FFD of 48.0 in., what should the new exposure time be so that the second x-ray is of the same intensity as the first?
10. An x-ray is taken with an FFD of 32.0 in. with an exposure time of 0.300 s. If another exposure is to be taken with an FFD of 24.0 in., what should the new exposure time be so that the second x-ray is of the same intensity as the first?
11. If the time in a second x-ray is changed from 0.200 s to 0.350 s, what should the new FFD be if the original FFD was 30.0 cm?
12. If the time in a second x-ray is changed from 0.250 s to 0.125 s, what should the new FFD be if the original FFD was 45.0 cm?
13. If the current used to make an x-ray exposure is changed from 30.0 mA for 3.00 s to 200 mA, what should the new exposure time be to maintain the same intensity?
14. The current used to make an x-ray exposure was changed from 20.0 mA for 1.00 s to 40.0 mA. What should the new exposure time be to maintain the same intensity?

15. An x-ray is taken at a distance of 6.00 ft using a current of 10.0 mA. What should the current setting be changed to if the distance is increased to 8.00 ft?

16. An x-ray is taken at a distance of 4.25 ft using a current of 5.00 mA. What should the current setting be changed to if the distance is increased to 6.00 ft?

17. If it is decided to change the exposure time of an x-ray from 2.00 s to 0.500 s, what should the current setting be if it was originally planned to be 50.0 mA?

18. It has been decided to change the exposure time of an x-ray from 1.50 s to 0.500 s. What should the current setting be if it was originally planned to be 12.0 mA?

19. Using an FFD of 80.0 cm, a technician found the biparietal diameter of an unborn child's head to be 10.2 cm on the film. If the OFD for this exposure was 16.0 cm, what is the actual biparietal diameter of the child's head?

20. Using an FFD of 65.0 cm, a technician found the biparietal diameter of an unborn child's head to be 9.25 cm on the x-ray film. If the OFD for this exposure was 25.0 cm, what is the actual biparietal diameter of the child's head?

21. A doctor determines that a certain pregnant woman may have difficulty with the delivery of the child if the child's biparietal diameter exceeds 9.00 cm. At the full term of her pregnancy, x-rays are taken and the baby's biparietal diameter is measured to be 10.5 cm. In the same x-ray, a measuring rod whose length is known to be 10.0 cm is seen to have a length of 12.6 cm on the x-ray film. Should the doctor prepare for complications in the delivery?

22. An OB-GYN has decided that a certain woman may have trouble having a normal delivery if her baby's biparietal diameter exceeds 8.8 cm. On an x-ray taken with an FFD of 100.0 cm and on OFD of 25.0 cm, the biparietal diameter is measured to be 11.6 cm. Will this woman have difficulty in delivery?

23. The image of the biparietal diameter of an unborn child measures 11.5 cm on the x-ray film. A 10.0-cm measuring rod on the same x-ray film measures 13.5 cm. What is the actual biparietal diameter of the child's head?

24. Using an FFD of 90.0 cm, an x-ray technician measured the biparietal diameter on the film of an unborn child's head to be 10.4 cm. If the OFD is 18.0 cm, what is the actual biparietal diameter of the baby's head?

25. Why are x-ray images usually magnified compared to the actual measurements?

SECTION 5.5 RATIOS AND PROPORTIONS RELATED TO INHALATION THERAPY

Respiratory therapists and respiratory therapy technicians work with doctors and other medical professionals to evaluate and care for patients with various lung disorders. Most respiratory therapists work in hospitals, but nursing homes and home health care agencies are employing more of these workers as demand grows.

To evaluate patients, respiratory therapists first perform limited physical examinations and conduct several types of diagnostic tests. First, to test a patient's lung capacity, the therapist will have a patient breathe into an instrument called a *spirometer* that measures the volume and flow of air during inhalation and exhalation. These results are then compared with a set of established norms and a determination is made about any lung deficiencies the patient may have. To analyze the concentration of oxygen in the patient's blood as well as levels of carbon dioxide and the pH level, therapists draw a blood sample, place it in a blood gas analyzer, and report the results to a doctor who will then recommend a treatment plan for the patient.

In a hospital, respiratory therapists may be assigned to care for patients on life support in the intensive care unit. Additionally, they may be required to set up and monitor ventilator equipment, or assist patients having chronic lung diseases with chest physiotherapy. For example, if a patient cannot breathe on his own, a therapist will connect him to a ventilator that delivers pressurized oxygen into his lungs. This is done by inserting a tube into the patient's trachea, connecting it to the ventilator, and setting the rate, volume, and oxygen concentration of the oxygen mixture entering the patient's lungs. If a patient can breathe on his own but is experiencing low oxygen levels in his blood, a therapist can increase the patient's concentration of oxygen by placing an oxygen mask, or nasal cannula, on the patient and setting the oxygen flow at the level prescribed by the physician. Patients who have mucus in their lungs resulting from the anesthesia during surgery or from chronic lung disorders such as cystic fibrosis receive rehabilitative therapy or chest physiotherapy from respiratory therapists. Therapists work with patients to try and loosen the mucus found in the lungs so that it can be expelled and patients can breathe easier. Respiratory therapists also educate patients about the proper administration of aerosol medications. Patients with breathing conditions such as asthma need to learn how to use inhalers effectively.

Your lungs and diaphragm essentially act as a pump to move air into and out of your lungs. The variables in this system include the **volume** of air involved, the **pressure** in the lungs, and the **temperature** of the air. Imagine that you have some air trapped in a container with a movable plunger—like a bicycle pump, for example. As the plunger is pushed down to "squeeze" the air, the pressure increases and the volume decreases. At the same time, the temperature of the air in the cylinder will increase. If you have ever used a bicycle pump, you may have noticed that, after being used for a time, the cylinder is warm to the touch.

Still using the bicycle pump example, you may have noticed that the air being pushed out of the pump feels cool to the touch. Similarly, you may have noticed that spray deodorant always feels cool on your skin. As the air leaves the pump or spray can, its volume rapidly increases (it spreads out), the pressure rapidly decreases, and as a result, the temperature of the air drops. These same relationships are true for lungs as well as bicycle pumps:

Pressure increases → Volume decreases → Temperature rises

Pressure decreases → Volume increases → Temperature falls

These variations in pressure, volume, and temperature may be studied separately or as a unified whole. In your chemistry or physics class, Charles' Law and Boyle's Law are used to calculate these values in specific problems. In most real-world situations, all three variables must be considered.

Pressures are measured in a variety of units, including pounds per square inch (psi), Pascals (Pa), inches of mercury (inHg), or millimeters of mercury (mmHg). Generally speaking, mmHg is used in the medical field. Volumes are also measured in one of several units, such as cubic inches (in.^{3}), cubic centimeters (cm^3 or cc), or milliliters (mL). In medical fields, milliliters (mL) are used for volumes most of the time. Only one temperature scale is used in this formula and that is the Kelvin temperature scale. (Recall from an earlier chapter that the Kelvin scale is an *absolute temperature scale* and has no negative temperature values.) If the temperature is measured on any other scale (Fahrenheit or Celsius), it must be converted to the Kelvin scale before being used in any calculation involving pressures and volumes. The following proportion combines all of these variables.

Charles' and Boyle's Laws Combined

If we let P_1 be the initial pressure, V_1 the initial volume, and T_1 the initial Kelvin temperature, and further let P_2 be the new pressure desired, V_2 the new volume, and T_2 the new Kelvin temperature, then the relationship of pressure, volume, and temperature can be stated as follows:

$$\frac{P_1 V_1}{T_1} = \frac{P_2 V_2}{T_2}$$

Note: Both T_1 and T_2 must be Kelvin temperatures. Remember, to convert a Celsius temperature to the equivalent Kelvin temperature, use the following formula:

$$T_K = T_C + 273.15$$

EXAMPLE 17: Calculating with All Six Variables—No Constants

Suppose that initially you have 1250 mL of nitrogen gas that is under a pressure of 730 mmHg and at a temperature of 18°C. If the pressure were changed to 800 mmHg and the temperature were changed to 10°C, what would the new volume be?

Solution

First, list the given information, making sure that the temperatures are in the correct scale:

Initial pressure = P_1 = 730 mm Hg
Initial volume = V_1 = 1250 mL
Initial temperature = T_1 = 18°C
New pressure = P_2 = 800 mm Hg
New volume = V_2 =?
New temperature = T_2 = 10°C

First convert the given temperatures from Celsius to Kelvin:

$$T_K = T_C + 273.15$$
$$T_1 = 18 + 273.15 = 291.15 \text{ K}$$
$$T_2 = 10 + 273.15 = 283.15 \text{ K}$$

$$\frac{P_1 V_1}{T_1} = \frac{P_2 V_2}{T_2}$$ Start with the basic formula.

$$\frac{(730 \text{ mmHg})(1250 \text{ mL})}{291.15 \text{ K}} = \frac{(800 \text{ mmHg})(V_2)}{283.15 \text{ K}}$$ Substitute known values.

$$(800)(V_2)(291.15) = (730)(1250)(283.15)$$ Cross multiply.

$$232{,}920 V_2 = 258{,}374{,}375$$ Simplify.

$$\frac{232{,}920 V_2}{232{,}920} = \frac{258{,}374{,}375}{232{,}920}$$ Use the Division Property of Equality.

$$V_2 = 1109.283736\ldots \text{ mL}$$ Simplify and round.

$$= 1109 \text{ mL}$$

Thus, the new volume will be about 1109 mL of nitrogen gas.

In some instances, not all of the quantities in the basic formula will change. For example, the pressure and volume may change slowly enough that no great temperature change occurs. It is also possible to set up situations where one of the three variables is carefully maintained at a constant value. The basic formula can be used in these situations as well by leaving the constant value out of the calculation entirely.

EXAMPLE 18: Calculating with Temperature Held Constant

If you have 150 mL of oxygen at a pressure of 750 mmHg, what would the volume be if the pressure were changed to 200 mmHg? (Assume that the temperature is constant.)

Solution

First list the given information:

P_1 = 750 mmHg	P_2 = 200 mmHg
V_1 = 150 mL	V_2 = ?
T is constant here.	

When we write down the formula for this situation, we will just ignore the portion that deals with temperature, since it is constant.

$$P_1 V_1 = P_2 V_2$$

$(750 \text{ mmHg})(150 \text{ mL}) = (200 \text{ mmHg})(V_2)$	Substitute known values.
$112500 = 200 V_2$	Simplify.
$\dfrac{112500}{200} = \dfrac{200 V_2}{200}$	Use the Division Property of Equality.
$562.5 \text{ mL} = V_2$	Simplify.

So the new volume will be about 563 mL of oxygen.

PRACTICE PROBLEM SET 5.5

1. As the pressure of a confined gas is increased, the volume occupied by the gas _____.

2. As the temperature of a confined gas increases, the volume occupied by the gas _____.

3. Pressure and volume are _____ (directly or inversely) related.

4. Pressure and temperature are _____ (directly or inversely) related.

5. If 250.0 mL is the volume of gas under a pressure of 800.0 mmHg, what would the volume be if the pressure were changed to 500.0 mmHg (assume that the temperature is held constant)?

6. If 325 mL is the volume of a container of oxygen at a pressure of 725 mmHg, what would the volume be if the pressure were increased to 950.0 mmHg?

7. When the pressure is 225 mmHg, the volume of a certain container of nitrogen is 165 mL. If the volume were to change to 325 mL, what would the pressure be?

8. If 345 mL of gas is under a pressure of 125 mmHg, then what would the pressure need to be to decrease the volume by one-third?

9. If a confined gas has a temperature of 25.0°C at a pressure of 800.0 mmHg, what will the pressure be if the temperature is raised to 60.0°C (assume that the volume is unchanged)?

10. If the pressure on a confined gas is 255 mmHg at a temperature of 15.0°C, what would the pressure be if the temperature were lowered to 0.0°C?

11. The pressure on a confined gas started out at 285 mmHg, at which point the temperature of the gas was 22.0°C. If the pressure were to be changed to 315 mmHg, what would the Celsius temperature be then?

12. A confined gas starts out at a temperature of 20.0°C and a pressure of 455 mmHg. If the pressure were to drop to 375 mmHg, what would the Celsius temperature be then?

13. If a gas occupies a volume of 125 mL at a temperature of 30.0°C, what temperature would be required to increase the volume to 500.0 mL (assume that the pressure is unchanged in this process)?

14. If 425 mL of nitrogen, originally at a temperature of 20.0°C, were rapidly squeezed so that the volume were to decrease by one-eighth, what would the temperature change to?

15. If some nitrogen occupies a volume of 285 mL when its temperature is 25.0°C, what would its volume be if the temperature were changed to −10.0°C?

16. Some oxygen occupies 500.0 mL when its temperature is 40.0°C. If you wished to decrease the volume by 100.0 mL, to what temperature Celsius would you need to lower the gas?

17. A quantity of helium occupies 2.50 L at a temperature of 18.0°C and is at a pressure of 760 mmHg. What would the new pressure be if the temperature was changed to 37.0°C and the volume lowered to 2.00 L?

18. A volume of 425 mL of oxygen is at a temperature of 15.0°C and a pressure of 125 mmHg. If the volume was increased to 475 mL and the temperature decreased to 12.0°C, what would the pressure be then?

19. Originally, $P = 415$ mmHg, $T = 15.0$°C, and $V = 25.0$ mL. If the pressure were changed to 455 mmHg, and the temperature increased to 20.0°C, what would the volume be?

20. To begin with, some oxygen is stored at a pressure of 55.0 mmHg and a temperature of 22.0°C and has a volume of 1.00 L. If the gas were to have its pressure changed to 25.0 mmHg and its temperature increased to 30.0°C, what would the volume change to?

21. Originally, $P = 115$ mmHg, $T = -25.0$°C, and $V = 185$ mL. If the pressure is changed to 75.0 mmHg and the volume were changed to 95.0 mL, what would the temperature Celsius be?

22. A volume of 250.0 mL of nitrogen is stored at a pressure of 750.0 mmHg and a temperature of 18.0°C. If the volume were reduced by half and the pressure were doubled, what would the Celsius temperature be then?

SECTION 5.6   RATIOS AND PROPORTIONS IN PREPARATION OF SOLUTIONS

In this section we will discuss the basics of solution preparation. While it is true that most solutions used in medical applications are prepared in the pharmacy by a trained pharmacist, nurses and other health and lab practitioners need to understand the concepts and basic preparation of solutions. This is especially true for allied health workers in home care circumstances.

A **solution** can be defined as a mixture of two or more substances. The substance that is dissolved to make the solution is called the **solute** and the substance that dissolves it is known as the **solvent**. Pharmacy workers and most lab technicians will call a solvent **diluent** (pronounced "DIL-u-ent"). Drugs are manufactured and distributed in pure and in diluted forms. The diluted forms generally have the pure drug (the solute) dissolved in or mixed with sterile water or normal saline (the solvent).

It is important to know or to be able to measure the concentration (strength) of solutions involving drugs and dosages. The **concentration** or **strength** of a solution is defined to be the amount of one substance in a solution relative to the amounts of the other substances in a solution. Concentration values are generally given in a ratio, such as grams per milliliter (g/mL); milligrams per deciliter (mg/dL); in fractional form, such as 1:2 or $\frac{1}{2}$ (both of which are read as "1-to-2" not "one-half"); part-to-part, or as a percent. There are several other concentration units used by chemists but these are not commonly used in allied health applications and will not be discussed here.

The use of the term **part-to-part** gives the relationships of substances in a solution without specifying particular units of measure. For example, mix 1 part A with 2 parts B could mean to mix 1 mL A with 2 mL B or 10 g A with 20 g B.

A concentration expressed as a **percent** is defined as the number of parts of solute per 100 parts of solution. Pure drugs from which solutions are to be made may be in either solid or liquid form to begin with. Generally, the final solution will be in liquid form that results from the mixing of a liquid drug and a liquid solvent or the dissolving of a solid drug in a liquid solvent. It is important to know what form the various parts of a solution were originally. Look at the following percents expressed as ratios of parts:

$$5\%\,^{W/V} = \frac{5\text{ g}}{100\text{ mL}} \qquad 5\%\,^{V/V} = \frac{5\text{ mL}}{100\text{ mL}} \qquad 5\%\,^{W/W} = \frac{5\text{ g}}{100\text{ g}}$$

Note the "tags" on the percent symbols. The **W/V** tag indicates that the original drug was a solid and was weighed out in grams and the solvent used was a liquid. The **V/V** tag indicates that the original drug and the solvent are both liquids. The **W/W** tag indicates that the drug and its solvent are both solids. Solid pills, such as aspirin tablets are manufactured with a specific number of grams of acetylsalicylic acid mixed with a certain number of grams of cornstarch to make the tablets. We will not work any problems using the **W/W** designation.

These ratios can be used to calculate the parts needed to make a particular volume of solution whose concentration is stated as a %. It is important to note that the denominator in these ratios represents the total volume of the final solution, so that 5% $^{W/V}$ means 5 g solute in 100 mL total solution.

In Chapter 1, we reviewed percents and looked at expressions of concentration (strength) in percent form. Remember, if the parts that comprise the solution are known, the percent (%) concentration can be easily calculated. The following examples give two methods for determining the percent concentration. Use the one that makes sense to you.

EXAMPLE 19: A Percent V/V (volume-to-volume) Solution—Ratio/Proportion Method

A solution contains 15 mL of alcohol in 250 mL of solution. What is the percent concentration of the alcohol?

Solution

Change to % using ratio/proportion:

$$x\% ^{V/V} = \frac{x}{100 \text{ mL}} = \frac{15 \text{ mL}}{250 \text{ mL}} \quad \text{Set up the proportion.}$$

$$250x = 1500 \qquad\qquad\quad \text{Cross-multiply.}$$

$$x = \frac{1500}{250} \qquad\qquad\quad \text{Use the Division Property of Equality.}$$

$$x = 6 \text{ mL} \qquad\qquad\quad \text{Simplify.}$$

The concentration of the solution is then $\dfrac{6 \text{ mL}}{100 \text{ mL}} = 6\% ^{V/V}$ alcohol.

EXAMPLE 20: A Percent V/V (volume-to-volume) Solution—Decimal Percent Method

A solution contains 15 mL of alcohol in 250 mL of solution. What is the percent concentration of the alcohol?

Solution

$$\frac{15 \text{ mL}}{250 \text{ mL}} = 15 \div 250 = 0.06 \qquad \text{Change ratio to a decimal.}$$

$$0.06 \times 100 = 6\% \qquad \text{Change the decimal to a percent.}$$

The concentration of the solution is 6% $^{V/V}$ alcohol, just as in Example 19.

As you start to solve applied problems with drugs, solutions, and dosages, you will use many of the techniques of dealing with percents that you reviewed in Chapter 2 of this text. You may wish to refer to that chapter if you are having trouble with percents here. It is also important that you know whether the original drug is a solid, to be measured in grams, or a liquid, to be measured in milliliters.

Making Solutions with Pure Stock Supplies

To solve applied problems involving the preparation of solutions, we will set up a *proportion*. One ratio will reflect the concentration that we desire to make, and the other will be the ratio of the original drug compared to the total volume we wish to make.

EXAMPLE 21: Preparing a Solution from a Pure Stock

How many grams of sodium chloride (NaCl, or common table salt) would be needed to make 250 mL of 15% sodium chloride solution?

Solution

Since NaCl is in dry form it will be measured in grams and the 15% should have a tag of W/V.

First, rewrite the desired percent concentration as a fraction with proper units as follows:

$$15\% \, ^{W/V} = \frac{15 \text{ g}}{100 \text{ mL}}$$

Now set up a proportion with the desired concentration (15%) as one fraction and the actual amount you want to make as the other fraction:

$$\frac{15 \text{ g}}{100 \text{ mL}} = \frac{x}{250 \text{ mL}} \qquad \text{Set up the proportion.}$$

$$100x = (15)(250) \qquad \text{Cross-multiply.}$$

$$100x = 3750 \qquad \text{Simplify.}$$

$$\frac{100x}{100} = \frac{3750}{100} \qquad \text{Use the Division Property of Equality.}$$

$$x = 37.5 \text{ g} \qquad \text{Simpify.}$$

Thus if you weigh out 37.5 g of sodium chloride and mix it with sterilized water until the total amount is equal to 250 mL, you will have made 250 mL of 15% salt solution, as required.

EXAMPLE 22: Making a Urinary Antiseptic Solution

You are asked to make 2 L of 2% urinary tract antiseptic solution using Neosporin tablets that contain 5.0 g of Neosporin each.

Solution

First note that the Neosporin is in dry form. A 2% solution would then contain 2 g of Neosporin in each 100 mL of solution that you make. Here you must find out how many grams of Neosporin will be required and then convert that into the number of 5-g tablets needed.

Convert the desired percent concentration into a fraction as part of your proportion:

$$2\% \, ^{W/V} = \frac{2 \text{ g}}{100 \text{ mL}}$$

Since we normally use milliliters in our proportions, convert the 2 L to 2000 mL. Set up the proportion with the desired concentration (2%) as one fraction and the amount you need to make as the other:

$$\frac{2 \text{ g}}{100 \text{ mL}} = \frac{x}{2000 \text{ mL}} \qquad \text{Set up the proportion.}$$

$$100x = (2)(2000) \qquad \text{Cross-multiply.}$$

$$100x = 4000 \qquad \text{Simplify.}$$

$$\frac{100x}{100} = \frac{4000}{100} \qquad \text{Use the Division Property of Equality.}$$

$$x = 40 \text{ g of Neosporin are needed.} \qquad \text{Simplify.}$$

Now figure out how many tablets you need:

$$\frac{1 \text{ tablet}}{5 \text{ g}} = \frac{x}{40 \text{ g}} \qquad \text{Set up the proportion.}$$

$$5x = (1)(40) \qquad \text{Cross-multiply.}$$

$$5x = 40 \qquad \text{Simplify.}$$

$$\frac{5x}{5} = \frac{40}{5} \qquad \text{Use the Divison Property of Equality.}$$

$$x = 8 \text{ tablets} \qquad \text{Simplify.}$$

Thus you need to dissolve 8 of the 5-g Neosporin tablets in enough sterilized water to make 2000 mL (2 L) of solution.

Making Solutions with Diluted Stock Supplies

Another common task related to solutions is the further dilution of solutions that have already been prepared in advance. If an order is written for a solution and you find some in stock that is diluted (not pure) but is more concentrated (stronger) than you need, you can simply dilute it to get the concentration that you need. However, if only weaker solutions are available, then you will need to make an entirely new solution using the pure drug or substance, as was shown in the previous examples.

Assuming that most solutions that fall into this category are liquids, there are several ways to approach this type of dilution. One of the simplest is to set up a proportion comparing volumes and concentrations. This proportion can be turned into the following formula.

Formula for Dilution of Solutions

$$V_1 C_1 = V_2 C_2$$

To use this formula, let V_1 be the amount (volume) you would like to make and C_1 the concentration that you desire to make. Let C_2 be the concentration of the stock solution that you are starting with and V_2 the amount of stock solution that you need to measure out to start with. Be sure that both volumes are in the same units and the concentrations are also in the same units.

EXAMPLE 23: Diluting a Solution

How would you make 1 L (1000 mL) of 5% saline solution from a stock supply that is 20%?

Solution

Let V_1 and C_1 equal the volume and concentration that you wish to make. Let V_2 and C_2 be the volume and concentration of the stock supply. You need to calculate the amount of stock supply that you need to start with.

$$V_1 C_1 = V_2 C_2 \qquad \text{Basic Formula}$$

$$(1000 \text{ mL})(5\%) = (V_2)(20\%) \qquad \text{Substitute the given values.}$$

$$V_2 = \frac{(1000)(5)}{20} \qquad \text{Use the Division Property of Equality.}$$

$$V_2 = 250 \text{ mL} \qquad \text{Simplify.}$$

So, measure out 250 mL of the 20% stock solution and then add enough water to make the total volume equal 1000 mL. This will give you 1 L of 5% saline solution.

EXAMPLE 24: Diluting a Stock Solution

How would you make 250 mL of 15% saline solution starting with a stock supply that is 10%?

Solution

The short answer here is "You can't." Notice that you are asked to make a "stronger" solution from a "weaker" one. This cannot be done. To make the required solution, you would either need to start with pure sodium chloride or find a stock solution with a concentration higher than 15%.

EXAMPLE 25: Making an Eye Wash Solution

You are asked to make 500 mL of 1:10 boric acid solution from a 40% stock supply.

Solution

Here V_1 = 500 mL and C_1 = 1:10, but the stock supply concentration is given as a percent. You may either change 1:10 to a percent or change 40% to a ratio.

$$C_1 = 1{:}10 = \frac{1}{10} = 0.1 = 10\%$$

V_2 is unknown and C_2 = 40%.

$$
\begin{array}{ll}
V_1 C_1 = V_2 C_2 & \text{Basic Formula} \\
(500 \text{ mL})(10\%) = (V_2)(40\%) & \text{Substitute the given values.} \\
5000 = 40 V_2 & \text{Simplify.} \\
\dfrac{5000}{40} = \dfrac{40 V_2}{40} & \text{Use the Division Property of Equality.} \\
V_2 = 125 \text{ mL} & \text{Simplify.}
\end{array}
$$

Thus you need to measure out 125 mL of the 40% stock and add enough water to make the total volume 500 mL. This will give you 500 mL of 10% (1:10) boric acid solution.

PRACTICE PROBLEM SET 5.6

1. A solution is made up of two components, a _____ and a _____.
2. Another name for solvent is _____.
3. The directions on a box of pesticide read: "Mix 1 part bug killer to 5 parts water." How much of the concentrated bug killer should be mixed with 2.5 L of water?
4. A procedure calls for a mixture of 1 part liquid soap to 10 parts water. If you have 250 mL of water, how much soap will be needed for this mixture?
5. A solution of alcohol and water contains 225 mL of alcohol in 400 mL of solution. What is the percent concentration of the alcohol? Of the water?
6. Ringer's solution (not Lactated Ringer's) contains three salts as follows: 8.6 g NaCl, 0.33 g $CaCl_2$, and 0.3 g of KCl_2 per liter of solution. What is the percent concentration of each of these three salts?
7. If you use 25 g of NaCl to make 1 L of solution, what percent concentration have you made?
8. If you dissolve 0.75 g of KCl_2 in 1500 mL of water, what percent concentration is the solution?
9. An isopropyl alcohol solution is labeled 18% $^{V/V}$ alcohol. How many cubic centimeters of pure alcohol would be in 500 cc of this solution?
10. In 3 L of 45% $^{V/V}$ isopropyl alcohol solution, how many milliliters of alcohol are present?

11. How many milliliters of alcohol are needed to make 240 mL of 75% $^{V/V}$ alcohol solution?

12. How many cubic centimeters of acetic acid are needed to make 600 cc of 7.5% $^{V/V}$ acetic acid solution?

13. You are given 200 g of dextrose and told to make the largest volume of the 5% $^{W/V}$ that you can. How many milliliters can you make?

14. How many milliliters of 7.5% $^{W/V}$ solution can be made with 250 g of NaCl?

15. Twenty grams of NaOH (a solid) are contained in 500 mL of a solution. What is the percent concentration of this solution?

16. You have 8 g of solute. If it takes 2 g to make 20 mL of solution, then the entire 8 g will make _____mL of solution altogether, and its percent concentration will be _____%.

17. You have 3 g of sucrose ($C_{12}H_{22}O_{11}$). You need to make a 1.5% $^{W/V}$ sucrose solution. How much solution will be produced using the entire 3 g?

18. How many grams of sodium chloride are there in 2.5 L of a 0.4% $^{W/V}$ solution?

19. How many grams of salt (NaCl) would be required to make the following?

   a. 500 mL of a 15% solution
   b. 150 mL of a 5% solution
   c. 75 mL of an 8% solution

20. Give the percent concentration of the following solutions:

   a. 12 g NaCl dissolved in 2000 mL of water
   b. 1300 mg $CaCl_2$ mixed in 50 mL of water
   c. 1.6 mL of HNO_3 mixed with 0.1 L of water
   d. 20 mL of HCl + 90 mL H_2O

21. How many 0.5-g tablets of aluminum acetate are needed to make 1250 mL of 1:500 aluminum acetate solution?

22. How many 1.0-g tablets of potassium permanganate will be needed to make 5.0 L of 1:50 potassium permanganate antiseptic solution?

23. How many 5.0-g tablets of Neosporin would be needed to make 5000 mL of 1.5% $^{W/V}$ antiseptic solution?

24. How many 0.5 g tablets of aluminum acetate would you need in order to make 750 mL of 10% aluminum acetate solution (sometimes called Burrow's solution)?

25. A doctor wants you to make 75 mL of 5% tincture of iodine from pure iodine crystals. How would you do this? (A tincture is a solution in which alcohol is used as the solvent.)

26. How would you make 100 mL of 3.5% tincture of iodine?

27. You are asked to dilute 2.0 L of 25% alcohol solution to make some 10% alcohol solution. How much 10% solution can you make?

28. A certain hospital's dishes are sterilized with a 4% bleach solution. How many gallons of water must be added to 5 gal of 8% bleach to make the 4% bleach solution required?

29. A hospital pharmacist needs some 6% $^{W/V}$ dextrose for an IV. How many cubic centimeters of pure sterilized water should be added to 500 cc of the 10% $^{W/V}$ stock to make the required solution?

30. How would you make 500 mL of 5% $^{V/V}$ alcohol solution from a 25% stock?

31. How much 15% saline solution can be made from 300 mL of 8.0% stock?

32. How would you make 350 mL of 1:20 boric acid solution from some 50% stock?

SECTION 5.7   ANGLE MEASUREMENTS AND PHYSICAL THERAPY

Measuring angles is an integral part of a physical therapy assistant's job. The angles measured are those created by bones of the human body at its various joints and flexure points. Finding the range of motion that a particular patient has at a particular joint is an important task. Such angle measurements can be very useful in evaluating the function of a joint and the surrounding tissue including muscles and ligaments. The results of such measurements can be used to determine whether a person has a possible problem or not. Often, repeated measurements are made over a period of time to track the progression of degenerative conditions such as rheumatoid arthritis, or to check on the progress or lack thereof for a patient undergoing physical rehabilitation.

Measuring Angles

Angles are measured as part of a circle. A full circle is divided into 360 equal size pie slices called **degrees**. Thus one full circle equals 360°, a half-circle equals 180°, and a quarter of a circle would equal 90°. An analog clock has 12 numbers on its face. The angle between each successive number would be one-twelfth of a circle: $\frac{1}{12} \times 360° = 30°$. This is shown in Figure 5.3.

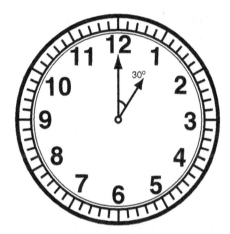

Figure 5.3 An Analog Clock

Angles are traditionally named using points on each ray (side) and the point at the corner which is called the vertex. The angle in Figure 5.4 can be named $\angle$ ABC, $\angle$ CBA, or $\angle$ B. Angles are commonly measured in degrees using a **protractor** such as the one shown in Figure 5.5. Angles that measure between 0° and 90° are called acute angles and those measuring between 90° and 180° are called obtuse angles. Right angles measure exactly 90° and straight angles measure exactly 180°.

To measure an angle using a protractor, lay the straight line at the bottom of the protractor along one side of the angle, align the center mark on the protractor with the vertex of the angle, and then read the number of degrees where the second side of the angle crosses the protractor. This is illustrated in Figure 5.6.

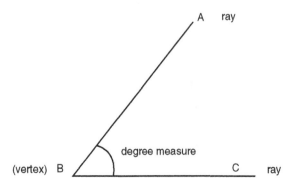

Figure 5.4

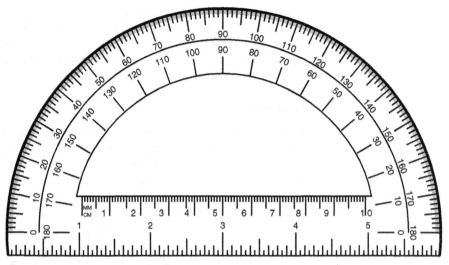

Figure 5.5 Protractor

In Figure 5.6, angle AOB is 45°, as read on the outer (clockwise) scale of the protractor. Angle AOC is 90° (called a *right* angle). Angle AOD, read on the clockwise scale, is 120°. Angle EOD, read on the inner (counterclockwise) scale is 60°. Angle AOE is 180° (called a *straight* angle). Angle EOB on the counterclockwise scale is 135°. Angle EOC is 90°.

Physical Therapy Measurements

Several methods of making measurements of joint ranges of motion are available for use by physical therapists. All have their advantages and disadvantages. Some use mechanical or electrical devices, computer animation, and other such methods. Here we will consider only one of the commonly used direct measurement methods using an

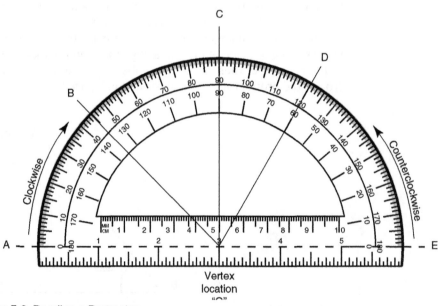

Figure 5.6 Reading a Protractor

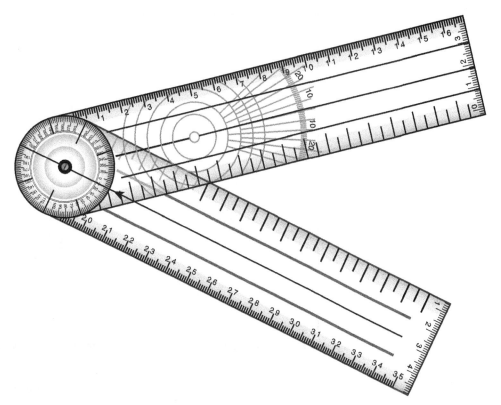

Figure 5.7 Goniometer

instrument called a **goniometer** (Figure 5.7), which is an adaptation of the common *protractor* that you may have used to measure angles in your high school geometry class. **Goniometry** is the name given to measuring the position of a particular joint and its range of motion.

The use of a goniometer is relatively straightforward. However, getting truly accurate measurements requires much practice and training in the fundamentals of muscle, bone, and joint structure and function. For example, to measure the range of motion of a hip joint, the body or fulcrum of the goniometer is placed over the hip joint, the stationary arm is placed on the side of the body above the hip joint, and the moving arm is aligned with the midline of the thigh. The patient's leg is then moved at the hip joint until it reaches its full flexure and the angle is then measured by the goniometer. This is pictured in Figure 5.8.

The result is compared with a chart showing the normal range of motion for the hip joint. Table 5.1 gives the normal number of degrees for the range of motion for some of the major joints of the body.

The table below is far from complete. Many joints are capable of several different motions. For example the ankle joint can be flexed up or down, the foot can be turned in or out, and rotated as well. Fingers can bend and flex, each by slightly differing amounts. Shoulder, hip, and elbow joints commonly rotate by various amounts. All of these motions have their own normal ranges of motion. A complete survey of all such motions is well beyond the scope of this text and will be left to your classes in physical therapy.

If extremely precise measurements are needed then radiographic techniques may be used. Generally x-rays will be taken of the joint and measurements are made directly on the pictures of the bones involved. This is not always necessary and care needs to be taken so that patients are not exposed to unnecessary radiation.

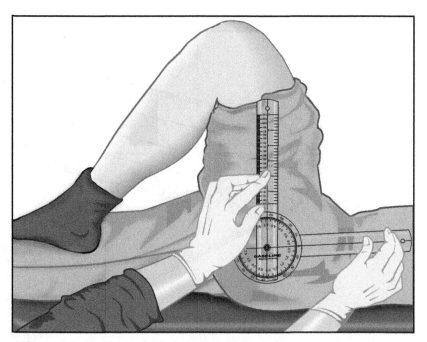

Figure 5.8 Measuring a Hip Joint's Range of Motion Using a Goniometer

Table 5.1 Normal Ranges of Motion for Joints of the Body

Joint	Flexure Range	Extension Range
Wrist	$0° - 90°$	$0° - 70°$
Elbow	$0° - 145°$	$145° - 0°$
Shoulder	$0° - 180°$	$0° - 50°$
Hip	$0° - 120°$	$0° - 15°$
Knee	$0° - 125°$	$125° - 0°$

PRACTICE PROBLEM SET 5.7

Using a protractor, measure each of the following angles to the nearest whole degree.

1.

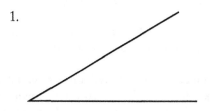

2.

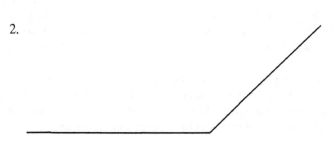

3.

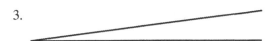

4.

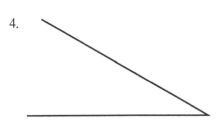

5.

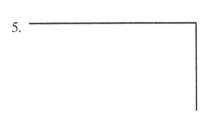

6.

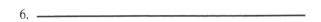

7.

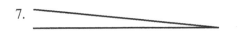

8.

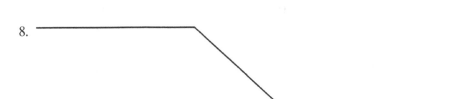

9.

10.

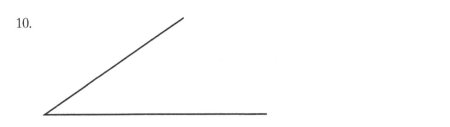

Using a protractor, draw angles of the following sizes.

11. 50°
12. 125°
13. 45°
14. 5°
15. 32°
16. 165°
17. 15°
18. 90°
19. 150°
20. 25°

If goniometers are available, measure the range of motion for several joints, knees or elbows for example, of your classmates and compare the results with Table 5.1. (Don't draw any conclusions about your results unless you are a licensed physical therapist.)

Chapter Summary

In this chapter we covered a variety of topics with applications requiring the use of ratios and proportions. It was not our intent to have you memorize a lot of formulas, terminology, drugs, or chemical formulas. Instead, we hope you will see that many apparently different areas have applied problems with very similar methods of solution. Even if you did not cover all of the sections of this chapter, you should have gotten a "taste" of several different allied health fields.

Important Terms and Formulas

concentration (strength)	pressure (mmHg or Pa)
cross-multiplication property	proportion
degrees	protractor
diluent	ratio
distance	solute
electrical current (mA)	solution
enteric (coated)	solvent
exposure time (t)	tablet
FFD	temperature
FOD	tincture
goniometer	V/V
goniometry	volume
OFD	W/V
part-to-part	W/W
percent concentration	

The cross-products of any true proportion are equal.

$$\text{If } \frac{a}{b} = \frac{c}{d}, \text{ then } ad = bc, \text{ where } b \neq 0 \text{ and } d \neq 0.$$

A Basic Dosage Calculation Formula

$$\frac{\text{Amount of "drug" in the stock}}{\text{Per volume or weight}} = \frac{\text{Amount of "drug" prescribed}}{\text{Volume or weight of stock needed}}$$

Body Surface Area Formulas

Metric Units:

$$BSA = \sqrt{\frac{\text{Weight in kg} \times \text{Height in cm}}{3600}}$$

U.S. Customary Units:

$$BSA = \sqrt{\frac{\text{Weight in lb} \times \text{Height in in.}}{3131}}$$

Note: BSA is measured in m².

Current-to-Distance Proportion

$$\frac{\text{Original mA}}{(\text{Original FFD})^2} = \frac{\text{New mA}}{(\text{New FFD})^2}$$

Time-to-Distance Proportion

$$\frac{\text{Original } t}{(\text{Original FFD})^2} = \frac{\text{New } t}{(\text{New FFD})^2}$$

Current-to-Time Proportion

$$\frac{\text{Original mA}}{\text{New } t} = \frac{\text{New mA}}{\text{Original } t}$$

Image Magnification Proportion Using Measured Distances

$$\frac{\text{Image length}}{\text{Object length}} = \frac{\text{Focus-to-film distance}}{\text{Focus-to-object distance}}$$

$$\frac{\text{Image length}}{\text{Object length}} = \frac{\text{FFD}}{\text{FOD}}$$

Note: FOD = FFD – OFD.

Image Magnification Proportion Using a Measuring Rod

$$\frac{\text{Measuring rod's image length}}{\text{Measuring rod's actual length}} = \frac{\text{Image length}}{\text{Object's length}}$$

Charles' and Boyle's Laws Combined

$$\frac{P_1 V_1}{T_1} = \frac{P_2 V_2}{T_2}$$

Note: Both T_1 and T_2 must be Kelvin temperatures.

$$T_K = T_C + 273.15$$

Formula for Dilution of Solutions

$$V_1 C_1 = V_2 C_2$$

Due to the nature of this chapter and the fact that individual sections may be covered without covering the entire chapter, the practice set is broken down by section number.

Section 5.2: Ratios and Proportions in Dosage Calculations

Find the appropriate label for the medication prescribed in Problems 1–12, and use the information on the label to answer the questions. The labels follow Problem 12.

1. A doctor orders that a patient be given 15 mg of olanzapine. How many tablets should be taken?

2. You are to give a patient a single dose of 80 mg of liquid Prozac. How many milliliters should be administered?

3. A physician orders 2 mg of trandolopril for a patient. How many tablets should be given if the label shown represents the only available supply of this drug?

4. How many grams of medication are in 5 Zithromax tablets?

5. The maintenance dosage of sulfasalazine for adults with ulcerative colitis is 2 g daily in evenly divided doses. How many tablets per day will a patient take?

6. In order to give 400 mg acyclovir to a patient, how many milliliters should you administer? How many teaspoons is this?

7. If a patient is given 10 mL Diflucan®, how many milligrams of medication were administered in that dose?

8. For a child at a weight of 9 kg, the recommended dose of cefaclor is $\frac{1}{2}$ t. How many milligrams of medication are in this dose?

9. A patient with bronchitis is prescribed 500 mg clarithromycin to be taken twice a day for 7 days. How many tablets will the patient take in one day?

10. A patient is prescribed 2 mg of Diazepam Oral Solution® twice a day. How many milliliters should this patient take for each dose?

11. To help a patient with incontinence, a doctor prescribes 4 mg of Detrol LA® to be taken once daily. How many capsules should this patient take as a daily dose?

12. If you inject 20 mL of lymphocyte immune globulin into a patient's IV, what dose in milligrams are you administering to the patient?

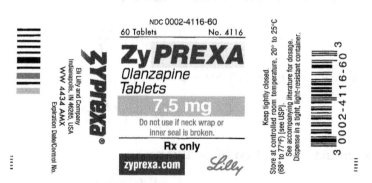

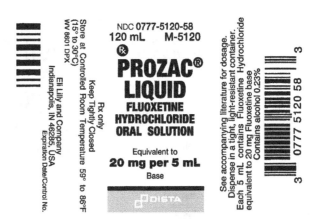

Source: Copyright Eli Lilly & Co. All rights reserved. Used with permission.

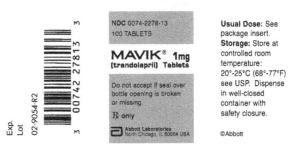

Source: Label © Abbott Laboratories. Used with permission.

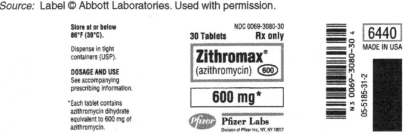

Source: Reproduced with permission of Pfizer, Inc. All rights reserved.

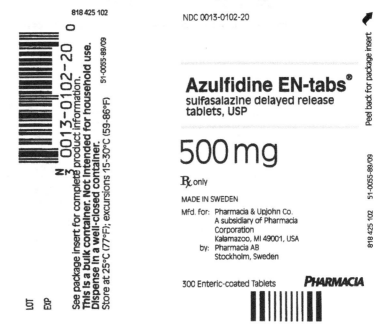

Source: Reproduced with permission of Pfizer, Inc. All rights reserved.

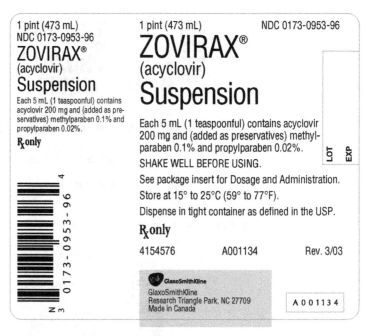

1 pint (473 mL)
NDC 0173-0953-96

ZOVIRAX®
(acyclovir)
Suspension

Each 5 mL (1 teaspoonful) contains
acyclovir 200 mg and (added as preservatives) methylparaben 0.1% and
propylparaben 0.02%.

R͟x only

1 pint (473 mL)   NDC 0173-0953-96

ZOVIRAX®
(acyclovir)

Suspension

Each 5 mL (1 teaspoonful) contains acyclovir
200 mg and (added as preservatives) methylparaben 0.1% and propylparaben 0.02%.

SHAKE WELL BEFORE USING.

See package insert for Dosage and Administration.

Store at 15° to 25°C (59° to 77°F).

Dispense in tight container as defined in the USP.

R͟x only

4154576   A001134   Rev. 3/03

gsk **GlaxoSmithKline**
GlaxoSmithKline
Research Triangle Park, NC 27709
Made in Canada

A 0 0 1 1 3 4

Source: Reproduced by permission of GlaxoSmithKline.

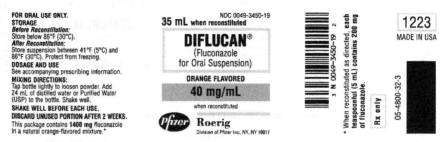

FOR ORAL USE ONLY.
STORAGE
Before Reconstitution:
Store below 86°F (30°C).
After Reconstitution:
Store suspension between 41°F (5°C) and
86°F (30°C). Protect from freezing.
DOSAGE AND USE
See accompanying prescribing information.
MIXING DIRECTIONS:
Tap bottle lightly to loosen powder. Add
24 mL of distilled water or Purified Water
(USP) to the bottle. Shake well.

SHAKE WELL BEFORE EACH USE.
DISCARD UNUSED PORTION AFTER 2 WEEKS.
This package contains **1400 mg** fluconazole
in a natural orange-flavored mixture.*

NDC 0049-3450-19
35 mL when reconstituted

DIFLUCAN®
(Fluconazole
for Oral Suspension)

ORANGE FLAVORED

40 mg/mL

when reconstituted

Pfizer **Roerig**
Division of Pfizer Inc, NY, NY 10017

* When reconstituted as directed, each
teaspoonful (5 mL) contains 200 mg
of fluconazole.

R͟x only

05-4800-32-3

1223
MADE IN USA

Source: Reproduced with permission of Pfizer, Inc. All rights reserved.

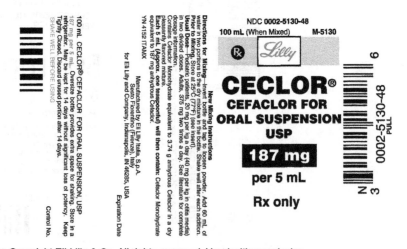

NDC 0002-5130-48
100 mL (When Mixed)   M-5130

Lilly

CECLOR®
CEFACLOR FOR
ORAL SUSPENSION
USP

187 mg

per 5 mL

Rx only

Source: Copyright Eli Lilly & Co. All rights reserved. Used with permission.

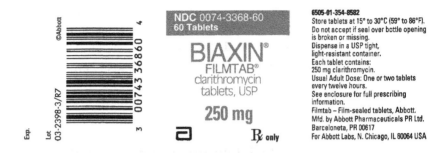

NDC 0074-3368-60
60 Tablets

BIAXIN®
FILMTAB®
clarithromycin
tablets, USP

250 mg

℞ only

6505-01-354-8582
Store tablets at 15° to 30°C (59° to 86°F).
Do not accept if seal over bottle opening
is broken or missing.
Dispense in a USP tight,
light-resistant container.
Each tablet contains:
250 mg clarithromycin.
Usual Adult Dose: One or two tablets
every twelve hours.
See enclosure for full prescribing
information.
Filmtab – Film-sealed tablets, Abbott.
Mfd. by Abbott Pharmaceuticals PR Ltd.
Barceloneta, PR 00617
For Abbott Labs, N. Chicago, IL 60064 USA

Source: Label © Abbott Laboratories. Used with permission.

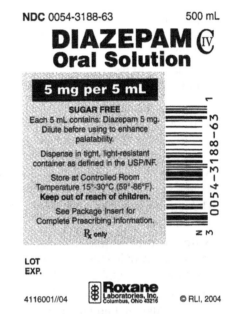

NDC 0054-3188-63   500 mL

DIAZEPAM ℞ IV
Oral Solution

5 mg per 5 mL

SUGAR FREE
Each 5 mL contains: Diazepam 5 mg.
Dilute before using to enhance
palatability.

Dispense in tight, light-resistant
container as defined in the USP/NF.

Store at Controlled Room
Temperature 15°-30°C (59°-86°F).
Keep out of reach of children.

See Package Insert for
Complete Prescribing Information.

℞ only

LOT
EXP.

4116001//04   **Roxane**
                Laboratories, Inc.
                Columbus, Ohio 43216   © RLI, 2004

Source: Label © Roxane Laboratories. Used with permission.

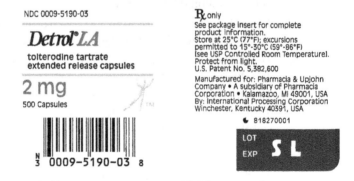

NDC 0009-5190-03

Detrol®*LA*

tolterodine tartrate
extended release capsules

2 mg
500 Capsules

3 0009-5190-03 8

℞ only
See package insert for complete
product information.
Store at 25°C (77°F); excursions
permitted to 15°-30°C (59°-86°F)
[see USP Controlled Room Temperature].
Protect from light.
U.S. Patent No. 5,382,600

Manufactured for: Pharmacia & Upjohn
Company • A subsidiary of Pharmacia
Corporation • Kalamazoo, MI 49001, USA
By: International Processing Corporation
Winchester, Kentucky 40391, USA

818270001

LOT
EXP   **S L**

Source: Reproduced with permission of Pfizer, Inc. All rights reserved.

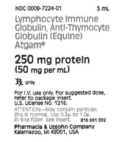

NDC 0009-7224-01   5 mL

Lymphocyte Immune
Globulin, Anti-Thymocyte
Globulin (Equine)
Atgam®

250 mg protein
(50 mg per mL)

℞ only

For I.V. use only. For suggested dose,
refer to package insert.
U.S. License No. 1216.
ATTENTION—May contain particles:
this is normal. Use 0.2μ to 1.0μ
in-line filter. See insert.   816 661 002
Pharmacia & Upjohn Company
Kalamazoo, MI 49001, USA

Source: Reproduced with permission of Pfizer, Inc. All rights reserved.

Modeling Health Applications with Ratios and Proportions   179

13. Kefzol® is given to children to treat infections. A dosage of 20 mg/lb/day is recommended. If a child weighs 40 lb, how much daily medication should he receive? If the label recommends 2 doses per day, how much medication will be contained in each dose?

14. The doctor has ordered 200 mg Amoxil® oral suspension to be given 2 times a day for a child weighing 10.2 kg. If the label states that the usual child dosage is 20 to 40 mg/kg/day, calculate the per dose dosage range. Is the amount prescribed a correct dosage?

Section 5.3: Ratios, Proportions, Formulas, and Dimensional Analysis in Multistep Dosage Calculations

15. A patient's order is 40 mg of codeine phosphate by subcutaneous injection. Available in stock is 50 mg in 1 mL of liquid for SC injection. How many milliliters will you administer?

16. A patient is to be given 25 mg of frusemide intravenously. Ten milligrams in 1 mL of liquid for IV injection is available. How many milliliters should you administer?

17. A child is prescribed 500 mg daily of Depakene (valporic acid) by his physician to help control seizures. The medication is to be taken in 2 doses per day. The stock solution available contains 250 mg in 5 mL of syrup. How many teaspoons should be given to the patient for each dose?

18. A doctor orders tetracycline elixir qid for a child weighing 55 lb at a dosage of 8 mg/kg/day in equally divided doses. How many milligrams would 1 dose contain? The tetracycline in stock is labeled 50 mg per 7 mL. How many milliliters should be administered?

19. A doctor orders quinidine for an adult patient weighing 212 lb at a dosage of 25 mg/kg/day q6h. How many milligrams should each dose contain? The stock supply of quinidine is supplied as 300-mg tablets. How many tablets should be given?

20. The doctor orders ampicillin IVPB for a child weighing 75 lb at a dosage of 20 mg/kg/day in 4 equally divided doses. How many milligrams should be given per dose? The ampicillin is supplied as 250 mg in 1.5 mL after reconstitution. How many milliliters should be administered?

21. The order is for erythromycin 2000 mg p.o. q6h for a 192-lb patient. The safe range for this medication is 30–50 mg/kg/day. Is the ordered dose safe?

22. The pediatrician prescribes Cefadyl 5 mg qid IM for a child weighing 15 kg. The label lists the recommended dosage as 1–3 mg/kg/day. Is the ordered dose safe?

23. The doctor orders garamycin 50 mg IM q6h for a child weighing 64 lb. According to the label, the recommended dose is 6–7.5 mg/kg/day in 4 equally divided doses. Garamycin is supplied as 80 mg/mL. Is the order within the safe range? How many milliliters should be administered?

24. A child with a fever is ordered Tylenol® suspension $\frac{1}{2}$ tsp p.o. q4h prn. The child weighs 33 lb. The label states that the recommended dose is 25–35 mg/kg/day q4h prn. The medication is supplied as 325 mg per 10 mL. Is the ordered dose in the safe range? If so, how many milliliters should be administered?

25. Calculate the BSA of a patient who is 72 cm tall and weighs 11.6 kg.

26. Calculate the BSA of a patient who is 115 cm tall and weighs 23.5 kg.

27. Calculate the BSA of a patient who is 5 ft. 10 in. tall and weighs 150 lb.

28. Calculate the BSA of a patient who is 6 ft. 3 in. tall and weighs 300 lb.

29. The BSA of the patient is 1.95 m². The physician ordered indinavir 275 mg/m². How many capsules would you administer if the label reads 0.25 g/capsule?

30. The recommended dosage of a particular medication is 150 mcg/m². If the patient is 148 cm tall and weighs 53 kg, how much medication should be administered?

Section 5.4: Ratios and Proportions in X-Ray Applications

31. In a given examination, the current employed by a technician was 6.00 mA, and an FFD of 30.0 in. was used. If a new exposure is to be made at a distance of 40.0 in., what current should be used in order for the second exposure to have the same intensity as the first?

32. An x-ray of a patient is taken with an FFD of 20.0 in. with an exposure time of 0.100 s. If another exposure is to be taken with an FFD of 60.0 in., what should the new exposure time be so that the second x-ray is of the same intensity as the first?

33. If the time in a second x-ray is changed from 0.100 s to 0.250 s, what should the new FFD be if the original FFD was 25.0 cm?

34. If the current used to make an x-ray exposure is changed from 20.0 mA for 2.00 s to 150 mA, what should the new exposure time be to maintain the same intensity?

35. An x-ray is taken at a distance of 8.00 ft using a current of 8.00 mA. What should the current setting be changed to if the distance is increased to 12.0 ft?

36. If it is decided to change the exposure time of an x-ray from 1.00 s to 0.500 s, what should the current setting be if it was originally planned to be 75.0 mA?

37. Using an FFD of 60.0 cm, a technician found the biparietal diameter of an unborn child's head to be 11.2 cm. If the OFD for this exposure was 20.0 cm, what is the actual biparietal diameter of the child's head?

38. A doctor determines that a certain pregnant woman may have difficulty with the delivery of the child if the child's biparietal diameter exceeds 9.25 cm. At the full term of her pregnancy, x-rays are taken and the baby's biparietal diameter is measured to be 10.0 cm. In the same x-ray, a measuring rod whose length is known to be 10.0 cm is seen to have a length of 12.6 cm on the x-ray film. Should the doctor prepare for complications in the delivery?

39. An OB-GYN has decided that a certain woman may have trouble having a normal delivery if her baby's biparietal diameter exceeds 9.00 cm. On an x-ray taken with an FFD of 100.0 cm and an OFD of 25.0 cm, the biparietal diameter is measured to be 10.6 cm. Will this woman have difficulty in delivery?

Section 5.5: Ratios and Proportions Related to Inhalation Therapy

40. If 300.0 mL is the volume of gas under a pressure of 800.0 mmHg, what would the volume be if the pressure were changed to 400.0 mmHg?

41. When the pressure is 250 mmHg, the volume of a certain container of nitrogen is 200 mL. If the volume were to change to 325 mL, what would the pressure be?

42. If a confined gas has a temperature of 20.0°C at a pressure of 740.0 mmHg, what will the pressure be if the temperature is raised to 30.0°C?

43. The pressure on a confined gas started out at 400 mmHg, at which point the temperature of the gas was 25.0°C. If the pressure were to be changed to 300 mmHg, what would the Celsius temperature be then?

44. If a gas occupies a volume of 225 mL at a temperature of 35.0°C, what temperature would be required to increase the volume to 300.0 mL?

45. If some nitrogen occupies a volume of 450 mL when its temperature is 22.0°C, what would its volume be if the temperature were changed to –15.0°C?

46. A quantity of helium occupies 5.50 L at a temperature of 28.0°C and at a pressure of 760 mmHg. What would the new pressure be if the temperature was changed to 30.0°C and the volume lowered to 4.00 L?

47. A volume of 525 mL of oxygen is at a temperature of 45.0°C and a pressure of 125 mmHg. If the volume was increased to 275 mL and the temperature decreased to 12.0°C, what would the pressure be then?

48. A volume of 450.0 mL of nitrogen is stored at a pressure of 760.0 mmHg and a temperature of 15.0°C. If the volume were reduced by half and the pressure were doubled, what would the Celsius temperature be then?

Section 5.6: Ratios and Proportions in Preparation of Solutions

49. A solution of alcohol and water contains 300 mL of alcohol in 750 mL of solution. What is the percent concentration of the alcohol? Of the water?

50. If you use 20 g of NaCl to make 1.5 L of solution, what percent concentration have you made?

51. An isopropyl alcohol solution is labeled 20% $^{V/V}$ alcohol. How many cubic centimeters of pure alcohol would be in 750 cc of this solution?

52. How many milliliters of alcohol are needed to make 500 mL of 50% $^{V/V}$ alcohol solution?

53. You are given 250 g of dextrose and told to make the largest possible volume of the 10% $^{W/V}$ solution that you can. How many milliliters can you make?

54. Twenty-five grams of NaOH (a solid) are contained in 750 mL of a solution. What is the percent concentration of this solution?

55. You have 30 g of sucrose ($C_{12}H_{22}O_{11}$). You need to make a 2.5% $^{W/V}$ sucrose solution. How much solution will be produced using the entire 30 g?

56. How many grams of sodium chloride are there in 3.0 L of a 0.8% $^{W/V}$ solution?

57. How many 0.5-g tablets of aluminum acetate are needed to make 1500 mL of 1:250 aluminum acetate solution?

58. How many 5.0-g tablets of Neosporin would be needed to make 3.0 L of 2.0% $^{W/V}$ antiseptic solution?

59. How would you make 250 mL of 2.5% tincture of iodine?

60. You are asked to dilute 1.5 L of 40% alcohol solution to make some 10% alcohol solution. How much 10% solution can you make?

61. A hospital pharmacist needs some 4% $^{W/V}$ dextrose for an IV. How many cubic centimeters of pure sterilized water should be added to 250 cc of the 10% $^{W/V}$ stock to make the required solution?

62. How would you make 750 mL of 4% $^{V/V}$ alcohol solution from a 40% stock?

63. How would you make 550 mL of 1:30 boric acid solution from some 75% stock?

64. A doctor tells a patient to soak her feet in a 4% solution of Epsom salts. Your job is to tell the patient how many tablespoons of Epsom salts need to be dissolved in a gallon of water to make the 4% solution. What do you tell her?

Section 5.7: Angle Measurements and Physical Therapy

Using a protractor, measure each of the following angles to the nearest whole degree.

65.

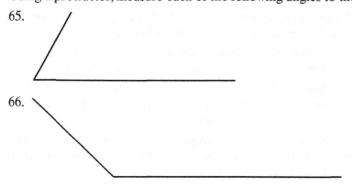

66.

67.

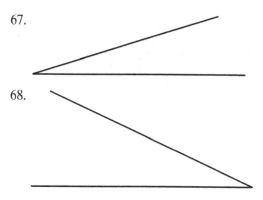

68.

Using a protractor, draw angles of the following sizes.

69. 75°

70. 40°

71. 145°

72. 170°

Chapter Test

Find the appropriate label for the medication prescribed in Problems 1, 2, and 4, and use the information on the label to answer the questions.

1. You are to give a patient 40 mg of liquid Prozac. How many milliliters should you give the patient? How many teaspoons is this?

2. A physician orders 500 mg of erythromycin for a patient. How many tablets should be given if the label included here represents the only available supply of this drug? May these tablets be split or crushed? Why or why not?

3. If a patient is given 18 mL of codeine phosphate, how many milligrams of medication were given if the supply is labeled "15mg per 5 mL" ?

4. If you administer 15 cc of Diflucan® to a patient, what dose of medication in milligrams will he receive?

5. Kefzol® is given to children to treat infections. A dosage of 15 mg/lb/day is recommended. If a child weighs 38 lb, how much daily medication shoulds she receive? If the

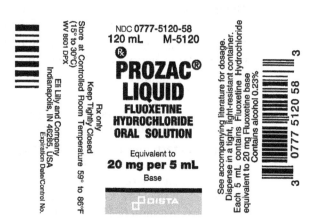

Modeling Health Applications with Ratios and Proportions

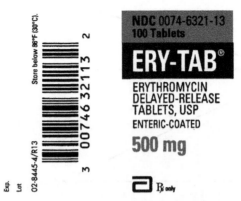

Source: Label © Abbott Laboratories. Used with permission.

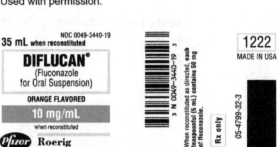

Source: Reproduced with permission of Pfizer, Inc. All rights reserved.

label recommends 2 doses per day, how much medication will be contained in each dose?

6. A patient's order is 40 mg of codeine phosphate by subcutaneous injection. Available in stock is 50 mg in 1 mL of liquid for SC injection. How many milliliters will you administer?

7. A doctor orders tetracycline elixir qid for a child weighing 44 lb at a dosage of 8 mg/kg/day in equally divided doses. How many milligrams would 1 dose contain? The tetracycline in stock is labeled 50 mg per 5 mL. How many milliliters should be administered?

8. For a child with a fever Tylenol® suspension 0.5 tsp p.o. q4h prn is ordered. The child weighs 33 lb. The label states that the recommended dose is 25–35 mg/kg/day. The medication is supplied as 325 mg per 10 mL. Is the ordered dose in the safe range? If so, how many milliliters should be administered?

9. Calculate the BSA of a patient who is 5 ft 8 in. and weighs 166 lb.

10. The BSA of the patient is 1.82 m². The physician ordered indinavir 275 mg/m². How many capsules would you administer if the label reads 0.25 g/capsule?

11. In a given examination, the current employed by a technician was 4.00 mA and an FFD of 30.0 in. was used. If a new exposure is to be made at a distance of 50.0 in., what current should be used in order for the second exposure to have the same intensity as the first?

12. If the current used to make an x-ray exposure is changed from 10.0 mA for 2.00 s to 50 mA, what should the new exposure time be to maintain the same intensity?

13. A doctor determines that a certain pregnant woman may have difficulty with the delivery of the child if the child's biparietal diameter exceeds 9.00 cm. At the full term of her pregnancy, x-rays are taken and the baby's biparietal diameter is measured to be 9.55 cm. In the same x-ray, a measuring rod whose length is known to be 10.0 cm is seen to have a length of 11.6 cm on the x-ray film. Should the doctor prepare for complications in the delivery?

14. When the pressure is 350 mmHg, the volume of a certain container of nitrogen is 200 mL. If the volume were to change to 225 mL, what would the pressure be?

15. If a confined gas has a temperature of 20.0°C at a pressure of 840.0 mmHg, what will the pressure be if the temperature is raised to 25.0°C?

16. A quantity of helium occupies 4.50 L at a temperature of 20.0°C and is at a pressure of 760 mmHg. What would the new pressure be if the temperature was changed to 35.0°C and the volume lowered to 3.75 L?

17. A solution of alcohol and water contains 250 mL of alcohol in 750 mL of solution. What is the percent concentration of the alcohol? Of the water?

18. If you use 15 g of NaCl to make 1.5 L of solution, what percent concentration have you made?

19. You are given 200 g of dextrose and told to make all of the 10%$^{W/V}$ solution that you can. How many milliliters can you make?

20. Twenty grams of NaOH (a solid) are contained in 750 mL of a solution. What is the percent concentration of this solution?

21. You are asked to dilute 1.0 L of 45% alcohol solution to make some 15% alcohol solution. How much 10% solution can you make?

22. A hospital pharmacist needs some 4%$^{W/V}$ dextrose for an IV. How many cubic centimeters of pure sterilized water should be added to 300 cc of the 5%$^{W/V}$ stock to make the required solution?

23. How would you make 1 L of 4%$^{V/V}$ alcohol solution from a 40% stock?

24. How would you make 550 mL of 1:40 boric acid solution from some 50% stock?

25. How would you make 450 mL of 15.0%$^{V/V}$ alcohol solution from a stock supply that is 10%$^{V/V}$?

26. What is the size of this angle?

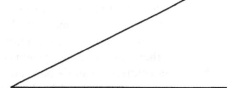

27. What is the size of this angle?

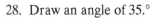

28. Draw an angle of 35.°

6

CALCULATIONS FOR BASIC IV THERAPY

Objectives for Chapter 6

After completing this chapter, the student will be able to:

1. Identify the abbreviations used for IV fluid orders and charting.

2. Calculate percentages in IV fluids.

3. Calculate IV flow rates and infusion times.

SECTION 6.1 INTRODUCTION TO IV FLUIDS

Doctors often order fluids and medications to be delivered to a patient intravenously during medical treatment. **Intravenous**, abbreviated IV, means through the veins. IV therapy is used to provide the patient with specific medications or additional fluid, nutrients, electrolytes, or minerals. There are estimated to be more than 200 different IV fluids manufactured today, and there are many additives that are used in combination with these fluids. This chapter will introduce you to some of the basic terms related to IV therapy and associated calculations.

Intravenous fluids are introduced into a patient's vein using a hollow needle called a **catheter** and a tubing system called an **administration set**. The tubing of the administration set connects to an IV bag and is hung on an IV stand. The enlarged part of the administration set is called a **drip chamber** that allows the nurse to count the number of drops per minute of fluid being infused. The chamber is filled with fluid to an indicator line to assist in counting the drops per minute. The chamber will be about half full. If it is too full, you cannot see the drops as they fall and if it is not full enough, there is a danger of air entering the tube during infusion. Just below the drip chamber is a **roller clamp** that allows changing the number of drops per minute by increasing or decreasing the pressure on the tubing. An **injection port** will also be located on the tubing. The port allows direct administration of medications into the line or the attachment of a second IV bag. See Figure 6.1.

IV fluids are prepared in volumes from 50 mL to 1000 mL. The most commonly used sizes are 500 mL and 1000 mL. Each bag is labeled with the complete name of the fluid and the exact amount of each component of the fluid. Most orders are written using abbreviations. It is important to understand what these letters and numbers represent. In IV fluids, **D** represents **dextrose**, **W** identifies **water**, **S** refers to **saline**, **NS** represents **normal saline**, and the numbers identify percent concentrations. Here are some examples of orders for commonly used fluids and their meanings:

- D5W, 5% D/W, and D5% W all represent orders for a 5% dextrose solution.

- 0.9% NS or 0.9NS represent orders for a 0.9% normal saline solution.

- 5% D 0.45% NS represents a solution that contains both 5% dextrose and 0.45% normal saline.

- **Ringer's Lactate (RL)** or **Lactated Ringer's Solution (LRS)** is a balanced electrolyte solution.

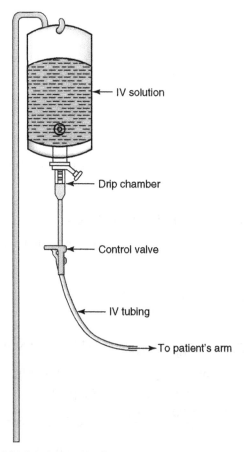

Figure 6.1 Gravity-Fed IV Administration Set

Other combinations of dextrose, saline, and Ringer's Lactate may be ordered and are interpreted in the same manner. For example, a D/5/RL is a fluid containing 5% dextrose and Ringer's Lactate. More complete information about IV fluids and their administration can be found in nursing and pharmacology textbooks.

Calculating Percentages in IV Fluids

The actual amount of each ingredient in IV fluid can be calculated with the same technique used for other medication dosages. You will not need to do this calculation often because the exact amounts of ingredients are listed on each bag of fluid in fine print under the name of the solution. However, understanding what the percents indicate will help you be aware of the amounts of saline, dextrose, and electrolytes a patient is receiving. The IV flow rate covered in the next section is vitally important to ensure that patients are receiving the desired amount of these ingredients during the prescribed time frame.

EXAMPLE 1: Concentration of IV Fluids

Determine the exact amount of dextrose in an order for 1000 mL of D20W.

Solution

The solution D20W is 20% dextrose in water so $20\% = \dfrac{20 \text{ g dextrose}}{100 \text{ mL solution}}$.

$$\frac{20 \text{ g dextrose}}{100 \text{ mL solution}} = \frac{x}{1000 \text{ mL}}$$ Set up a proportion.

$$20(1000) = 100x$$ Cross-multiply.

$$20{,}000 = 100x$$ Simplify.

$$\frac{20{,}000}{100} = \frac{100x}{100}$$ Use the Division Property of Equality.

$$200 = x$$ Simplify.

Therefore, there are 200 grams of dextrose in 1000 mL of D20W solution.

EXAMPLE 2: Concentration of IV Fluids

Determine the exact amount of dextrose and NaCl in an order for 500 mL 5% D/$\frac{1}{2}$S.

Solution

a. Dextrose: $5\% \text{D} = \dfrac{5 \text{ g dextrose}}{100 \text{ mL solution}}$

$$\frac{5 \text{ g dextrose}}{100 \text{ mL solution}} = \frac{x}{500 \text{mL}}$$ Set up a proportion.

$$5(500) = 100x$$ Cross-multiply.

$$2500 = 100x$$ Simplify.

$$\frac{2500}{100} = \frac{100x}{100}$$ Use the Division Property of Equality.

$$25 \text{ g} = x$$ Simplify.

Therefore, there are 25 grams of dextrose in 500 mL of this solution.

b. Salt: $\frac{1}{2}$S represents half strength saline. Normal saline has a concentration of 0.9%, so find the percent concentration by multiplying $\frac{1}{2}(0.9\%) = 0.45\%$.

$$0.45\% \text{NS} = \frac{0.45 \text{g NaCl}}{100 \text{ mL solution}}$$

$$\frac{0.45 \text{ g NaCl}}{100 \text{ mL solution}} = \frac{x}{500 \text{ mL}}$$ Set up a proportion.

$$0.45(500) = 100x$$ Cross-multiply.

$$225 = 100x$$ Simplify.

$$\frac{225}{100} = \frac{100x}{100}$$ Use the Division Property of Equality.

$$2.25 \text{ g} = x$$ Simplify.

Therefore, there are 2.25 g of NACl in 500 mL of this solution.

PRACTICE PROBLEM SET 6.1

Interpret the components and their concentrations for each of the following IV fluid orders in problems 1–10.

1. D/5/RL

2. 5% DNS

3. D5 0.22S

4. D5 $\frac{1}{2}$ NS

5. $2\frac{1}{2}$% D/W

6. RLS

7. D5 .9NS

8. 0.9% NS

9. D20W

10. D/5/0.45% NS

11. Determine the amount of dextrose in 500 mL 5% DW.

12. Determine the amount of dextrose in 1000 mL D5W.

13. Determine the amount of dextrose in 500 mL D20W.

14. Determine the amount of dextrose in 750 mL D10W.

15. Determine the amount of NaCl in 1000 mL 0.9% NS.

16. Determine the amount of NaCl in 850 mL 0.45% NS.

17. Determine the amount of dextrose and NaCl in 250 mL D5 0.22S.

18. Determine the amount of dextrose and NaCl in 750 mL D5 $\frac{1}{2}$ NS.

19. Determine the amount of dextrose and NaCl in 500 mL D/5/0.45% NS.

20. Determine the amount of dextrose and NaCl in 1000 mL D5 $\frac{1}{4}$ NS.

21. Determine the amount of dextrose in 1500 mL D5RL.

22. Determine the amount of dextrose in 500 mL D5RL.

SECTION 6.2   IV FLOW RATE CALCULATIONS

The rate of infusion of intravenous solutions is controlled by an electronic pump (Figure 6.2) or by gravity-fed hand controls. If an electronic pump is being used, the desired rate of infusion is set electronically. Pumps allow for a precise amount of fluid to be delivered over a period of time, and if there is an interruption of the flow, an alarm will sound alerting the nursing staff. However, if you are using a gravity-fed infusion set, you will need to calculate the **drip rate**, which is the rate at which fluid drips from the IV bag into the intravenous line. Intravenous fluids are most frequently ordered as mL/hr. Examples of orders would be 1000mL/6hr, 1200mL/16hr, or 125mL/hr.

The volume over time for a gravity-fed infusion set is controlled by adjusting the flow rate of the IV, which is counted in drops per minute, or **gtt/min**. The size of the drops is regulated by the size of the IV tubing. Not all tubings are the same size and therefore the size of drops will vary. IV tubings are calibrated in gtt/mL, called a **drop factor**, and this ratio will be needed for the calculation of the flow rate.

An IV solution set will be labeled with the number of drops that equal 1 mL. Be sure to look for this information when setting up any IV for a patient. Some common drop factors include: 10-, 12-, 15- and 20-drop sets. These sets are called **macrodrip sets**. In a 15-drop set, for example, the tubes are calibrated so that 15 drops = 1 mL. A **microdrip set** is used if there is a need to limit the volume of fluid infused. For example, a microdrip set would probably be used for a pediatric patient. The drop factor for any tubing calibrated in microdrips is 60μgtt = 1 mL (60 microdrips = 1 mL).

In order to determine how to adjust the drip set to administer the required amount of fluid over the prescribed time, we will use a mathematical formula. You will need three pieces of information for this calculation: the total volume to be infused in mL, the time (in minutes) ordered for the infusion, and the drip set of the IV bag being used.

Calculating Flow Rate in Drops/Minute (gtt/min)

$$\text{gtt/min} = \frac{\text{Volume to be infused} \times \text{Drip set}}{\text{Time (in min)}}$$

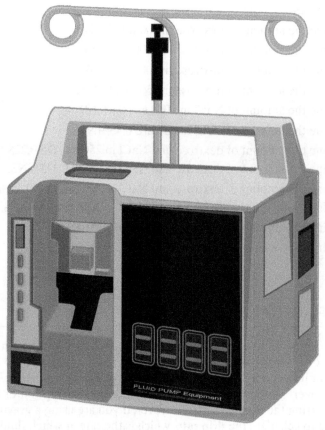

Figure 6.2 IV Fluid Pump

EXAMPLE 3: Calculating Flow Rate with a Formula

A doctor orders an IV infusion of D5W 1000 mL to infuse over the next 8 hours. The IV tubing that you are using delivers 20 gtt/min. What is the correct rate of flow?

Solution

We will first convert 8 hours to minutes by multiplying $8 \times 60 = 480$ min.

Next, substitute into the formula.

$$\text{gtt/min} = \frac{\text{Volume to be infused} \times \text{Drip set}}{\text{Time (in min)}}$$

$$\text{gtt/min} = \frac{1000 \text{ mL} \times 20 \text{ gtt/min}}{480 \text{ min}}$$

$$\text{gtt/min} = \frac{20{,}000}{480} = 41.667 = 42 \text{ gtt/min}$$

Flow rates are usually rounded off. Answers within 1 to 2 drops per minute are considered correct.

EXAMPLE 4: Calculating Flow Rates with a Formula

The physician orders 1000 cc NS from 6 A.M. to 6 P.M. The IV tubing delivers 15 gtt/min. Calculate the flow rate for this IV.

Solution

The orders from 6 A.M. to 6 P.M. cover 12 hours. Convert this time to minutes first.

$$12 \text{ hr} \times 60 \text{ min/hr} = 720 \text{ minutes}$$

Remember that 1000 cc = 1000 mL. Now use the formula to find the flow rate.

$$\text{gtt/min} = \frac{\text{Volume to be infused} \times \text{Drip set}}{\text{Time (in min)}}$$

$$\text{gtt/min} = \frac{1000 \text{ mL} \times 15 \text{ gtt/min}}{720 \text{ min}}$$

$$\text{gtt/min} = \frac{15,000}{720} = 20.8333 = 21 \text{ gtt/min}$$

Therefore, the flow rate for this IV is 21 drops per minute.

Once the flow rate has been calculated, it is regulated by counting the number of drops falling in the drip chamber during 15-second intervals. The roller clamp will be used to adjust the rate of the flow to the desired drops/minute. In Example 2, the required flow rate was 42 gtt/min. To calculate the number of drops in 15 seconds, we divide this number by 4 (15 seconds is $\frac{1}{4}$ minute). Therefore, $42 \div 4 = 10.5$, meaning you should adjust the flow rate to approximately 10–11 drops/15 s.

Another method of calculating flow rates is by using dimensional analysis. Follow these three steps. Set up the ratio of the volume/hour, multiply times the ratio of hours to minutes, finally multiply times the drop factor in drops/mL. This process is demonstrated in Example 5.

EXAMPLE 5: Calculating Flow Rates with Dimensional Analysis

The doctor's orders are for 2500 mL fluid to be infused in 24 hr. The IV set is calibrated at 10 gtt/mL. Calculate the flow rate for this IV.

Solution

Set up the following problem:

$$\frac{\text{Volume}}{\text{hr}} \times \frac{1 \text{ hr}}{60 \text{ min}} \times \frac{\text{Drops}}{\text{mL}} = \frac{2500 \text{ mL}}{24 \text{ hr}} \times \frac{1 \text{ hr}}{60 \text{ min}} \times \frac{10 \text{ gtt}}{1 \text{ mL}}$$

$$= \frac{25000}{1440} = 17.36 = 17 \text{ gtt/min}$$

The flow rate for this IV is 17 drops per minute.

Some IV infusions are prescribed based on a patient's body weight. For example, a doctor's order might state 0.005 mg/kg/min. This means that each minute the patient should receive 0.005 mg (5 mcg) of the drug for every kilogram of weight. The calculations involved in computing the correct flow rate based on body weight are illustrated in Example 6.

EXAMPLE 6: Calculating a Flow Rate Based on Body Weight in Drops/Minute

A doctor orders 500 mg medication in an IV infusion of 500 mL D5W, 0.006 mg/kg/min. The patient's weight is 180 lb. The drop rate is 20 gtt/min. Calculate the correct flow rate.

Solution

Since our medication is based on kilograms, we must first convert 180 lb to kg.

Remember that 1 kg = 2.2 lb, so

$$180 \text{ lb} \times \frac{1 \text{ kg}}{2.2 \text{ lb}} = \frac{180}{2.2} = 81.8 \approx 82 \text{ kg}$$

The order is 0.006 mg/kg/min, drop rate is 20 gtt/min, and there are 500 mg of medication in the 500-mL solution. Use this series of conversions as follows:

$$82 \text{ kg} \times \frac{0.006 \text{ mg}}{\text{kg} \times \text{min}} \times \frac{500 \text{ mL}}{500 \text{ mg}} \times \frac{20 \text{ gtt}}{1 \text{ mL}} = 9.6 \approx 10 \text{ gtt/min}$$

Therefore, the correct flow rate is 10 drops per minute.

If an infusion pump is used for an IV, you will need to calculate the flow rate in mL/hr. For example, if a doctor orders an IV of 500 mL fluid to be infused over 4 hours, you can calculate the flow rate by dividing 500 mL by 4 hr or $\frac{500 \text{ mL}}{4 \text{ hr}} = 125$ mL/hr. If the dosage is based on weight, you will need to set up a series of conversions, as demonstrated in Example 7.

EXAMPLE 7: Calculating a Flow Rate Based on Body Weight in mL/hr

A doctor orders 500 mg medication in an IV infusion of 500 mL D5W, 0.006 mg/kg/min. The patient's weight is 180 lb. Calculate the correct flow rate in mL/hr.

Solution

Using the conversion in Example 6, we know that 180 lb ≈ 82 kg.

Use this series of conversions to calculate the flow rate in mL/hr.

$$82 \text{ kg} \times \frac{500 \text{ mL}}{500 \text{ mg}} \times \frac{0.006 \text{ mg}}{\text{kg} \times \text{min}} \times \frac{60 \text{ min}}{1 \text{ hr}} = 29.52 \approx 30 \text{ mL/hr}$$

PRACTICE PROBLEM SET 6.2

1. The 15-second count of an IV flow rate is 8 gtt. A 33 gtt/min rate is required. Is this rate correct?

2. The 15-second count of an IV flow rate is 6 gtt. A 31 gtt/min rate is required. Is this rate correct?

3. You are to regulate an IV to deliver a flow rate of 45 gtt/min. Using the 15-second count, how would you set the flow rate?

4. How many drops will you count in 15 seconds if the flow rate is to be set at 50 gtt/min?

5. If the flow rate is calculated to be 17 gtt/min, how would you set the flow rate using the 15-second rule?

6. An IV is to run at 21 gtt/min. What should the drop rate be for a 15-second interval?

7. The doctor orders 1500 mL of Lactated Ringer's Solution to be administered intravenously over the next 12 hours. The IV tubing delivers 15 gtt/mL. Calculate the correct flow rate.

8. The doctor orders an IV infusion of D5W 1000 mL to infuse over the next 8 hours. The IV tubing delivers 15 gtt/mL. What is the correct flow rate?

9. An injured patient has an order to start D5NS 1000 mL at 30 mL/hr. The IV tubing has a calibration of 20 gtt/mL. What is the correct flow rate?

10. The doctor's orders are for an IV infusion of 100 mL of D5$\frac{1}{2}$NS with 40 MEq of KCl over the next hour. The set calibration is 15 gtt/mL. What is the correct flow rate?

11. You need to administer 500 mL NS over the next 2 hours. The set calibration is 15 gtt/mL. What is the correct flow rate?

12. The orders are to administer 350 mL of Lactated Ringer's Solution over the next 1.5 hours. The set calibration is 12 gtt/mL. What is the correct flow rate?

13. You need to administer an IV of 250 mL over 3 hours. The tubing delivers 15 gtt/mL. What is the correct flow rate?

14. You need to administer an IV of 75 mL over the next hour. The set is calibrated at 15 gtt/mL. What is the correct flow rate?

15. An IV of 2000 mL is to infuse in 10 hours. The tubing delivers 20 gtt/mL. What is the correct flow rate?

16. An IV of 3000 mL is to infuse in the next 24 hours. The tubing delivers 15 gtt/mL. What is the correct flow rate?

17. The doctor orders 250 mL 0.9% NS to be infused over a 4-hour period. The drop factor is 60 μgtt/mL. Calculate the correct flow rate.

18. The doctor orders 250 mL D5W to be infused over an 8-hour period. The drop factor is 60 μgtt/mL. What is the correct flow rate?

19. A physician orders 3 L of 5% dextrose and Lactated Ringer's Solution to be infused over the next 24 hours. The tubing delivers 10 gtt/mL. What is the correct flow rate?

20. A physician orders 875 mL of 5% D/W to be infused over 6 hours. The drop factor is 10 gtt/mL. What is the correct flow rate?

21. The patient is to receive 1000 mL of IV fluid over the next 8 hours. What flow rate in mL/hr would you set on an infusion pump?

22. The patient is to receive 500 mL of IV fluid over the next 3 hours. What flow rate in mL/hr would you set on an infusion pump?

23. The patient is to receive 100 mL of IV fluid over the next 30 minutes. What flow rate in mL/hr would you set on an infusion pump?

24. The patient is to receive 125 mL of IV fluid over the next 30 minutes. What flow rate in mL/hr would you set on an infusion pump?

25. A doctor orders 250 mg medication in an IV infusion of 500 mL D5W, 0.008 mg/kg/min. The patient's weight is 150 lb. The drop rate is 10 gtt/mL. Calculate the correct flow rate.

26. A doctor orders 500 mg lidocaine in an IV infusion of 500 mL D5W, 0.020 mg/kg/min. The patient's weight is 176 lb. The drop rate is 15 gtt/mL. Calculate the correct flow rate.

27. Calculate the flow rate in Problem 25 in mL/hr.

28. Calculate the flow rate in Problem 26 in mL/hr.

29. The patient's order states that 250 mg of medication should be added to 500 mL D5W to be given at a rate of 10 micrograms per kilogram per minute IV. What is the flow rate in mL/hr if the patient weighs 80 kg?

30. A doctor orders acyclovir sodium 5 mg/kg/hr. You are to add 500 mg (10 mL) to 100 mL D5W. If the patient weighs 180 lb, calculate the flow rate in mL/hr.

SECTION 6.3   CALCULATION OF INFUSION TIMES

The **infusion time** is the total amount of time required for a particular volume of fluid to infuse intravenously. Infusion times may be in minutes, hours, or days, depending on the treatment required by the patient's needs. Three factors will affect total infusion time: the drip rate, the total volume to be infused, and the drop factor or calibration of the set. Knowing the infusion time will allowing nursing staff to have the next solution prepared and ready to hang once the present bag has been completely infused.

The basic infusion time formula will compare the total volume to be infused with the rate of infusion. The first formula uses an infusion rate in mL/hr. The second formula expands this basic formula to use an infusion rate based on drops per minute (gtt/min).

Infusion Rate Formulas

$$\text{I. Infusion time} = \frac{\text{Total volume to infuse}}{\text{mL/hr being infused}}$$

$$\text{II. Infusion time} = \frac{\text{Total volume to infuse}}{\dfrac{\text{Flow rate in gtt/min}}{\text{Drop factor}} \times 60\dfrac{\text{min}}{\text{hr}}}$$

or

$$\text{Total volume to infuse} \div \left(\frac{\text{Flow rate in gtt/min}}{\text{Drop factor}} \times 60\frac{\text{min}}{\text{hr}} \right)$$

The information provided in each situation will determine the formula that you use. Examine how the formulas are used in each problem demonstrated in Examples 8–11.

EXAMPLE 8: Infusion Times Using mL/hr

An IV of 500 mL D5W is to infuse at a rate of 75 mL/hr. What is the infusion time for this IV?

Solution

Based on the information provided, use Formula I.

$$\text{I. Infusion time} = \frac{\text{Total volume to infuse}}{\text{mL/hr being infused}}$$

$$\text{Infusion time} = \frac{500 \text{ mL}}{75 \text{ mL/hr}} = 6.666\ldots \text{ hr}$$

Since $0.666\ldots = \frac{2}{3}$ hr, find the number of minutes by multiplying

$$\frac{2}{3}\text{ hr} \cdot 60 \text{ min/hr} = 40 \text{ min}$$

Therefore, the total infusion time is 6 hr 40 min.

EXAMPLE 9: Calculating the Time an Infusion Is Complete

An IV was started at 11 A.M. The medication order is 150 mL to infuse at a rate of 80 mL/hr. At what time will the infusion be complete?

Solution

Based on the information provided, use Formula I.

$$\text{I. Infusion time} = \frac{\text{Total volume to infuse}}{\text{mL/hr being infused}}$$

$$\text{Infusion time} = \frac{150 \text{ mL}}{80 \text{ mL/hr}} = 1.875 \text{ hr}$$

To calculate the number of minutes equal to 0.875 hr, multiply:

$$0.875 \text{ hr} \cdot 60 \text{ min/hr} = 52.5 \approx 53 \text{ min}$$

Therefore, the total infusion time is 1 h 53 min and the completion time is

$$11{:}00 \text{ A.M.} + 1 \text{ hr } 53 \text{ min} = 12{:}53 \text{ P.M.}$$

EXAMPLE 10: Calculating Infusion Time from Drops/Minute

A patient is given an IV of 500 mL D5W. The flow rate is 25 gtt/min and the set calibration (drop factor) is 15 gtt/mL. How long will it take this infusion to finish?

Solution

Based on the information provided, use Formula II.

$$\text{II. Infusion time} = \frac{\text{Total volume to infuse}}{\dfrac{\text{Flow rate in gtt/min}}{\text{Drop factor or set calibration}} \times 60\dfrac{\text{min}}{\text{hr}}}$$

$$\text{Infusion time} = \frac{500 \text{ mL}}{\dfrac{25 \text{ gtt/min}}{15 \text{ gtt/mL}} \times 60\dfrac{\text{min}}{\text{hr}}}$$

$$\text{Infusion time} = \frac{500 \text{ mL}}{100 \text{ mL/hr}} = 5.00 \text{ hr}$$

Therefore, the total infusion time is 5 hours.

EXAMPLE 11: Calculating Infusion Times from Drops per Minute

The doctor orders 750 mL D5RL to be given to a patient. The flow rate is 12 gtt/min and the drop factor (set calibration) is 10 gtt/mL. If the IV is started at 8:30 A.M., what time will the infusion be complete?

Solution

Based on the information provided, use Formula II.

$$\text{II. Infusion time} = \frac{\text{Total volume to infuse}}{\dfrac{\text{Flow rate in gtt/min}}{\text{Drop factor or set calibration}} \times 60\dfrac{\text{min}}{\text{hr}}}$$

$$\text{Infusion time} = \frac{750 \text{ mL}}{\dfrac{12 \text{ gtt/min}}{10 \text{ gtt/mL}} \times 60\dfrac{\text{min}}{\text{hr}}}$$

$$\text{Infusion time} = \frac{750 \text{ mL}}{72 \text{ mL/hr}} = 10.417 \text{ hr}$$

Convert 0.417 hr to minutes by multiplying:

$$0.417 \text{ hr} \cdot 60 \text{ min/hr} = 25.02 \approx 25 \text{ min}$$

Therefore, the infusion time is 10 hr 25 min and the completion time will be

$$8{:}30 \text{ A.M.} + 10 \text{ hr } 25 \text{ min} = 6{:}55 \text{ P.M.}$$

IV flow rate calculation and monitoring is an important part of patient care. Remember that changing a patient's position after an IV has been initiated may alter slightly the rate of flow, causing the infusion to run ahead of schedule or behind schedule. If this occurs, you may need to use the formulas in this chapter to recalculate the flow rate using the volume and time remaining. However, the ability of the patient to tolerate an increased rate of infusion and the type of fluid or medication involved must both be assessed before adjustments are made. Some hospitals have specific policies to follow when adjustments need to be made and you should be familiar with these policies before any changes are made.

PRACTICE PROBLEM SET 6.3

1. The doctor orders 25 mL medication to be added to 250 mL D5W and infused at a rate of 11 mL/hr. How long will it take for this infusion to be complete?

2. A doctor orders an infusion of 1000 mL of hyperalimentation at 80 mL/hr. How long will it take for this IV to infuse?

3. There are 150 mL left in an IV that is infusing at a rate of 25 mL/hr. How much longer will it take to complete this infusion?

4. A doctor orders an infusion of 250 mL of packed red blood cells at a rate of 20 mL/hr. How long will this infusion take?

5. A doctor ordered an IV containing morphine sulphate for a patient's pain. The volume of the IV was 300 mL and the flow rate was 60 mL/hr. If the IV was begun at 10 P.M., what time was the infusion completed?

6. An IV of 1000 mL of 0.45% NS is started at 7 A.M. If the flow rate is 42 mL/hr, at what time will the infusion be complete?

7. At 10:30 A.M., you note that there are 270 mL of fluid remaining in an IV. If the flow rate is 30 mL/hr, at what time will the infusion be complete?

8. An IV of 1000 mL of D5W is started at 8:15 P.M. If the order is for 125 mL/hr, at what time will the infusion be complete?

9. The order is for 1000 mL D5W to run at 100 mL/hr and the IV is hung at 12 P.M. How long will this IV last and when will the next bag need to be hung?

10. The order is for 500 mL NS to run at 60 mL/hr and the IV is hung at 2 P.M. How long will this IV last and when will the next bag need to be hung?

11. The doctor orders an IV for an infant of 25 mL of solution. The flow rate is 25 gtt/min using a microdrip set calibrated at 60 μgtt/mL. Calculate the infusion time for this IV.

12. An IV bag of D5W has 300 mL of solution remaining in the bag. If it is infusing at a rate of 20 gtt/min and the set calibration is 12 gtt/mL, how long will it take to complete this infusion?

13. The doctor orders an IV of 1000 mL 5% D/0.9% NS that is infusing at 25 gtt/min with a set calibration of 10 gtt/mL. How long will it take to complete this infusion?

14. A medication is added to 200 mL D5W resulting in a total volume of 232 mL to be infused. The flow rate is 116 gtt/min using a microdrip set calibrated at 60 µgtt/mL. How long will it take for this IV to infuse completely?

15. An infusion of 500 mL of Lactated Ringer's Solution was started at 2 P.M. The flow rate is 25 gtt/min and the set calibration is 15 gtt/mL. At what time will this infusion be complete?

16. A patient has an IV of 1000 mL of 5% D/W which is started at 3:30 P.M. The flow rate is 36 gtt/min and the drop factor is 10 gtt/mL. At what time will this infusion be complete?

17. There is 150 mL of fluid left in a patient's IV bag. The flow rate is 15 gtt/min and the set calibration is 10 gtt/mL. If the current time is 3:45 P.M., at what time will the infusion be completed?

18. A person is to receive 500 mL of blood. The drop factor is 10 gtt/mL and the flow rate is 21 gtt/min. If the IV was started at 11:30 A.M., what time should the infusion be completed?

19. A child is to receive 500 mL of IV fluid. The set calibration is 60 µgtt/mL and the flow rate is 75 µgtt/min. If the IV was started at 2:30 P.M., at what time will the infusion be complete?

20. A doctor orders 3000 mL D5NS to be administered to a patient. The set calibration is 15 gtt/mL and the flow rate is 31 gtt/min. If the IV was hung at noon, what time will the infusion be completed?

Chapter Summary

In this chapter, we have introduced the basic mathematics involved in IV therapy. More complicated procedures and calculations, including the addition of second IV lines and intravenous medications, are covered in detail in other courses. In this chapter, we examined the calculation of flow rates in mL/hr and gtt/min. Infusion pumps operate with settings in mL/hr; gravity-fed sets require the calculation of drops per minute as counted in the drip chamber. We have also calculated infusion times in order to be prepared to hang a new bag of fluid at the appropriate time.

Important Terms and Rules

administration set	gtt/min
catheter	infusion time
D5W	injection port
dextrose (D)	intravenous
drip chamber	Lactated Ringer's Solution (LRS)
drip rate	macrodrip set
drip set	microdrip set
drop factor	microdrops

normal saline (NS)

Ringer's Lactate (RL)

roller clamp

saline (S)

water (W)

Calculating Flow Rate in Drops/Minute (gtt/min)

$$\text{gtt/min} = \frac{\text{Volume to be infused} \times \text{Drip set}}{\text{Time (in min)}}$$

Infusion Rate Formulas

$$\text{I. Infusion time} = \frac{\text{Total volume to infuse}}{\text{mL/hr being infused}}$$

$$\text{II. Infusion time} = \frac{\text{Total volume to infuse}}{\dfrac{\text{Flow rate in gtt/min}}{\text{Drop factor}} \times 60 \dfrac{\text{min}}{\text{hr}}}$$

or

$$\text{Total volume to infuse} \div \left(\frac{\text{Flow rate in gtt/min}}{\text{Drop factor}} \times 60 \frac{\text{min}}{\text{hr}} \right)$$

Chapter Review Problems

Interpret the components and their concentrations for each of the following IV fluid orders.

1. 5% D $\frac{1}{4}$ NS

2. D5RL

Calculate the amount of dextrose and the amount of salt in each solution.

3. 500 mL D5NS

4. 1000 mL D5 0.22S

5. The 15-second count of an IV flow rate is 8 gtt. A 31 gtt/min rate is required. Is this rate correct?

6. You are to regulate an IV to deliver a flow rate of 17 gtt/min. Using the 15-second count, how would you set the flow rate?

7. The order is for 800 mL NS in 4 hours. If the set calibration is 10 gtt/mL, what is the correct flow rate in gtt/min?

8. You are to administer 100 mL NS using an IV with a set calibration of 15 gtt/mL. The infusion is to be completed in 60 minutes. What is the correct flow rate in gtt/min?

9. The order is to infuse 500 mL intralipids in 6 hours. The set calibration is 10 gtt/mL. What is the correct flow rate in gtt/min?

10. A patient is to receive 1000 cc of fluid over 12 hours. The drop factor is 12 gtt/mL. What is the correct flow rate in gtt/min?

11. A person is to receive 120 mL of fluid over 50 minutes. What rate would you use to set the infusion pump to the prescribed rate?

12. The doctor orders a patient to receive 100 mL of fluid in 30 minutes. What rate would you use to set the infusion pump to the prescribed rate?

13. The doctor orders 3000 cc of fluid to be delivered. The patient is to receive 125 cc/hr. How long will it take for the fluid to infuse completely?

14. A doctor orders a medicated solution labeled 250 mg/200 mL. He prescribes 4 mcg/kg/min for a 121-lb patient. The set calibration is 60 µgtt/mL. Calculate the flow rate in drops/min for this IV.

15. The physician orders Vancocin 1 g in 150 mL of D5W over 1.5 hours. The drop factor is 60 gtt/mL. Calculate the flow rate in drops/min.

16. If the IV in Problem 15 is infused by pump, calculate the flow rate in mL/hr.

17. The physician orders Albumisol 25% in a 50-mL vial over 30 minutes. The drop factor is 10 gtt/mL. Calculate the flow rate in gtt/min.

18. If the IV in Problem 17 is infused by pump, calculate the flow rate in mL/hr.

19. A doctor orders 250 mg medication in an IV infusion of 500 mL D5W, 0.008 mg/kg/min. The patient's weight is 198 lb. Calculate the correct flow rate in mL/hr.

20. A patient weighs 165 lb. The doctor orders 250 mL 5% DW with 60 mg medication, 0.006 mg/kg/min IV. The set calibration is 20 gtt/mL. Calculate the correct flow rate for this IV in gtt/min.

21. There are 300 mL of saline remaining in a bag, which is being infused at a rate of 15 drops per minute using a set with a drop factor of 12 gtt/mL. How long will the infusion take to complete at that rate?

22. The doctor orders an IV of 2000 mL 5% D/0.9% NS that is infusing at 17 gtt/min with a set calibration of 15 gtt/mL. How long will it take to complete this infusion?

23. A medication is added to 500 mL D5W, resulting in a total volume of 550 mL to be infused. The flow rate is 116 gtt/min using a microdrip set calibrated at 60 µgtt/mL. How long will it take for this IV to infuse completely?

24. An infusion of 500 mL of Lactated Ringer's Solution was started at 1 P.M. The flow rate is 25 gtt/min and the set calibration is 10 gtt/mL. What time will this infusion be completed?

25. A patient has an IV of 1000 mL of 5% D/W, which is started at 5:30 P.M. The flow rate is 31 gtt/min and the drop factor is 12 gtt/mL. What time will this infusion be completed?

Chapter Test

1. Interpret the components and their concentrations for the following IV fluid order: D5$\frac{1}{2}$NS.

2. Calculate the amount of dextrose and the amount of salt in this solution: 500 mL D5$\frac{1}{4}$NS.

3. You are to regulate an IV to deliver a flow rate of 33 gtt/min. Using the 15-second count, how would you set the flow rate?

4. Your orders are to give a 50-cc IVPB over 30 minutes using IV tubing with a set calibration of 10 gtt/mL. How many drops per minute should this IVPB be set for?

5. You have an IV of Keflex 2 g mixed in 50 mL of D5W. To infuse the IV in 20 minutes with 15 gtt/mL tubing, what is the flow rate in drops per minute?

6. The physician orders 1000 mL of D_5W over 8 hours. The drop factor is 12 gtt/mL.

   The IV is infused by gravity. Calculate the flow rate in gtt/min.

7. The physician orders 500 mL NS over 8 hours. The IV is infused by pump. Calculate the flow rate in mL/hr.

8. A patient is to receive 1000 cc of fluid over 12 hours. What is the correct flow rate in mL/hr?

9. The physician orders 2500 mL of D5 0.45NS over 24 hours. The drop factor is 15 gtt/mL. If the IV is infused by gravity, calculate the flow rate in gtt/min.

10. Assume the IV in Problem 9 is infused by pump. Calculate the flow rate in mL/hr.

11. A doctor orders a medicated solution labeled 250 mg/500 mL. He prescribes 5 mcg/kg/min for a 132-lb patient. The set calibration is 60 µgtt/mL. Calculate the flow rate in drops/min for this IV.

12. A doctor orders 200 mg medication in 250 mL D5W to be given at 0.012 mg/kg/min. The patient weighs 121 lb. How many mL/hr will the patient receive?

13. An IV of 1000 mL 5%D/0.9%NS is infusing at 17 gtt/min with a set calibration of 10 gtt/mL. How long will it take to complete this infusion?

14. A medication is added to 250 mL D5W, resulting in a total volume of 350 mL to be infused. The flow rate is 31 gtt/min using a macrodrip set calibrated at 15 gtt/mL. How long will it take for this IV to infuse completely?

15. An infusion of 1500 mL of Lactated Ringer's Solution was started at 10:15 A.M. The flow rate is 17 gtt/min and the set calibration is 10 gtt/mL. What time will this infusion be completed?

THE BASICS OF STATISTICS

Objectives for Chapter 7

After completing this chapter, the student should be able to:

1. Define the terms related to basic statistics, such as data, population, sample, average, normal curve, and outlier.

2. Calculate the value of the mean, median, midrange, and mode of a set of data.

3. Gather data and create appropriate graphs, such as line graphs and bar graphs, to display that data.

4. Read and interpret various types of graphs including pie charts.

5. Interpret the meaning of the range, standard deviation, and the coefficient of variation in applied situations.

6. Use the normal curve and empirical rule to understand control charts.

SECTION 7.1 INTRODUCTION TO STATISTICS

Data collection and statistics are an important part of the allied health field. Keeping patient records of intake and output, medications administered, and inventory on hand are all examples of data collection. In some professions, charting results and interpreting graphs may also be required. In this chapter, we will examine some of the uses of statistical methods in health care professions. The chapter is not intended to be a complete course in statistics; it will just introduce the topic and explore some of the fundamentals. We will cover the basics of data collection, presentation of data, and analysis of data. New terminology will be introduced, but even though the words may be unfamiliar, their meanings are usually fairly simple.

Statistics is the area of mathematics that is involved with the collection, summary, classification, and presentation of data. We are surrounded by data. Researchers in medicine collect volumes of data when field-testing new medications. Lab technicians use quality control techniques to ensure that the results being published by their lab are accurate. Medical assistants and nursing assistants collect data on patients and record results in their charts on a regular basis. A fundamental knowledge of statistics will allow you to deal with data in an honest and skillful manner. It will also help you to look objectively and critically at someone else's presentation of data and form your own conclusions if, as a health care worker, you need to read and understand reports and articles containing various health-related statistics. All of us must become good consumers of data in this modern world.

Statistics can be divided into two general categories, descriptive statistics and inferential statistics. **Descriptive statistics** summarizes data in a clear and understandable way with tables or graphs or with summary statistics such as averages and standard deviations. All the numerical information, such as temperatures recorded during a person's hospital stay could be classified as descriptive data.

While descriptive statistics has been around for centuries, inferential statistics is a twentieth-century development. **Inferential statistics** involves drawing conclusions about a population based on the information collected from a sample selected from that population. The sample data should be carefully chosen from the target population; results from the sample can then be used to generalize to the population. For example, when researchers are testing a new medication for female heart patients, it would be impossible to find all female heart patients to participate in the study. Therefore, a sample of female heart patients is used to test the medication. If the medication helps this sample of women, then by inference, the researchers conclude that this medication will help all female heart patients. This reasoning is the basis for inferential statistics. It is important that the sample be a fair sample that is representative of the target population. If is does not fairly represent the target population, an incorrect statistical conclusion or inference is highly likely.

Generally speaking, **data** are numerical facts or categorical information that is collected through experimentation or research. When you are gathering information for a statistical analysis, you must be aware of how this data will be used. Two commonly used terms in statistics that relate to data collection are **sample** and **population**. A population is a complete data set; a sample is a data set that is a subset of a given population. In recording patient data, we collect all facts and data to create a population of data. Sample data are generally used when it would be difficult or impossible to gather statistics on the entire population. In most situations involving medical research, we deal with samples of data and calculate sample statistical values. The formulas and rules used by statisticians are very similar for both sample and population statistics, but there are some differences in order to allow for the fact that sample values are based on incomplete information.

Definitions

Statistics—the area of mathematics that is involved with the collection, summary, classification, and presentation of data that has been collected

Descriptive Statistics—presents information about a population of data by classifying, sorting, graphing, and summarizing it

Inferential Statistics—uses a sample of data to draw conclusions about a similar target population based on the data collected

---

The data that we collect in a statistical study can be categorized as quantitative data or as qualitative data. **Quantitative data** is a set of numbers that indicate amounts, differences, or counts. This is the easiest type of data to deal with. Patients' heights, weights, and temperatures are some examples of quantitative data. **Qualitative data** is generally words or categories that indicate observations or characteristics. The classification of your body's frame—small, medium, or large—would be an example of qualitative data.

Before beginning to analyze a set of data it is important to know which type of data you have. We cannot deal with both types of data in the same way. For example, numerical averages can be found for quantitative data but it is not possible to get a numerical average for qualitative data. Certain graphs are appropriate for qualitative data whereas other types are more appropriate for quantitative data.

Definitions

Population—a complete data set

Sample—a subset of a given population

Data—numerical facts or categorical information that is collected through research or experimentation

Qualitative Data—a set of words or categories that indicate observations or characteristics

Quantitative Data—a set of numbers that indicate amounts, differences, or counts

---

EXAMPLE 1: Quantitative versus Qualitative Data

Suppose you are preparing questions for a patient in the hospital. If you ask questions to gain information about this patient, would you expect quantitative or qualitative data as a response to each of the following questions?

Solution

a. What is your age?

The data provided here should be numbers of years and is quantitative.

b. What are your symptoms?

The data here will be the name of a symptom such as sore throat or backache. This type of data is qualitative.

c. What are your height and weight?

The patient's height and weight are numerical data indicating amounts, so they typify quantitative data.

Misleading Statistics

As you study statistical methods, you will recognize the unfortunate fact that statistics can be used to mislead as well as to inform the public. A quote from Mark Twain relates to this idea: "Facts are stubborn, but statistics are more pliable." The purpose of this section is to help you learn how to interpret results and determine the reliability of these results.

One of the most important things to remember when choosing a sample for a survey or experiment is to select a sample of sufficient size to be representative of the target population. The nature of the group that is chosen for a poll or experiment can cause inaccurate conclusions if the group is biased in some way or if the sample size is too small. For example, if 2 out of 3 dentists recommend White Tooth Toothpaste, how many dentists were surveyed, 3 or 3000? If only 3 dentists were polled, then the results cannot be generalized to the entire population of dentists.

Misleading graphs can also be used to create false conclusions. For example, bar graphs and pie charts can be drawn in such a way as to exaggerate or understate the true nature of the data. The scales of graphs can be used quite easily to exaggerate. Three-dimensional pictographs can also create the illusion of a greater difference between numbers than is actually true. Look at the graph of the data in Figure 7.1. It appears that Thrifty Savings Bank wants you to believe that its rates are twice as good as the rates at Miserly Savings Bank. By varying the increments on the horizontal axis (1%, 2%, 3%, 3.25%, 3.5%, 3.6%), the difference in the bars exaggerates the actual difference in the rates being offered at each bank.

Many polls or surveys are deliberately misleading. For example, the way a question is asked in a survey can dramatically change the results. Respondents are primed to answer

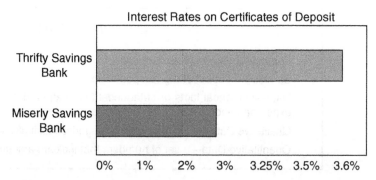

Figure 7.1 Misleading Bar Graph

the way a survey's sponsor wishes. These questions can then lead to false conclusions. Be sure to look at a copy of the questions used in a survey. Are they biased or loaded? Are they ordered in such a way as to be leading toward an agenda or conclusion? The refusal rate in a survey is also important. Be sure to determine how many people actually answered a survey. Ask who sponsored the survey. Do they have an interest in the outcome? We are likely to have different outcomes in the analysis of results if one survey on smoking is conducted by a cigarette manufacturer and another by the American Cancer Society.

Vague or ambiguous results may also confuse an issue. The word *average* is a statistical term that is used freely in general conversation, but with different interpretations. For example, a calculated average of salaries in a company will be changed greatly if Bill Gates comes to work! One very large or very small data item can greatly skew a calculated average. These extreme values are called **outliers**. The effect of outliers will be evident to those of you who have made good grades for an entire semester, only to have your calculated average ruined by one very low grade. For financial data, statisticians often use another statistic called the median because it gives a better representation of the "average" of a set of data. Remember that the average is just that—the measure of the center of the data set. There are always data items both higher than and lower than the average.

Percentages can be used to make facts seem more sensational. We know that 1 out of 1 is 100%, but this is not a large enough sample to be valid. On the other hand, you should also beware of numbers that seem too precise. We believe that if people are specific with their numbers (1,523,452 people believe the president is right), then they are stating precise facts.

Do numbers lie? Numbers are the basis of most statistical conclusions. The careless collection and use of data can sometimes lead us to false conclusions. Additionally, the intentional misinterpretation of data can be used to promote causes that may not truly be supported by the facts. When evaluating a statistical study, remember to judge the methods used to conduct the experiment for fairness, find out who conducted the survey or experiment to determine if it is a biased group, and find out how many items or individuals were in the sample. Numbers don't lie but they can be manipulated!

PRACTICE PROBLEM SET 7.1

1. Define *statistics* in your own words.

2. Explain, in your own words, the difference between inferential statistics and descriptive statistics.

3. What is a population? What is a sample?

4. What is the difference between quantitative data and qualitative data?

5. Name at least three ways that statistics can be misleading or used to create false conclusions.

6. Name at least three tasks that a health care worker does that involves statistics.

Classify each of the following as quantitative or qualitative data.

7. Your weight in kilograms
8. Your hair color
9. Your telephone number
10. Your Social Security number
11. Your current numerical average in this course
12. The letter grade you made in your English class
13. Your shoe size
14. The input and output data for a patient
15. The amount of food consumed by a patient in a 24-hour period
16. The level of pain rating on a scale of low, medium, high
17. The hourly wage earned by a CNA
18. The dosage of medication ordered by the doctor
19. The prescription number on a prescription
20. The pulse rate of a patient

For each of the following statements, tell why the stated conclusions may represent misinterpretations of the facts given.

21. The state of Arizona has the highest death rate in the United States for asthma. Therefore, people with asthma should not go to Arizona.
22. Snackwell Cookies® are fat-free. Therefore, you will not gain weight if you eat them.
23. Four out of five dermatologists recommend a new skin cream for acne. Therefore, this cream is the best topical treatment for acne.
24. Two out of three dentists surveyed recommended Whitey Toothpaste. Therefore, we should all buy Whitey Toothpaste.
25. In 2002, a survey of 8000 nurses in California found that the average annual salary was $52,500. Therefore, if I become a nurse, I will make $52,500 per year.
26. Adults average 2–5 colds per year. Therefore, if I have had 2 colds this year, I can expect to have 3 more before the year is over.
27. The majority of car accidents occur on Saturday night. Therefore, people drive carelessly on Saturday night.
28. Women are less likely to be in a car accident than men. Therefore, women are better drivers than men.
29. The new Healthwise Chips state on the package that they have no cholesterol. Therefore, you can eat as many as you want and still be healthy.
30. Orange juice contains vitamin C, and vitamin C helps prevent colds. Therefore, if I drink orange juice, I will not have colds.

SECTION 7.2   CONSTRUCTING AND INTERPRETING GRAPHS

Americans are confronted with numbers on a daily basis. Facts and figures are in almost every article or report you find in newspapers and magazines and on television. The presentation of these facts and figures is important in statistical analysis. Charts and graphs assist readers in understanding the meaning of the data collected and allow them to draw valid conclusions. Though charts are helpful organizational tools, graphs can really give a visual impact and allow the consumer to look at trends in the data. Remember, however, that graphs can be altered to make the results seem better or worse than they are. Pay attention to the scales used on the graphs to ensure the data is being fairly represented.

Line Graphs

We begin the construction of a **line graph** by drawing a horizontal axis and a vertical axis. Each axis will have equally spaced points with numbers or categories assigned to them. The horizontal axis generally represents the data categories that we are graphing. The vertical axis will be the frequency or percent frequency of each item. When axes are labeled with numbers, it is important to remember to label in equal increments. You do not have to start at 0 each time, but if you start at 100 and count by 50s, then your numbering should be consistent along the axis.

Line graphs may be useful when comparing two sets of data. Upward and downward trends are easily visible when using a line graph to display data sets. Look at the construction of the line graph in Example 2.

EXAMPLE 2: Construction of a Line Graph

Table 7.1 gives statistics from the years 1992–2002 collected by the Centers for Disease Control (CDC) that represent the infant mortality rates for children under 1 year of age.

We can use a line graph to chart the information given for comparison of the data. The years from 1992 to 2002 will be represented on the horizontal axis and we will count by 1s since there are only 11 years being displayed. The chart values go from a low of 5.8 to a high of 16.8, so to determine a scale for the vertical axis, we use these values as a reference. The number 0 is placed at the bottom of the axis and we count in increments of 5 up to a maximum value of 20. This range of label values ensures that all chart values will be represented. Each individual value from the chart is plotted on the graph and then the values are connected with lines. See Figure 7.2. It is easy to see that the trend in infant deaths has moved down during this period but the number of deaths for African-American mothers remains consistently higher than the rate for white mothers.

Table 7.1 Numbers Representing Deaths per 1000 Live Births

Year	Race of Mother: White	Race of Mother: Black of African-American
1992	6.9	16.8
1993	6.8	16.5
1994	6.6	15.8
1995	6.3	15.1
1996	6.1	14.7
1997	6.0	14.2
1998	6.0	14.3
1999	5.8	14.6
2000	5.7	14.1
2001	5.7	14.0
2002	5.8	14.4

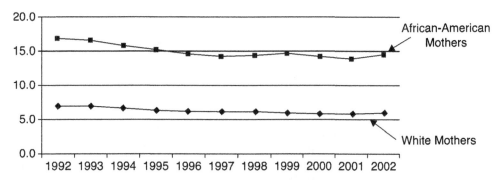

Figure 7.2 Example 2

Bar Graphs

Bar graphs display data in a form that is easy to read and use. Data that might otherwise be difficult to analyze in a table is easily analyzed when viewing a bar graph. Newspapers, reports, and magazines have bar graphs in almost every issue to display statistics of some type. A bar graph can be horizontal or vertical. A bar graph with bars representing several subcategories in one category may be called a double bar graph. See Figures 7.3 and 7.4.

It is easy to see from the graph in Figure 7.3 that the adjusted death rate for women with coronary heart disease in 2000 was lower than that of men. The different-color bars also allow you to subdivide the population by race so that the graph gives information about race and gender at the same time. The horizontal graph in Figure 7.4 gives the age-adjusted death rates for heart failure by gender and country for the year 1999. The United States ranked seventh highest for heart failure mortality in females and ninth highest for males. Remember to pay attention to the scale on any bar graph to make sure that the picture represents the data fairly. The width or height of bars can be easily manipulated to exaggerate differences.

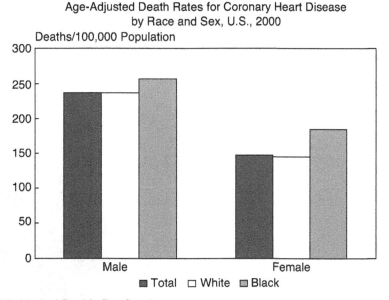

Figure 7.3 Vertical Double Bar Graph
(*Source: 2002 Chart Book*, National Institute of Health)

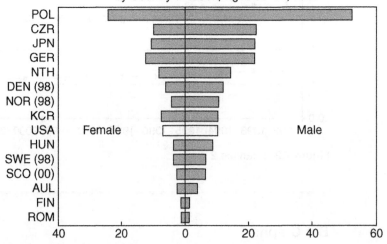

Figure 7.4 Horizontal Bar Graph

(*Source: 2002 Chart Book*, National Institute of Health)

Circle Graphs

Circle graphs or **pie charts** are a very popular method of displaying data that is in percent form. The total of the percents represented in the graph must always equal 100%. To draw a circle graph, we use a protractor and the fact that the number of degrees in a circle is 360°. By using the percents for the problem, we can calculate the number of degrees that should be in each angle of the pieces of pie in the chart. For example, if we are trying to represent 20% of the pie chart as a particular category, multiply $20\%(360°) = (0.2)(360) = 72°$. Draw a circle and, using the center of the circle as the vertex of the angle, draw a 72° angle, extending the sides of the angle to intersect the circle. See Figure 7.5. This "piece of pie" represents 20% of the circle.

Few of us will be required to construct a pie graph and if we are required to do so, it is likely that we would use software to assist us. However, most of us will be required to

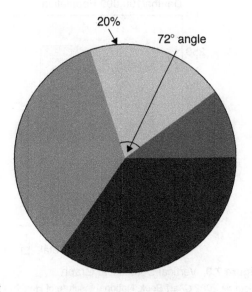

Figure 7.5 Pie Chart

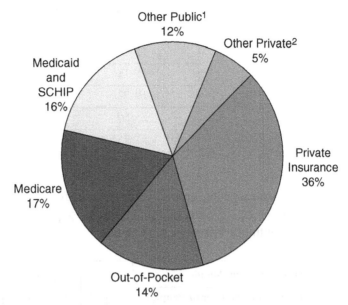

Figure 7.6 Example 3

(*Source*: Centers for Medicare & Medicaid Services, Office of the Actuary, National Health Statistics Group.)

read and understand the material presented in various pie charts. Examine the problem in Example 3.

EXAMPLE 3: Where the Nation's Health Dollar Came from in 2003

The graph in Figure 7.6 was published by the Centers for Medicare and Medicaid Services on their Web site. It illustrates the different sources of funds paid for health care in the United States in the year 2003. If \$15,450,000 was spent on health care in Beaufort County in 2003, based on this circle graph, how much was paid for by private insurance? by Medicare?

Solution

a. Private insurance represents 36% of the funds.

$36\% (\$15,450,000) = (0.36)(15,450,000) = \$5,562,000$

b. Medicare represents 17% of the funds.

$17\% (\$15,450,000) = (0.17)(15,450,000) = \$2,626,500$

Therefore, in Beaufort County, private insurance paid approximately \$5,562,000 for health care in 2003 and Medicare paid approximately \$2,626,500.

PRACTICE PROBLEM SET 7.2

1. Construct a line graph to represent the following information.

---

[1] "Other Public" includes programs such as workers' compensation, public health activity, Department of Defense, Department of Veterans Affairs, Indian Health Service, and state and local hospital subsidies and school health.

[2] "Other Private" includes industrial in-plant, privately funded construction, and nonpatient revenues, including philanthropy.

Daily Calories Needed to Maintain Weight for Females at These Age Intervals.

11–14	2200 calories
15–18	2100 calories
19–22	2050 calories
23–50	2000 calories
51–75	1800 calories
75+	1500 calories

2. Construct a line graph to represent the following information.

   This table contains the weight loss by 50 patrons at a weight-loss clinic after one month of a new workout program.

Weight Loss in Pounds	0	1	2	3	4	5	6	7	8	9	10
Frequency (Number of People)	2	3	3	5	2	8	5	6	2	9	5

3. Many of the states in the northeastern part of the United States have minimum wage laws that set the minimum wage in their states higher than the current U.S. minimum wage of $5.15. Use the following table to construct a line graph illustrating the minimum wages in each of these states.

State	New York	Maine	Rhode Island	Delaware	Massachusetts	Vermont
Minimum Wage	$6.75	$6.35	$6.75	$6.15	$6.75	$7.00

(*Source*: U.S. Department of Labor, Employment Standards Administration Wage and Hour Division.)

4. Construct a line graph to represent the following information.

Influenza Vaccination Among Adults 65 and Over in the U.S., 1997–2002

Year	Percent
1997	63.5
1998	63.6
1999	65.9
2000	64.5
2001	63.1
2002	65.8

(*Source*: Centers for Disease Control and Prevention, National Center for Health Statistics, National Health Interview Survey.)

5. Construct a bar graph to display the number of new cases of diagnosed diabetes among U.S. adults aged 20 years or older. In the year 2002, there were about 195,000 new cases among people aged 20–39 years; 568,000 new cases among people aged 40–59 years; and 492,000 among people aged 60 years and older.
   (*Source*: 1999–2001 National Health Interview Survey estimates projected to 2002.)

6. Construct a bar graph to display percentage of U.S. adults aged 20 years or older who had diabetes in the year 2002. The percentage of adults with diabetes

was 2.2% among those aged 20–39 years, 9.7% among those aged 40–59 years, and 18.3% among those aged 60 years and older.

(*Source:* 1991–2001 National Health Interview Survey and 1999–2000 National Health and Nutrition Examination Survey estimates projected to 2002.)

7. Construct a double bar graph to display the data given in the table.

Current Cigarette Smoking Among High School Students by Sex and Grade Level, United States 2003

Grade	Male Current Smoker Percent	Female Current Smoker Percent
9	16.0	18.9
10	21.7	21.9
11	23.2	24.0
12	29.0	23.3

(*Source*: Centers for Disease Control and Prevention, National Center for Chronic Disease Prevention and Health Promotion, Youth Risk Behavior Study.)

8. Construct a double bar graph to display the data given in the table.

High School Students Not Engaging in Recommended Amounts of Physical Activity (neither moderate nor vigorous) by grade and sex: United States, 2003

Grade	Male Students Percent	Female Students Percent
9	23.8	32.7
10	25.6	35.9
11	27.0	46.2
12	32.1	48.4

(*Source*: Centers for Disease Control and Prevention, National Center for Chronic Disease Prevention and Health Promotion, Youth Risk Behavior Study.)

Use the bar graph in Figure 7.7 to answer Questions 9–12.

9. During which month in 2001 was the average gas price the highest?

10. During which month in 2001 was the average gas price the lowest?

11. During which months was the average price higher than $1.50 per gallon?

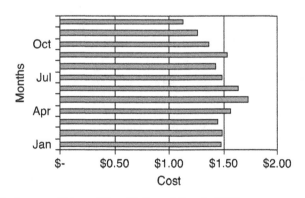

Figure 7.7 Average Price of One Gallon of Gas in 2001

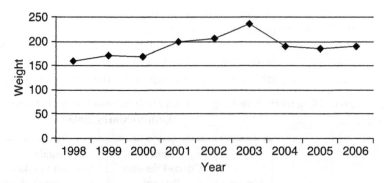

Figure 7.8 Julio's Weight on New Year's Day

12. How many months had an average gas price lower than $1.25? Which months?

Each New Year's Day, Julio records his weight. He graphs his weights to compare the yearly values and look for trends. Use the line graph in Figure 7.8 to answer Questions 13–16.

13. In what year did Julio record the highest weight on New Year's Day?

14. In what year did Julio record the lowest weight on New Year's Day?

15. During how many years does it appear his weight was at least 200 lb?

16. During what year would you guess that Julio went on a diet/physical fitness plan?

Use the circle graph of expenditures for local government to answer Questions 17–22.

17. On which sector does local government spend the least?

18. Approximately how many times the expenditure on highways is the expenditure that is spent for education?

19. If the local government has $1,825,000 in revenue for the year, how much will be spent on public welfare?

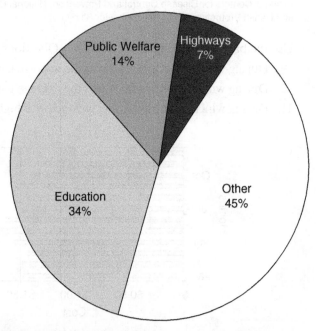

Figure 7.9 Expenditures of Local Government

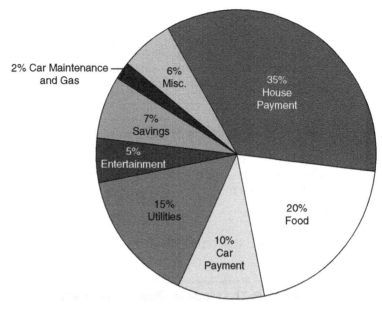

Figure 7.10 Household Budget

20. If the local government has $5,355,750 in revenue for the year, how much will be spent on education?

21. If 45% of the "Other" revenues category represents the amount spent on the police department, what percent of the total budget is spent on the police department? If the budget is $2,500,000, how much would that be?

22. If 15% of the "Other" revenues category represents the amount spent on the fire department, what percent of the total budget is spent on the fire department? If the budget is $2,500,000, how much would that be?

Pictured in Figure 7.10 is the household budget for the Fredrickson family. Each piece of the pie chart represents the percent of monthly income spent on various bills. Use Figure 7.10 to answer Questions 23–28.

23. Which financial obligation represents the smallest part of the family budget?

24. Which financial obligation represents one-fifth of the total budget?

25. If the family take-home income per month is $4200, how much is their house payment?

26. If the family take-home income per month is $4200, how much is the family saving each month?

27. If the family income per month is $3500, determine the amount of money budgeted for each category.

28. If the family income per month is $5000, determine the amount of money budgeted for each category.

SECTION 7.3   MEASURES OF CENTRAL TENDENCY

In this section, we will explore some of the common manipulations that can be performed on data once it has been collected. One of the most often-stated statistics is the "average" of a set of data. As stated in Section 7.1, there can be several different averages for a given set of data. This means that we cannot just use the word **average** to represent all of them. All averages are called **measures of central tendency**. There are four commonly used measures of central tendency for data: the mode, the median, the mean, and the midrange.

The Mode

The mode of a set of data is the most often repeated observation or item. If there are two data items repeated at the same rate, then the data has two modes and is said to be **bimodal**. If no data item is repeated more than another, the data set has no mode.

EXAMPLE 4: The Mode of Qualitative Data

In a recent survey done at a nursing home, 45 patients had brown eyes, 21 had blue eyes, 8 had green eyes, and 15 had hazel eyes. What is the mode for this set of data (i.e., the modal eye color)?

Solution

The most often repeated observation is brown eye color, so the mode = brown.

EXAMPLE 5: The Mode of Quantitative Data

Find the mode of the following sets of measurements:

    a. 1.5 cc, 4 cc, 6.5 cc, 8 cc, 8 cc, 10.5 cc, 12 cc

    b. 2.0 mg, 2.0 mg, 7.5 mg, 4.0 mg, 4.0 mg, 6.0 mg, 6.0 mg, 6.0 mg

    c. 81 lb, 92 lb, 101 lb, 102 lb, 125 lb, 140 lb

Solution

    a. In this set of numbers, 8 is the only repeated number, so the mode = 8 cc.

    b. The numbers 2, 4, and 6 are all repeated but 6 is repeated more than any of the others, so the mode = 6.0 mg.

    c. Since this list of values contains no repeated data items, there is no mode.

The second type of "average" is the **median**. To find a median, place the data items in order from lowest to highest (or highest to lowest). Determine the item in the middle of this ordered set of data, and that value will be the median. The median separates the upper half of the data from the lower half of the data and is the same thing as the 50th percentile of a set of data. For example, the 50th percentile of a height-weight chart represents the median height or weight for each age group so that 50% of children of a particular age will be above this point and 50% will be below it.

The Median

The median for a set of observations is the observation in the center or middle of a list of items after they have been placed in some kind of meaningful order.

EXAMPLE 6: The Median of Qualitative Data

In a recent survey done at a nursing home, 45 patients had brown eyes, 21 had blue eyes, 8 had green eyes, and 15 had hazel eyes. What is the median for this set of data?

Solution

For a set of data to have a median, it must be data that can be placed in a meaningful order. There is no meaningful order for eye color, so there is no median here.

EXAMPLE 7: The Median of Quantitative Data

Find the median for the following sets of data:

    a. 1.5 cc, 4 cc, 6.5 cc, 8 cc, 8 cc, 10.5 cc, 12 cc
    b. 4.0 mg, 6.0 mg, 3.5 mg, 2.0 mg, 4.0 mg, 2.0 mg, 6.0 mg, 6.0 mg
    c. 81 lb, 92 lb, 101 lb, 102 lb, 125 lb, 140 lb

Solution

    a. Since these numbers are already in a meaningful order, simply find the middle of the list. There are seven numbers in the list, so the fourth one (counting from either end) would be in the middle of the list.

$$\text{The median} = 8 \text{ cc}$$

    b. First sort the numbers into numerical order as follows: 2.0 mg, 2.0 mg, 4.0 mg, 4.0 mg, 6.0 mg, 6.0 mg, 6.0 mg, 7.5 mg.

Finding the number in the middle is not so easy this time. There are eight numbers in this list. Counting four from each end places the middle *between 4.0 and 6.0*. When this happens, the median must be calculated by adding the two numbers on either side of the middle and then dividing by 2.

$$\text{The median} = \frac{4.0 \text{ mg} + 6.0 \text{ mg}}{2} = 5.0 \text{ mg}$$

    c. 81 lb, 92 lb, 101 lb, 102 lb, 125 lb, 140 lb

Since these numbers are already in a meaningful order, simply find the middle of the list. With an even number of data items,

$$\frac{101 \text{ lb} + 102 \text{ lb}}{2} = 101.5 \text{ lb}$$

so this is the median.

Note in Examples 7b and c that the median is not a member of the original data set but it does divide the set into an equal number of items above its value and below its value. Whenever a set of numerical data has an even number of items, the median will be between two of the items. If there is an odd number of items in the list, then the median will be one of the data items—the one in the middle.

The most common meaning of the word *average* is the mean. The **mean** includes all data items in its calculation and is therefore a very useful statistic. It represents the balancing point for a set of data.

The Mean Average

The mean average is found by totaling the observations in a set of data and then dividing that total by the number of items in the original list. This average has its own symbol, called *x*-bar, $\bar{x}$. The formula is

$$\bar{x} = \frac{\Sigma x}{n}$$

where
Σx represents the sum of the data items and n represents the number of items in the data set.

For a set of data to have a mean average, it must be numerical data so that the amounts may be added. Therefore, there is no mean average for qualitative data. For example, there is no meaningful answer to the problem blue + brown divided by 2!

Example 8: The Mean of Quantitative Data

Find the mean average for the following sets of data:

    a. 1.5 cc, 4 cc, 6.5 cc, 8 cc, 8 cc, 10.5 cc, 12 cc

    b. 4.0 mg, 6.0 mg, 3.5 mg, 2.0 mg, 4.0 mg, 2.0 mg, 6.0 mg, 6.0 mg

    c. 81 lb, 92 lb, 101 lb, 102 lb, 125 lb, 140 lb

Solution

    a. First, add the numbers then divide by 7, which is the number of items in this list of numbers:

$$\bar{x} = \frac{\Sigma x}{n} = \frac{1.5\ cc + 4\ cc + 6.5\ cc + 8\ cc + 8\ cc + 10.5\ cc + 12\ cc}{7}$$

$$= \frac{50.5}{7} = 7.21 = 7\ cc$$

The final average is 7 cc. It has been rounded using the rounding rules for measurements discussed in Chapter 3.

    b. Again add, and this time divide by 8 and use the rounding rules:

$$\bar{x} = \frac{\Sigma x}{n} = \frac{4.0\ mg + 6.0\ mg + 3.5\ mg + 2.0\ mg + 4.0\ mg + 2.0\ mg + 6.0\ mg + 6.0\ mg}{8}$$

$$= \frac{33.5}{8} = 4.1875 = 4.2\ mg$$

    c. Add the numbers then divide by 6, which is the number of items in this list of numbers:

$$\bar{x} = \frac{\Sigma x}{n} = \frac{81\ lb + 92\ lb + 101\ lb + 102\ lb + 125\ lb + 140\ lb}{6}$$

$$= \frac{641}{6} = 106.833\ldots = 107\ lb$$

The final average is 107 lb. It has been rounded using the rounding rules for measurements discussed in Chapter 3.

The **midrange** is the value halfway between the lowest value in a data set and the highest value in the data set. It is an easily calculated value. However, its usefulness as a measure of center can be compromised if there is an outlier (a data item that is much higher or much lower than the rest of the data). Outliers affect both the value of the midrange and the mean of the data, sometimes increasing them or decreasing them significantly so that they will not represent the true center of the data.

Midrange

The midrange is the value halfway between the highest and lowest values in the data set. Its formula is

$$Midrange = \frac{Lowest\ value + Highest\ value}{2}$$

Example 9: The Midrange of Quantitative Data

Find the midrange of the following sets of data:

    a. 1.5 cc, 4 cc, 6.5 cc, 8 cc, 8 cc, 10.5 cc, 12 cc

    b. 4.0 mg, 6.0 mg, 3.5 mg, 2.0 mg, 4.0 mg, 2.0 mg, 6.0 mg, 6.0 mg

    c. 81 lb, 92 lb, 101 lb, 102 lb, 125 lb, 140 lb

Solution

    a. The lowest value in the data set is 1.5 cc and the highest is 12 cc.

$$\text{Midrange} = \frac{\text{Lowest value} + \text{Highest value}}{2}$$

$$\text{Midrange} = \frac{1.5 \text{ cc} + 12 \text{ cc}}{2} = \frac{13.5 \text{ cc}}{2} = 6.75 \text{ cc} = 7 \text{ cc}$$

        The answer is rounded based on the rounding rules for measurements.

    b. The lowest value is 2.0 mg and the highest is 6.0 mg.

$$\text{Midrange} = \frac{\text{Lowest value} + \text{Highest value}}{2}$$

$$\text{Midrange} = \frac{2.0 \text{ mg} + 6.0 \text{ mg}}{2} = \frac{8.0 \text{ mg}}{2} = 4.0 \text{ mg}$$

    c. The lowest value in the data set is 81 lb and the highest is 140 lb.

$$\text{Midrange} = \frac{\text{Lowest value} + \text{Highest value}}{2}$$

$$\text{Midrange} = \frac{81 \text{ lb} + 140 \text{ lb}}{2} = \frac{221 \text{ lb}}{2} = 110.5 \text{ lb} = 111 \text{ lb}$$

        The answer is rounded based on the rounding rules for measurements.

As a matter of practice in everyday life, we use the word *average* to refer to all four of these measures of central tendency. But a builder who builds houses for the "average American family" is interested in the most common family size, or the mode. The median is often used to report financial information because it is not subject to extreme data values, or outliers. An example of the use of the median is in a Mayo Clinic study published in the *Journal of the American Medical Association* that concluded the nine-year median costs for persons with AD/HD compared to those without AD/HD were more than double ($4,306 versus $1,944). By using the median, they are eliminating the few instances where costs were unusually high or unusually low. When computing a "grade point average," the mean average is used in order to reflect *all* grades made by that student during the course. The midrange is used when a quick measure of center needs to be calculated. Again, extreme values can make this measure of central tendency invalid.

PRACTICE PROBLEM SET 7.3

1. Describe in your own words the meaning of the mode of a set of data. Give an example where the mode would be an appropriate measure of central tendency.

2. Describe in your own words the meaning of the median of a set of data. Give an example where the median would be an appropriate measure of central tendency.

3. Describe in your own words the meaning of the mean of a set of data. Give an example where the mean would be an appropriate measure of central tendency.

4. Describe in your own words the meaning of the midrange of a set of data. Give an example where the midrange would be an appropriate measure of central tendency.

Find all possible averages—mode, median, mean, and midrange—for each of the following sets of data (Problems 5–14).

5. 2 oz, 3 oz, 4 oz, 6 oz, 2 oz, 3 oz, 8 oz, 2 oz, 7 oz, 9 oz

6. 2.3 mL, 4.5 mL, 6.8 mL, 2.2 mL, 5.8 mL, 9.0 mL, 2.5 mL, 4.5 mL

7. 130 lb, 95 lb, 96 lb, 172 lb, 104 lb, 88 lb, 199 lb, 289 lb, 135 lb, 257 lb

8. 350 mL, 250 mL, 300 mL, 200 mL, 300 mL, 300 mL, 250 mL

9. 1850 calories, 1775 calories, 1500 calories, 2250 calories, 1800 calories, 2000 calories, 1950 calories

10. 98.6°F, 97.6°F, 99.2°F, 98.6°F, 99.8°F, 101.2°F, 96.4°F, 97.6°F

11. $6.64/hr, $7.50/hr, $6.60/hr, $7.70/hr, $12.50/hr, $6.50/hr, $7.70/hr, $6.65/hr

12. 16.0 g, 15.0 g, 10.5 g, 12.5 g, 10.5 g, 8.0 g, 10.5 g, 12.5 g, 11.5 g, 6.5 g

13. 350 cc, 300 cc, 325 cc, 250 cc, 300 cc, 200 cc

14. $110.50, $85.00, $125.75, $225.00, $250.00, $25.75

15. John had his cholesterol checked 4 times last year. The numbers were 200, 186, 207 and 210. Find his mean cholesterol level last year. What was the midrange of these levels? How does it compare to the mean?

16. Mariana is diabetic and must check her blood sugar level 6 times a day. Monday, her blood sugar readings were 101, 155, 210, 124, 180, and 145. Find her mean blood sugar level on Monday. What was the midrange of these readings? How does it compare to the mean?

Would you use the mean, median, or mode to give a fair representation of the "average" in Problems 17–26?

17. The buyer for shoes at the department store considers the "average" woman's shoe size as she contemplates the number of each size shoe to order for the spring season.

18. The "average" nursing student is a white female.

19. The grade point "average" for medical assisting students at Alamance Community College is 3.54.

20. In a 2000 census report, it was stated that the "average" number of children in households with children was 1.89.

21. The "average" cost of a hospital stay for a heart patient at Cook County Memorial Hospital is $45,000.

22. An article in the *Journal of the American Medical Association* in 2004 reported that obese patients' "average" prescription costs were $357.65, compared to $157.86 for nonobese patients.

23. The "average" nursing home resident is at high risk for breaking a bone.

24. An article in *USA Today* in March 2004 reported that "today's average premium for a family insurance policy—$9,086 a year—already represents 21% of the national median household income of $42, 409."

25. Joan is on a diet, so she calculated the "average" number of calories she ate per day this week to be 1352.

26. My "average" monthly drug cost in 2004 was $165.90.

27. The mean is the "most sensitive" average since it is affected by any change in the data. Determine the mean, median, midrange, and mode for 1, 2, 3, 4, 4, 7, 9. Now change the 9 to a 20 in the same list. Which averages will be affected by this change? How are they affected?

28. The business magazine *Forbes* estimates (November 6, 1995) that the "average" household wealth of its readers is either about $800,000 or about $2.2 million, depending on which "average" it reports. Which type of "average" do you believe the $800,000 represents?

29. Which of the measures of central tendency must be one of the data items?

30. The following data set represents shirts sizes for a girls' soccer team:

    S, S, S, M, M, M, M, M, M, M, M, M, M, M, M, L, L, L, L, XL, XL, XL.

    Select the most appropriate measure of central tendency (average) for the data described.

31. What measure of central tendency is associated with the 50th percentile?

32. In 1998, the Bureau of Labor Statistics reported that half of all registered nurses earned more than $40,690. Is this number an example of a mean, median, mode, or midrange? Explain your answer.

33. A CDC survey reports that in 2002, the median percentage of smokers in the nation was 23%. This number was based on surveys from 54 states and territories of the United States. Interpret this number using the definition of the word *median.*

34. A CDC survey reports that in 2002, the median percentage of the population in the nation that was obese based on Body Mass Index (BMI) was 22.1%. This number was based on surveys from 54 states and territories of the United States. Interpret this number using the definition of the word *median.*

The following statistics represent the salaries of registered respiratory therapists in central North Carolina:

Mean—$45,867   Median—$45,648   Mode—$45,500

35. What is the most common salary of those surveyed?

36. What salary did half of these respiratory therapists surpass?

37. Use the salary wizard at http://salary.hotjobs.com to research the median salary for a dental assistant in your area of the country. Then enter your chosen health care field and your zip code to research the median salary for your profession.

SECTION 7.4   UNDERSTANDING RANGE, STANDARD DEVIATION, AND THE COEFFICIENT OF VARIATION

Measures of variation in a set of data are an important tool in statistical analysis. While large variability among items in some data sets might not be unusual (a set of a students' grades in a statistics course), large variability in the amount of liquid in a 2-L cola might cause consumers to buy another brand of cola. Although the average amount of cola in all bottles might be 2 L, the variability in individual bottles makes the product undesirable.

Consider the following set of statistics derived from three different sets of weights:

Table 7.2

Number Set	Mean Avg.
Group X	165 lb
Group Y	165 lb
Group Z	165 lb

Table 7.3

Number Set	Data			
Group X	165 lb	165 lb	165 lb	165 lb
Group Y	166 lb	165 lb	165 lb	164 lb
Group Z	167 lb	166 lb	164 lb	163 lb

Looking at Table 7.2, it would be easy to assume that the sets of numbers were identical and not really three sets at all. However, if you look at the actual sets of numbers in Table 7.3, it is obvious that there are differences.

Averages or measures of central tendency give us information about numbers near the middle of a set. If more information is needed about the data items and the consistency of those items, then other statistics must be calculated. If we are interested in how similar or different the numbers in a data set are to each other, we are interested in the variability of the data in the set. The difference between and among numbers in a set of data is called **variation** or **dispersion** in statistics. Measures of variation or dispersion tell us about the consistencies or inconsistencies among numbers within a set of observations. There are two commonly used measures of variation: the **range** and the **standard deviation** of the set of data.

Range

The range of a set of data is the difference between the highest and the lowest number in the data set.

R = Highest number − Lowest number

Example 10: Calculating the Range

Refer to Table 7-3 and calculate the range of each set of data.

Group X: R = 165 lb − 165 lb = 0 lb
Group Y: R = 166 lb − 164 lb = 2 lb
Group Z: R = 167 lb − 163 lb = 4 lb

It can be seen from the calculations in Example 10 that all three sets of numbers are *not* the same because all three have different ranges. When the value of the range is reported along with the measures of central tendency, it is easy to see that there are differences in the sets of numbers.

The best characteristic of the range is its ease of calculation. However, because it uses only the highest and the lowest data items to give an answer, it can be unreliable if an outlier, either high or low, is in the data set. One extreme value can create a large and misleading value of the range even if the majority of the numbers are relatively consistent. Consider the set of blood glucose numbers 80 mg/dL, 82 mg/dL, 220 mg/dL, 86 mg/dL. Although the range is 140, three of the four blood sugar levels are fairly close together. So, the range in this case is a misleading indicator of the consistency of the data.

Another measure of variability not so strongly affected by outliers or extreme values is more commonly used in statistical analysis to describe the variation that occurs within a set of data. It is known as **standard deviation.**

The standard deviation is a statistic that tells you how tightly all the various data items are clustered around the mean of the set. It is symbolized either by the Greek letter σ (sigma) or the letter s. The σ is used when the standard deviation of a population of data is being calculated. The letter s is used for the standard deviation when the data being analyzed is a sample taken from a population. In health care, the majority of statistics gathered are sample data, so we will assume that the data we are analyzing in our problems represents sample data.

When the standard deviation of a set of data is small, most of the data items are close to the mean. In Table 7.3, the standard deviation of Group X is 0, of Group Y is 0.8, and of Group Z, having the largest standard deviation, 1.8. If you look at these data sets, it is evident from the numbers in each list that the data in Group Z was more variable.

The importance of the size of the standard deviation of a set of data varies according to the problem being assessed. IQ scores in the general population, for example, have a relatively large standard deviation. However, a small standard deviation is important in quality control procedures used by many industries and laboratories. If a company manufactures medication, it strives to have consistency in its product. For example, although each pill in a batch will contain slightly different amounts of an active ingredient, all products should be extremely close in value to the desired dosage. This requires little variation and, therefore, a small standard deviation in the amount of active ingredient in each pill produced. When a lab runs a series of blood tests, control samples are included in each run for quality control during the test. Small standard deviation numbers help the technician ensure that the test is being run correctly and that the results of the unknown samples are reliable and accurate. Generally, results should be within 2 standard deviation units of the mean of the sample in order for the process to be "in control."

The calculation of the standard deviation is a cumbersome process, especially with a large data set. We will use a relatively small data set of whole numbers to demonstrate the process of finding the average deviation of the data from the mean.

To Find the Sample Standard Deviation of a Set of Data:

1. Find the mean, $\overline{x}$, of the data.
2. Make a chart having three columns:

   Data x Data $-$ Mean $x - \overline{x}$ (Data $-$ Mean)^2 $(x - \overline{x})^2$
3. List the data vertically under the column marked Data.
4. Complete the Data $-$ Mean column for each piece of data.
5. Square the values obtained in the Data $-$ Mean column and record these values in the (Data $-$ Mean)^2 column.
6. Find the sum of the (Data $-$ Mean)^2 column.
7. Divide the sum in step 6 by $n - 1$ (the number of data items minus 1).
8. Find the square root of quotient in step 7. This is the standard deviation number.

These steps are summarized by the standard deviation formula (Σ is the mathematical symbol for a summation of numbers):

$$s = \sqrt{\frac{\Sigma(x - \bar{x})^2}{n - 1}}$$

EXAMPLE 11: Calculating the Standard Deviation

Find the standard deviation of the following set of data:

$$6, 5, 2, 9, 0, 3, 3$$

Solution

a. Find the Mean: $\bar{x} = \dfrac{6 + 5 + 2 + 9 + 0 + 3 + 3}{7} = 4$

b. Chart the data:

Data	Data − Mean	(Data − Mean)^2
6	6 − 4 = 2	$2^2 = 4$
5	5 − 4 = 1	$1^2 = 1$
2	2 − 4 = −2	$(-2)^2 = 4$
9	9 − 4 = 5	$5^2 = 25$
0	0 − 4 = −4	$(-4)^2 = 16$
3	3 − 4 = −1	$(-1)^2 = 1$
3	3 − 4 = −1	$(-1)^2 = 1$

$$\Sigma(\text{data} - \text{mean})^2 = 4 + 1 + 4 + 25 + 16 + 1 + 1 = 52$$

$$s = \sqrt{\frac{\Sigma(x - \bar{x})^2}{n - 1}} = \sqrt{\frac{52}{6}} = \sqrt{8.667} = 2.94$$

Determining the calculation of standard deviation by hand involves a long series of calculations, even with the shortcut formulas available. With large data sets, this is a tedious process and the possibility of arithmetic errors is great. Using a calculator or computer program is the best way to derive the standard deviation.

Using a Calculator to Derive the Standard Deviation

■ A *standard scientific calculator* can be used to find the standard deviation, but there are many different ways of entering the initial data. In a regular scientific calculator, use the $\Sigma+$ or the **M**+ button to enter the data. You may need to put your calculator into Statistics Mode. (See your instructions for specific information.) Then locate the standard deviation button (s_x or σ_{n-1}) to complete the calculations.

■ A *graphing calculator* (TI-83+ or TI-84) will find the standard deviation very efficiently as follows: Press STAT. Choose EDIT from the menu. You should now be looking at a screen that will allow you to enter lists of numbers. Enter each number in the data set and then press the ENTER key after each number. After entering the last number, press STAT. Use the arrow key to move over to CALC. Choose 1-VarStats by pressing ENTER. Press ENTER a second time. You should now see a list of statistical values. The ones that you are most interested in are $\bar{x}$ = the mean average, **s** = sample standard deviation, σ = population standard deviation, **n** = the number of items in the list, **Med** = the median, and **minX** and **maxX** are the smallest and largest numbers that you entered.

In the lab, if you are working in a quality control area, the computers will give standard deviation readings for the data being collected and analyzed. It will be up to you to determine the meaning and applications of these numbers. For all sets of data, more than half of the data set will be within 1 standard deviation of the mean and a majority of the data will be within 2 standard deviations of the mean. In a data set that is normally distributed, there are specific percents that apply. We will examine this idea more closely in the next section.

EXAMPLE 12: Interpreting Standard Deviation

Assume that the duration of a normal human pregnancy can be described with a mean of 270 days and a standard deviation of 15 days. A majority of the babies will be delivered after how many days?

Solution

Based on statistical data, we know that most babies will arrive within 2 standard deviations of the mean. Therefore, most will arrive $270 \pm 2(15) = 270 \pm 30$ days or after a pregnancy of 240–300 days.

Deviations in sizes among children as they grow can be analyzed and standardized to develop growth charts such as the one shown in Figure 7.11. Doctors use these charts to compare a child's measurements with those of other children his or her age. These charts are developed by the National Center for Health Statistics and published by the Centers for Disease Control (CDC). There are various types of charts that provide information about a child's height for age, weight for age, and body mass index (BMI) for age. There are separate charts for boys and girls since they grow at different rates. On the graph, there are seven curves in all, each labeled with a number—5th, 10th, 50th, 75th, 90th, and 95th. The dark curve in the center of the graphs, labeled 50th, is the mean average weight for a boy at a particular age. The other numbers are percentile ranks and are related to the standard deviation of the data. If your son's weight falls on the 75th line, then his weight is more than 75% of boys his same age in the United States and less than 25% of boys his age. Children with weights above the 95th percentile line are considered overweight and children with weights below the 5th percentile line are considered underweight. Doctors primarily use these charts to plot a child's growth over time, looking for any unusual trends in the child's growth patterns.

Coefficient of Variation

The **coefficient of variation (CV)** for a sample set is calculated by dividing the standard deviation by the mean average and multiplying the result by 100. The coefficient of variation is a dimensionless number that allows comparison of samples that have different means and standard deviations. Suppose you want to compare the variation in the data sets of the exam grades of two classes. Since you expect to have a different class average on the exam for each class and a different standard deviation, you can use the CV to compare the amount of variation in each class.

Coefficient of Variation

$$CV = \frac{\text{Standard deviation}}{\text{Mean average}} \times 100\% = \frac{s}{\bar{x}} \times 100\%$$

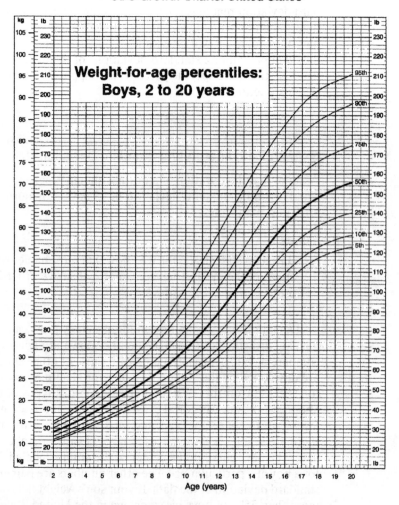

Figure 7.11 CDC Growth Charts: United States

Source: Developed by the National Center for Health Statistics in collaboration with the National Center for Chronic Disease Prevention and Health Promotion (2000).

The coefficient of variation is used in many laboratory tests and is preferred when the standard deviation increases in proportion to concentration. The Centers for Disease Control (CDC) has set a CV of 3% as the nationwide standard for all measurements of cholesterol values by all clinical and testing laboratories. The CDC sends a controlled sample of cholesterol to all testing labs and requires that they are within ±3% of the stated target value. If a lab's results do not fall in this range, the lab personnel must examine all lab procedures and make corrections in the process and instrumentation so that the results will fall within this range.

EXAMPLE 13: Calculating a Coefficient of Variation

A single sample of cholesterol was tested repeatedly, with the following concentration results in mg/dL:

$$187, 182, 201, 208, 188$$

a. Give the mean and standard deviation for these readings.

b. Calculate the coefficient of variation (CV).

c. Is the CV within CDC standards?

Solution

a. Mean $= \dfrac{187 + 182 + 201 + 207 + 188}{5} = 193$

Standard Deviation

Data	Data − Mean	(Data − Mean)^2
187	$187 - 193 = -6$	$(-6)^2 = 36$
182	$182 - 193 = -11$	$(-11)^2 = 121$
201	$201 - 193 = 8$	$8^2 = 64$
207	$207 - 193 = 14$	$14^2 = 196$
188	$188 - 193 = -5$	$(-5)^2 = 25$

$$\sqrt{\dfrac{\Sigma(x - \bar{x})^2}{n - 1}} = \sqrt{\dfrac{442}{4}} = \sqrt{110.5} = 10.51$$

(The authors recommend that you use your calculator functions to find the standard deviation but the formula has been provided for practice.)

b. $\text{CV} = \dfrac{\text{Standard deviation}}{\text{Mean average}} \times 100\% = \dfrac{s}{\bar{x}} \times 100\%$

$\dfrac{10.51}{193} \times 100\% = 5.4\%$

c. Since the calculated CV is >3%, these results are not within CDC standards.

Another advantage of the coefficient of variation is that it provides a general "feeling" about the performance of a method. CVs of 5% or less generally give us a feeling of good method performance, whereas CVs of 10% and higher sound bad. However, look carefully at the mean value before judging a coefficient of variation. At very high concentrations, the CV may be low, and at low concentrations the CV may be high. For example, a bilirubin test with a standard deviation of 0.1 mg/dL at a mean value of 0.5 mg/dL has a CV of 20%, whereas a standard deviation of 1.0 mg/dL at a concentration of 25 mg/dL corresponds to a CV of 4.0%.

PRACTICE PROBLEM SET 7.4

1. What does it mean if the standard deviation of a set of data is 0? What does it mean if the range of a set of data is 0?

2. Why is the range not the best measure of the variation of a set of data?

3. John and Mario are diabetic and both had mean average blood sugar readings this week of 128 mg/dL. However, John's readings had a standard deviation of 25.2 mg/dL and Mario's readings had a standard deviation of 52.1 mg/dL. Which patient has better blood sugar control? Why?

4. The mean average of Patient A's cholesterol readings during the last 12 months was 175 with a standard deviation of 55.5 points. Patient B had a mean over the last 12 months of 175 with a standard deviation of 22.3 points. Whose cholesterol is more consistently close to 175? Why?

5. Without actually calculating the standard deviation, can you tell which of the following sets of data has the greater standard deviation? Explain.

$$53, 56, 59, 62, 65 \qquad\qquad 213, 216, 219, 222, 225$$

6. Without actually calculating the standard deviation, can you tell which of the following sets of data has the greater standard deviation? Explain.

$$12, 14, 16, 18, 20 \qquad\qquad 22, 24, 24, 24, 26$$

Using your calculator or the formulas, find the mean, range, and standard deviation for each of the following data sets.

7. 0, 1, 2, 3, 4, 5, 6, 7, 8, 9

8. 2, 4, 6, 8, 10, 12, 14, 16, 18, 20

9. 0, 0, 2, 5, 6, 9, 11, 15, 18, 18

10. 2, 2, 2, 2, 2, 2, 2, 2, 2, 2

11. 6, 6, 10, 12, 3, 5

12. 120, 121, 122, 123, 124, 125, 126

13. 4, 0, 3, 6, 9, 12, 2, 3, 4, 7

14. 22, 36, 28, 24, 12, 6, 40, 26, 18, 28

15. If you are doing urine tests in a lab and control samples are included in each run, would you want a small standard deviation or a large standard deviation in your quality control measurements? Why?

16. A patient is diabetic and checks his blood sugar levels 4 times a day. When he submits his record to the doctor, his mean blood sugar level for the last month is 101. Would the doctor be pleased to see a small standard deviation from this set of numbers or a large standard deviation? Why?

17. You see an advertisement for a battery (Brand X) that has an average life of 155 hours with a standard deviation of 5 hours. Another brand (Brand Y) also has a mean life of 155 hours but it has a standard deviation of 15 hours. Which brand would you buy and why?

18. Brite-Lite light bulbs have a mean expected lifetime of 750 hours with a standard deviation of 25 hours. Shiny-White light bulbs have a mean expected lifetime of 750 hours with a standard deviation of 20 hours. Which brand would you buy and why?

19. The nurses in a doctor's office have monthly salaries as follows: $3500, $3600, $3700. Each receives a $50 monthly raise. How does this raise affect the mean salary? How does this raise affect the standard deviation of these salaries?

20. The nurses in a doctor's office have monthly salaries as follows: $3500, $3600, $3700. Each receives a 2% monthly raise. How does this raise affect the mean salary? How does this raise affect the standard deviation of these salaries?

21. Assume that a series of glucose concentration measurements has been done. The mean average for this series was determined to be 84 mg/dL with a standard deviation of 2.7 mg/dL. What is the coefficient of variation for these measurements?

22. Assume that a series of BUN measurements has been done. The mean average for this series was determined to be 17.2 mg/dL with a standard deviation of 1.26 mg/dL. What is the coefficient of variation for these measurements?

23. A series of tests for glucose concentrations has been done and the mean average for this series is 103 mg/dL with a standard deviation of 3.5 mg/dL. What is the coefficient of variation for this series?

24. The results of a quality control test for sodium give a mean of 150 mEq/L with a standard deviation of 2.2 mEq/L. What is the coefficient of variation for these results?

SECTION 7.5   THE NORMAL DISTRIBUTION AND CONTROL CHARTS

Large sets of quantitative data are difficult to analyze without being organized into a chart or graph. These data sets can be sorted into a table called a **frequency distribution.** The tables have classes or categories into which data is sorted by 5s, 10s, or any other amount that is relevant to the data. In general, there will be 5 to 15 categories or classes of numbers.

Once the data has been tallied and sorted into classes, this frequency distribution becomes the basis for a bar graph called a **histogram**. Each category or class is represented by one bar. The height of the bar represents the frequency of data items for that category.

EXAMPLE 14: Creating a Frequency Distribution and Histogram

The medical assisting class (MED 101) at the community college measured the pulse rates of its 30 students. The rates in beats per minute are given below. Construct a frequency distribution and histogram of this data.

88 90 81 85 88 78 84 90 66 75 74 85 86 88 82

80 79 79 88 81 78 85 91 85 87 84 82 81 82 74

The highest number in the data set is 91 and the lowest is 66. Therefore, the classes must be chosen so that all items will be included. Generally it is easiest to count by 5s, 10s, 25s, or some other "easy-to-count" number. Therefore, we will begin with the lowest class at 65 and count by 5s. That will give us six classes which is an adequate number.

Classes **Beat per Minute**	*Frequency* **Number of Students**
65–69	1
70–74	2
75–79	5
80–84	9
85–89	10
90–94	3

Once we have tabulated the data and completed the frequency distribution, draw the graph by putting the classes on the horizontal axis and the frequency units on the vertial axis. Remember to count in equal increments. The bars will touch because the width of each bar covers 5 numbers (65–69, 70–74, etc.). See Figure 7.12.

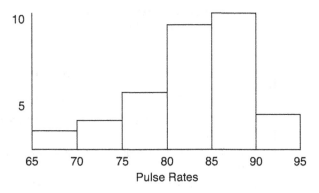

Figure 7.12 Pulse Rates of Students in MED 101

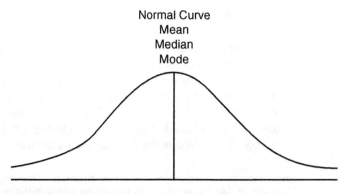

Figure 7.13 The Normal Curve

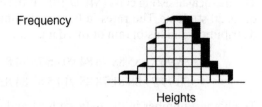

Figure 7.14 Six-Year-Old Girls' Heights

Many types of data will form a graph that is shaped like a **normal curve** (or **bell curve**). The normal curve has applications in many areas of science and allied health. A sample graph is shown in Figure 7.13.

Data sets that include measurements are usually from populations that are normally distributed. Suppose that you were to gather a set of data on the heights of 6-year-old girls. You would expect to find a few very tall girls and a few very short girls. However, you would expect to find that the vast majority of 6-year-old girls were of approximately the same height. If you were to build a graph of this data set, you would plot each height onto the graph. The shape of the graph would slowly emerge as more and more data is added. Eventually, there would be enough data plotted to see the true bell shape of the data emerge. (See Figure 7.14.) Data about the heights of children is used to draw similar graphs that are then used to develop the growth charts and graphs, such as the one in Figure 7.11, that are used in doctors' offices.

In laboratories and industry, normal distributions and other statistical analyses are done as part of quality control operations. Many laboratory workers are part of the quality assurance departments of their labs, so some familiarity with normal curves and their common characteristics will be very useful to lab technicians.

Most things that are measured are normally distributed, including heights, weights, speeds of cars down the highway, and IQ scores. Once a set of data has been collected and is known to be approximately normally distributed, then the **Empirical Rule** can be applied to the analysis of the data.

The Empirical Rule

For a distribution that is symmetrical and normally distributed:

1. Approximately 68.2% of all data values will lie within 1 standard deviation on either side of the mean.
2. Approximately 95.5% of all data values will lie within 2 standard deviations on either side of the mean.
3. Approximately 99.7% of all data values will lie within 3 standard deviations on either side of the mean.

These percentages are based on the amount of area under the normal curve between the standard deviation locations specified in the empirical rule. These divisions and the corresponding percents are shown in Figure 7.15. The area under the curve is theoretically 100%, though we are never 100% sure about anything when we are using inferential statistics. Note that the curve is symmetric, with 50% of the area above the mean and 50% below the mean.

One medical application of the Empirical Rule is blood screening. Blood screening is the testing of blood for the presence of different elements. The levels of these elements are measured and recorded for each patient. Based on these levels, different diseases can be diagnosed and preventative action can be prescribed if needed.

The diagnosis is made by comparing the levels of these elements in a patient's blood to an interval called the reference balance. The reference balance is found by adding and subtracting 2 standard deviations from the mean for each element. For example, the reference range for blood glucose is 70 mg/dL–125 mg/dL. This represents the average blood glucose reading for a healthy patient plus or minus 2 standard deviations. Based on the Empirical Rule, we would expect 95% of healthy patients to fall within this range. If a patient's blood glucose falls outside this range, more investigation is needed to determine if it is a chance occurrence or a medical problem.

Control Charts

In modern laboratories, **control charts**, based on the properties of the normal curve, are commonly used. The Levey-Jennings chart is one of the charts commonly used in the lab. It is based on a normal curve turned on its side. The centerline of the chart represents the value of the mean average for the data you are charting. Each of the lines above and below the mean represents 1 standard deviation unit. Figure 7.16 shows a Levey-Jennings chart for charting cholesterol levels using a particular commercial product with a mean of 200 mg/dL and a standard deviation of 4 mg/dL (CV 2.0%). Heavy lines are drawn at the $\pm 2s$ and $\pm 3s$ locations to draw attention to the upper and lower control limits for this data.

Once the control chart has been set up, you start plotting the new control values that are being collected as part of your routine work. The idea is that for a stable testing process, the new control measurements should show the same distribution as the past control measurements. That means it will be somewhat unusual to see a control value that exceeds a $2s$ control limit and very rare to see a control value that exceeds a $3s$ control limit. If the method is unstable and has some kind of problem, then there should be a higher chance of seeing control values that exceed the control limits. Therefore, when the control values fall within the expected distribution, you classify the run to be "in control,"

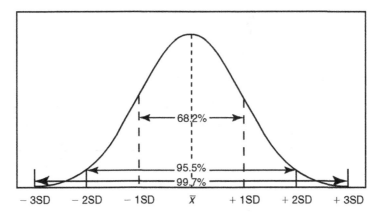

Figure 7.15 The Empirical Rule

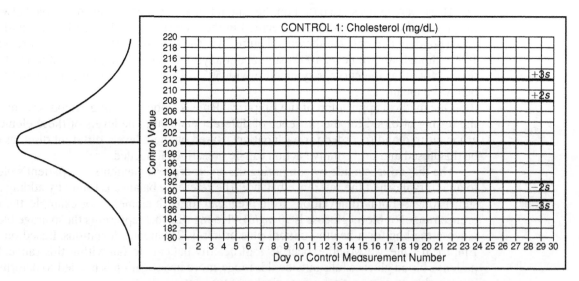

Figure 7.16 Levey-Jennings Chart for Cholesterol

accept the results, and report patient test results. When the control values fall outside the expected distribution, you classify the run as "out of control," reject the test values, and do not report patient test results. Figure 7.17 illustrates a control chart where three values exceed the control line.

The Westgard multirule system is a set of rules for quality control used by many laboratories. It is used in conjunction with Levey-Jennings charts and gives quality assurance staff rules to use when monitoring a testing process. An out-of-control process can occur when the value is outside of the 2s range or the 3s range, as previously stated. You can also have a shift of the average, a trend downward or upward with the values, and many other indications of an out-of-control process. The most important thing is that the results are monitored so that results reported by a lab are accurate and reliable.

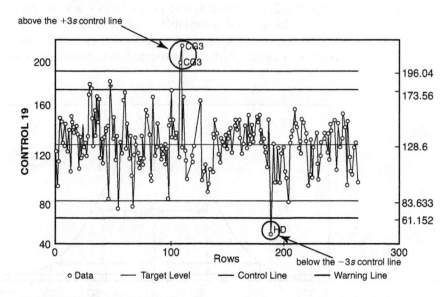

Figure 7.17 Completed Control Chart

PRACTICE PROBLEM SET 7.5

1. The cholesterol readings of 50 patients were reported as follows:

    227 213 202 182 143 194 235 136 180 225
    230 202 152 191 180 141 145 229 227 173
    209 182 175 225 329 306 258 237 285 199
    238 326 330 225 227 255 340 325 221 325
    151 183 241 318 148 203 165 196 210 230

    Classify these data into a grouped frequency distribution (lowest class 135–154). What is the class with the highest frequency? How many values are 195 or above?

2. The body temperature of 30 healthy patients was recorded. Classify these temperatures into a grouped frequency distribution (lowest class 96.5°–96.9°).

    97.0 97.6 97.5 98.8 98.4 98.2 97.7 97.3 97.5 97.1 98.6 98.6 97.8 98.7 97.9

    97.8 97.8 97.6 96.8 97.0 98.0 98.8 97.9 98.4 99.1 98.8 98.7 98.3 98.5 97.8

    What is the class with the highest frequency? Does this make you wonder if the "normal" body temperature of 98.6° is accurate?

3. Use the frequency distribution given to draw a histogram of the data.

Systolic Blood Pressure of Men and Women	Frequency
80–99	10
100–119	45
120–139	22
140–159	2
160–179	0
180–199	1

    Does this graph approximate the shape of a normal curve?

4. Refer to the table in Problem 3 to answer the following questions. How many people were in this sample? What percent of men and women in the sample had systolic blood pressures between 120–139?

5. Use the frequency distribution given to draw a histogram of the data.

Body Mass Index of Women	Frequency
15.0–19.9	9
20.0–24.9	12
25.0–29.9	25
30.0–34.9	6
35.9–39.9	2
40.0–44.9	1

    If women with a BMI below 25 are considered to be normal weight, how many of these women would be classified as overweight?

6. Refer to the table in Problem 5 to answer the following questions. How many women were included in this sample? What percent of the women have a BMI between 25.0 and 29.9?

7. Data was collected in a lab and the mean of the data was 7.6 mmol/L with a standard deviation of 0.1 mmol/L. What are the $+2s$ and $-2s$ control limits for this data?

8. Data was collected in a lab and the mean of the data was 7.0 mg/dL with a standard deviation of 0.25 mg/dL. What are the $+2s$ and $-2s$ control limits for this data?

9. Data was collected in a lab and the mean of the data was 112 mg/dL with a standard deviation of 18 mg/dL. What are the $+2s$ and $-2s$ control limits for this data?

10. Data was collected in a lab and the mean of the data was 8.6 mmol/L with a standard deviation of 0.7 mmol/L. What are the $+2s$ and $-2s$ control limits for this data?

Use the table of blood glucose readings to answer Questions 11–16.

Blood Glucose Readings in mg/dL

Day	1	2	3	4	5	6	7	8	9	10	11	12	13	14	15
mg/dL	102	99	99	97	101	101	100	99	103	100	102	99	100	103	98

11. Use a frequency distribution to sort the data. Put one number in each class and record the frequencies.

Blood Glucose	Frequency
97	
98	
99	
100	
101	
102	
103	

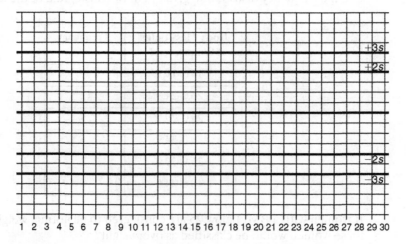

Figure 7.18

12. Draw a histogram of this frequency distribution. Does it approximate a normal curve?

13. Find the mean, median, mode, range, standard deviation, and CV of this data set.

14. Use the mean and standard deviation to determine the upper and lower control limits for this normal glucose control.

15. Use the Levey-Jennings chart in Figure 7.18 and label the upper control limits ($+2s$ and $+3s$) and the lower control limits ($-2s$ and $-3s$).

16. The blood glucose readings of a patient were obtained for 10 consecutive days. Use the Levey-Jennings chart to plot these readings and determine if they fall within the control limits.

Day	1	2	3	4	5	6	7	8	9	10
mg/dL	101	98	99	113	97	100	108	103	99	86

Chapter Summary

In this chapter, we have provided a brief introduction to statistics. Data is gathered and analyzed continually in the allied health field. Everything from charting a patient's temperatures to checking for quality assurance in a clinical laboratory will involve the use of statistics. Understanding graphs and terminology such as mean, standard deviation, and coefficient of variation can help you make sound decisions in your job as a health care worker and in your daily life. Quality control in the clinical laboratory is crucial to the reliability of test results. The use of the normal curve and Levey-Jennings charts can assist technicians in monitoring the quality of the testing process.

Important Terms, Rules, and Formulas

average
bar graph
bell curve
bimodal
circle graph
coefficient of variation (CV)
control charts
data
descriptive statistics
dispersion
Empirical Rule
frequency distribution
histogram
inferential statistics
Levey-Jennings chart
line graph

mean($\bar{x}$)
measures of central tendency
median
midrange
mode
normal curve
outlier
pie chart
population
qualitative data
quantitative data
range
sample
standard deviation (σ, s)
statistics
variation

Mean Average:

$\bar{x} = \dfrac{\Sigma x}{n}$, where Σx represents the sum of the data items and n represents the number of items in the data set.

Median:

The median for a set of observations is the observation in the center or middle of the list of items after they have been placed in some kind of meaningful order.

Mode:

The mode of a set of data is the most often repeated observation or item. If there are two data items repeated at the same rate, then the data has two modes and is said to be bimodal. If no data item is repeated more than another, the data set has no mode.

Midrange:

$$\dfrac{\text{Lowest value } + \text{ Highest value}}{2}$$

Standard Deviation:

$$s = \sqrt{\dfrac{\Sigma(x-\bar{x})^2}{n-1}}$$

The Empirical Rule:

For a distribution that is symmetrical and normally distributed:

1. Approximately 68.2% of all data values will lie within 1 standard deviation on either side of the mean.
2. Approximately 95.5% of all data values will lie within 2 standard deviations on either side of the mean.
3. Approximately 99.7% of all data values will lie within 3 standard deviations on either side of the mean.

Chapter Review Problems

1. Define the term *statistics* in your own words.
2. Explain, in your own words, the difference between inferential statistics and descriptive statistics.
3. What is a population? What is a sample?
4. What is the difference between quantitative data and qualitative data?
5. Name at least two ways that statistics can be misleading or used to create false conclusions.

If you were to collect the following data, would it be quantitative or qualitative data?

6. The bacteria count in your house drinking water
7. The occupation of several hundred of your college classmates
8. The marital status of members of your immediate family
9. The number of students in math classes at your college
10. Tell why the stated conclusion may represent a misinterpretation of the facts given.

   The median cost of a house in the United States is $170,000. Since I can't afford to pay $170,000 for a house, I can't afford to buy a house in the United States.

11. Consider the following sets of data:

    Data set A: 2, 4, 6, 8, 10   Data set B: 1, 3, 5, 7, 19

    Without calculating any numerical values, which group will have the largest standard deviation? Why?

Calculate the mean average, median, mode, range, and standard deviation for each of the following sets of data.

12. 32 lb, 33 lb, 33 lb, 35 lb, 35 lb, 36 lb, 36 lb, 36 lb, 40 lb, 42 lb, 44 lb
13. 12.3 g, 2.5 g, 16.8 g, 23.5 g, 36.1 g, 3.9 g, 16.2 g, 24.2 g, 5.5 g
14. 102 mg/dL, 115 mg/dL, 135 mg/dL, 89 mg/dL, 106 mg/dL, 100 mg/dL, 115 mg/dL
15. $8, $8, $8, $8, $8, $8, $8, $8
16. Wesley is diabetic and must check his blood sugar level 4 times a day. Sunday, his blood sugar readings were 189, 165, 215, and 104. Find his mean blood sugar level on Sunday. What was the median of these readings? How does it compare to the mean?

Would you use the mean, median, or mode to give a fair representation of the "average" in each of the following statements (Problems 17–19).

17. The "average" yearly college cost of enrollment at a four-year private university is $27,677.
18. The "average" amount of cheese eaten by Americans is 31 pounds per person.
19. The "average" American likes chocolate ice cream.
20. Assume that a series of BUN measurements has been done. The mean average for this series was determined to be 16.9 mg/dL with a standard deviation of 1.16 mg/dL. What is the coefficient of variation for these measurements?
21. Find the mean median, mode, standard deviation, and coefficient of variation for the following set of blood glucose measurements. All measurements are in mg/dL.

    125, 136, 108, 89, 160, 210, 251, 286, 165, 144, 98, 101

Use the circle graph in Figure 7.19 to answer Questions 22–24.

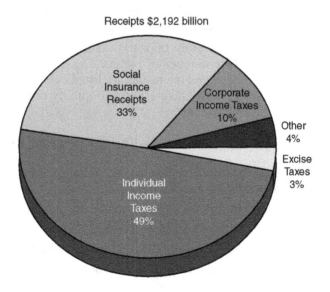

Receipts $2,192 billion

Figure 7.19 Sources of Revenue for the Federal Government in 2002
(*Source*: http://www.whitehouse.gov/omb/budget/fy2002)

22. What is the largest source of revenue for the federal government?

23. If receipts were $2,192 billion in 2002, how much was collected in corporate income taxes?

24. If receipts were $2,192 billion in 2002, how much was collected for Social Security?

25. Create a line graph to show Marie's weights for the last two months. Is the trend upward or downward? What is the percent change from January 1 to February 26?

Date	1–1	1–8	1–15	1–22	1–29	2–5	2–12	2–19	2–26
Weight	198	195	194	196	194	191	192	192	190

26. Plot a Levey-Jennings chart for the following data. Assume that these numbers are concentrations in g/L. Use a mean of 0.72 g/L and a standard deviation of 0.03 g/L to find the upper and lower control limits for your chart. Then plot these values. Are any values out of control?

0.75, 0.72, 0.64, 0.78, 0.70, 0.70, 0.68, 0.74, 0.71, 0.70, 0.71, 0.79, 0.69

Chapter Test

1. What is data?

2. Is a Social Security number quantitative or qualitative data? Why?

3. Is a patient's temperature quantitative or qualitative data? Why?

4. Which "average" is associated with the 50th percentile, the mean, median, mode, or midrange?

5. What is an outlier? How does it affect the mean average?

6. The "average" sports car is red. Is this use of the word *average* an example of mean, median, mode, or midrange?

7. The "average" number of children in an American household today is 1.89. Is this use of the word *average* an example of mean, median, mode, or midrange?

8. When bottles of aspirin are manufactured, machines fill each bottle with a specific number of tablets. The number of tablets in 10 bottles of 100 tablets is counted and the results are listed below. What is the standard deviation of this data? Does this indicate that the quality control of this process is adequate or needs improvement?

95, 100, 101, 108, 99, 105, 92, 100, 100, 100

Find the mean, median, mode, midrange, range, and standard deviation of the following data sets (Problems 9–11).

9. 25 mg, 36 mg, 12 mg, 19 mg, 26 mg, 25 mg, 12 mg, 32 mg, 12 mg, 46 mg, 16 mg

10. $5.15, $5.75, $6.55, $5.15, $6.75, $6.50

11. 1.58 μg, 2.32 μg, 0.05 μg, 2.06 μg, 1.54 μg, 3.05 μg, 3.25 μg, 1.86 μg

12. Consider the following sets of data:

Data set A: 100, 105, 110, 115   Data set B: 1, 3, 5, 7, 9

Without calculating any numerical values, which group will have the largest standard deviation? Why?

13. June's doctor checked her cholesterol level 4 times last year. The results were total cholesterol numbers of 220, 210, 196, and 188. What is the mean average of these readings? What is the range of her results?

14. Assume that a series of BUN measurements has been done. The mean average for this series was determined to be 19.9 mg/dL with a standard deviation of 1.45 mg/dL. What is the coefficient of variation for these measurements?

15. Find the mean, median, mode, standard deviation, and coefficient of variation for the following set of blood glucose measurements. All measurements are in mg/dL.

202, 155, 168, 88, 70, 101, 186, 200, 168, 120

Use the circle graph in Figure 7.20 to answer Questions 16–18.

16. What is the largest expenditure of the federal government?

17. If $2.0 trillion dollars was spent in 2002, how much was spent for Medicare?

18. If $2.0 trillion dollars was spent in 2002, how much was spent for Medicaid?

19. This chart is from a recent magazine advertisement for a Canadian drug company soliciting business in the United States. It compares costs of some well-known drugs in the United States and Canada. Create a double bar graph to illustrate this data.

Drug	Lipitor	Celebrex	Synthroid	Zocor	Premarin	Fosamax
U.S. cost	$205	$291	$50	$358	$110	$214
Canadian Company	$145	$147	$28	$195	$76	$57

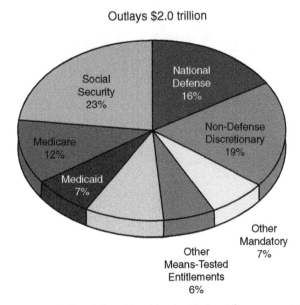

Figure 7.20 How Your Tax Dollars Were Used by the Federal Government in 2002
(*Source*: http://www.whitehouse.gov/omb/budget/fy2002)

20. Plot a Levey-Jennings chart for the following data. Assume that these numbers are concentrations in g/L. Use a mean of 1.2 g/L and a standard deviation of 0.15 g/L to find the upper and lower control limits for your chart. Then plot these values. Are any values out of control?

1.5, 1.2, 1.4, 1.8, 1.7, 1.3, 1.6, 1.4, 0.7, 1.0, 1.1, 1.9, 0.9

LOGARITHMS, IONIC SOLUTIONS, AND pH

Objectives for Chapter 8

After completing this chapter, the student should be able to:

1. Calculate common logarithms and antilogarithms.

2. Understand the pH scale and its values as they relate to the acidity of a solution.

3. Calculate pH values from hydrogen ion concentrations.

4. Calculate hydrogen ion concentrations given the pH of a solution.

SECTION 8.1 AN INTRODUCTION TO LOGARITHMS AND ANTILOGARITHMS

In the equation $y = b^x$, the base b is raised to the power x to give a value of y. The value of y, therefore, is a function of (or depends on) the value of x. This type of equation is known as an exponential function. If the base, b, and the exponent, x, are given, we use the given power to calculate the value of y. However, if we know the value of y and the value of b and we are asked to find the value of x (the exponent), we are being asked to find a **logarithm**. A logarithm is not a number in the usual sense, but is an **exponent**. Although the base for these problems can be any positive number, in a **common logarithm**, the base for the exponent will always be the number 10. These are the types of logarithms that will be needed for work in the allied health field. In working with equations or formulas that use logarithms, certain standard abbreviations are used. The word *logarithm* and the phrase *logarithm of* when used for logarithms are abbreviated **log**.

Logarithms are used frequently in the chemistry lab. The pH, pOH, and pK scales, plotting of standard curves, radioactive decay rates and half-life calculations for radioactive tracers and elements, and population growth rates are all examples of areas where logarithms are used. In this chapter, you will learn the basic manipulations and procedures that are necessary for dealing with logarithms. In solving problems and doing basic calculations in this chapter, it is assumed that you will have access to a scientific calculator that has logarithm function keys. To be sure that your calculator can be used, look for a key labeled *log*. If your calculator has this key, then you are ready to do all of the problems and applications in this chapter.

Let's begin our study by analyzing the definition of a logarithm as an exponent with a base of 10. When trying to determine the common logarithm of any number, we express the given number as 10^x and the value of x is the logarithm. For example, to find the logarithm of the number 1000, first write 1000 as a power of 10. Since $1000 = 10^3$, the required exponent is $x = 3$. Therefore, the answer to the problem log 1000 $= x$ is $x = 3$ (log 1000 $= 3$).

EXAMPLE 1: Finding a Common Logarithm Using the Definition

Find log 100.

Solution

We are trying to find the exponent that is used on the number 10 to give an answer of 100. Since $10^2 = 100$, log 100 = 2.

EXAMPLE 2: Finding a Common Logarithm Using the Definition

Find log 0.001.

Solution

Remember that $0.001 = \frac{1}{1000}$. When finding the logarithm of decimal numbers between 0 and 1, we will use negative exponents on the base of 10. By definition, $\frac{1}{1000} = 10^{-3}$. Therefore, log 0.001 = -3.

Verify your answer by entering 10^{-3} on your calculator. $10^{-3} = 0.001$.

Notice that there are three decimal places in this problem and the exponent needed is a -3.

Many numbers that end in zeroes can be easily written as powers of 10. However, not all numbers can be easily converted to common logarithms. For example, how do we find log 1225? We cannot easily determine an exponent to use on the base of 10 to generate the number 1225. In this case, you will need to use your calculator to find the logarithm. There are many different brands of calculators available, but they will work using one of the two methods shown in Example 3. Find out which one works for your particular calculator and then follow the same procedure each time.

EXAMPLE 3: Finding a Common Logarithm Using the Calculator

Find log 1225.

Solution

Locate the key labeled *log* on your calculator. On many standard calculators, you must first enter the number whose log you are calculating. Enter 1225 and press the *log* key (the sequence is 1225 log). Your calculator should display the number 3.088136089. . . . (Other calculators may be direct entry calculators and you can enter log 1225 as it is written.) Most logarithms must be rounded when doing computations in applied problems. We can round this answer to 3.088.

In order to check your answer, use your logarithm as the exponent for 10. If we use the rounded answer, we get $10^{3.088} = 1224.616199$. . . . This value is a little lower than 1225 because the answer was rounded. If we use the exact exponent, the answer will be exactly 1225 when we check it. Therefore, log 1225 = 3.088 (rounded value).

You cannot find the log of a negative number because the base used for a common logarithm is positive 10. If you try to find log(-10) using a calculator, it will display E, indicating that an error has occurred.

Antilogarithms

As mentioned earlier in this section, the pH scale is one example of a logarithmic scale. The pH numbers assigned to a solution indicate its level of acidity. These numbers are actually common logarithms or exponents that indicate the concentration of hydrogen ions in a solution. If a logarithm is known, such as the pH of a solution, the corresponding value is found by raising the number 10 to this logarithm exactly as we did to check the answer in Example 3. This is called finding the **antilogarithm**, or **antilog**. So, if we need to calculate the concentration of hydrogen ions in a solution from the pH number, we use a formula that involves the antilogarithm function. This formula will be explored more extensively in Section 8.3. The following examples demonstrate the steps to follow when finding the antilogarithm of a number.

EXAMPLE 4: Finding an Antilogarithm Using the Definition

Solve $\log x = 5$.

Solution

Because we are using a common log, the base number is 10 and the log always equals the exponent that is to be placed on that base. Therefore, we have a base of 10 with an exponent of 5, $10^5 = 100,000$.

EXAMPLE 5: Finding an Antilogarithm Using the Calculator

Solve $\log x = 5$.

Solution

To get our calculator to calculate the value of x here, we must do an antilog. On your calculator you must find the *second function* key (or its equivalent on your calculator). The key may be marked 2nd or 2nd f. To find the antilog, enter the following sequence: 5 2nd f log =. (Notice that above the log button you see 10^x.) As with the log function, if you have a direct entry calculator, you may be required to do the 2nd f log buttons first, followed by the number (2nd f log 5 =).

The calculator should display the number 100,000.

EXAMPLE 6: Finding an Antilogarithm Using the Calculator (Different Notation)

Solve $\log^{-1} 1.138$.

Solution

In your calculator enter: 1.138 2nd f log (or for direct entry, 2nd f log 1.138). The result is 13.74047975. . . . Thus, $x = 13.74047975 \approx 13.74$.

PRACTICE PROBLEM SET 8.1

Find each of the following common logs without your calculator.

1. $\log 10 =$
2. $\log 1,000,000 =$
3. $\log 0.01 =$
4. $\log 0.1 =$
5. $\log 100,000 =$
6. $\log 0.00001 =$

Find each of the following common logs using your calculator.

7. log 35 =

8. log 40 =

9. log(−1) =

10. log(−0.1) =

11. log 0.012 =

12. log 0.16 =

13. log 55,000 =

14. log 2000 =

15. $\log \frac{3}{8}$ =

16. $\log \frac{4}{5}$ =

17. log 641 =

18. log 195 =

19. log 0.0000001 =

20. log 0.001 =

21. $\log 3.5 \times 10^4$ =

22. $\log 1.25 \times 10^{-3}$ =

Find each of the following antilogs with your calculator (i.e., solve for x in each case).

23. log x = 2

24. log x = 0

25. log x = −0.05

26. log x = −5

27. $\log^{-1} 0.375 = x$

28. $\log^{-1} 0.25 = x$

29. $\log^{-1} 2 = x$

30. $\log^{-1} 5 = x$

31. $\log^{-1} 1.35 = x$

32. $\log^{-1} 3.75 = x$

33. antilog −2 = x

34. antilog −1 = x

35. antilog 1 = x

36. antilog 4 = x

37. antilog 2.53 = x

38. antilog 4.15 = x

39. antilog −2.5 = x

40. antilog −1.75 = x

SECTION 8.2   IONIC SOLUTIONS

Logarithms have many applications in health fields, especially for work in laboratories. In a previous chemistry course you should have studied ions and ionic bonds, so we will briefly review some basic facts here. Ions are attracted to each other in a compound due to their opposite electrical charges. If ionically bonded molecules are dissolved in a solvent, they will **ionize** or **dissociate** because the ionic bonds are broken. The solution then contains ions of both positive charge and negative charge from the original molecules.

Generally, there are three categories of ionic compounds—**acids, bases, and salts**. Acids are compounds that contribute free protons in the form of hydrogen ions (H^+) to a solution in which they are dissolved. Bases accept protons from a solution and generally contribute hydroxyl ions (OH^-) to the solution. Salts are compounds that contribute neither free protons (H^+) nor hydroxyl ions (OH^-) to a solution in which they are dissolved. An acidic solution contains more H^+ ions than OH^- ions. A basic or alkaline solution has more free OH^- ions than it does H^+ ions. In a neutral solution, the numbers of H^+ and OH^- ions are equal.

There are many ways to express the concentration of solutions. The primary one that we have examined earlier in this textbook is percent concentration. However, there are other expressions of concentration used for many solutions in a laboratory. Two of these are **molarity** and **normality**.

A **mole** is a unit of measurement for an extremely large number of items. Its value is 6.022×10^{23} which is called Avogadro's number. The mole is one of the seven base units in the International System. Another way of defining a mole is as an amount of a substance containing the same number of formula units as there are atoms in exactly 12 g of carbon-12. In other words, 1 mole of carbon = 6.022×10^{23} atoms of carbon, which have an atomic mass of 12 g. Therefore, we can state that the mass of 1 mole of substance = the weight of 6.022×10^{23} atoms of that substance = its atomic mass.

Molarity is a numerical expression of concentration that indicates the number of moles of a solute in 1 liter of solution (mol/L). A 2 M saline solution contains 2 moles of salt per liter of solution. Since we know that the atomic mass of salt is 58.5 g, this is the weight of 1 mole of salt. Therefore, a 2 M solution contains $2 \times 58.5 \text{ g} = 117 \text{ g}$ of salt per liter of solution.

In all aqueous solutions, whether acid, base, or neutral, the molar concentration of the hydrogen ions multiplied by the molar concentration of the hydroxyl ions will always be equal to 1×10^{-14}. Brackets are used around the ion symbols to represent molar concentration. $[H^+]$ indicates the molar concentration of hydrogen ions in a solution and $[OH^-]$ the molar concentration of hydroxyl ions.

Important Fact

In all aqueous solutions, the molar concentration of the hydrogen ions multiplied by the molar concentration of the hydroxyl ions will always be equal to 1×10^{-14}. This relationship is described by the formula

$$[H^+] \times [OH^-] = 1 \times 10^{-14}$$

If the concentration of hydrogen ions in a particular solution is known, we can use this relationship to determine the concentration of hydroxyl ions in the solution. See Example 7.

EXAMPLE 7: Finding the Concentration of Hydroxyl Ions in a Solution

An aqueous solution has a hydrogen concentration $[H^+]$ of 0.005 mol/L. Find the concentration of hydroxyl ions $[OH^-]$ in this solution.

Solution

$$\text{Equation: } [H^+] \times [OH^-] = 1 \times 10^{-14}$$

Since $[H^+] = 0.005$, substitute this into the equation and solve.

$$0.005 \times [OH^-] = 1 \times 10^{-14}$$

$$[OH^-] = \frac{1 \times 10^{-14}}{0.005} = 2 \times 10^{-12}$$

Therefore, the concentration of hydroxyl ions is 2×10^{-12} mol/L.

The concentration of many acids is given in normality. **Normality** is a concentration unit that is based on a unit of mass called the **equivalent weight**, instead of the gram molecular weight used for molarity.

The weight of an **equivalent** of solute is the mass of that substance that will combine with or replace 1 mole of hydrogen.

In a 2 N solution, there are 2 equivalents of solute per liter of solution. Generally, equivalent weight can be calculated by dividing the gram molecular weight of the substance by its positive valence.

The hydrogen ion concentration in a given solution depends upon the percent of ionization or degree of dissociation that occurs in the solution. In strongly acidic or basic solutions, the percent of ionization is usually known, and $[H^+]$ can be determined from the normality, N, using the formula shown here.

We know that strong acids readily dissociate in water (100% ionization). Examples of strong acids are hydrochloric acid (HCl) and sulfuric acid (H_2SO_4). Similarly, strong bases such as sodium hydroxide (NaOH) readily dissociate in water, giving up hydroxyl (OH^-) ions. Weak acids, such as acetic acid (CH_3COOH), release hydrogen ions less readily in solution, and weak bases also release hydroxyl ions less readily in solution.

EXAMPLE 8: Finding the Hydrogen Ion Concentration of an Acid

What is the hydrogen ion concentration of a 0.3 N solution of H_2SO_4?

Solution

Strong acids will completely dissociate (100% ionization). Use the formula to calculate the molar concentration of hydrogen in this solution as follows:

$$N \times \% \text{ ionization} = [H^+]$$
$$(0.3\,N)(100\%) = [H^+]$$
$$(0.3)(1) = [H^+]$$
$$0.3 = [H^+]$$

Therefore, $[H^+] = 0.3$ mol/L H^+ in a 0.3 N H_2SO_4 solution.

EXAMPLE 9: Finding the Hydrogen Ion Concentration of an Acid

What is the hydrogen ion concentration of a 1.5 N solution of acetic acid?

Solution

Weak acids will not completely dissociate in solution. Acetic acid will only slightly dissociate into H^+ ions and acetate ions. Assume that this dissociation is 1%. Calculate the hydrogen ion concentration of a 1.5 N solution of acetic acid.

$$N \times \% \text{ ionization} = [H^+]$$
$$(1.5\,N)(1\%) = [H^+]$$
$$(1.5\,N)(0.01) = [H^+]$$
$$0.015 = [H^+]$$

Therefore, $[H^+] = 0.015$ mol /L H^+ in a 1.5 N acetic acid solution.

PRACTICE PROBLEM SET 8.2

Round all concentrations to 3 significant figures.

1. An aqueous solution has a hydrogen concentration $[H^+]$ of 0.5 mol/L. Find the concentration of hydroxyl ions $[OH^-]$ in this solution.

2. An aqueous solution has a hydrogen concentration $[H^+]$ of 0.00012 mol/L. Find the concentration of hydroxyl ions $[OH^-]$ in this solution.

3. An aqueous solution has a hydrogen concentration $[H^+]$ of 1.3×10^{-5} mol/L. Find the concentration of hydroxyl ions $[OH^-]$ in this solution.

4. An aqueous solution has a hydrogen concentration $[H^+]$ of 3.2×10^{-8} mol/L. Find the concentration of hydroxyl ions $[OH^-]$ in this solution.

5. An aqueous solution has a hydroxyl concentration $[OH^-]$ of 0.0002 mol/L. Find the concentration of hydrogen ions $[H^+]$ in this solution.

6. An aqueous solution has a hydroxyl concentration $[OH^-]$ of 0.00015 mol/L. Find the concentration of hydrogen ions $[H^+]$ in this solution.

7. An aqueous solution has a hydroxyl concentration $[OH^-]$ of 1.75×10^{-7} mol/L. Find the concentration of hydrogen ions $[H^+]$ in this solution.

8. An aqueous solution has a hydroxyl concentration $[OH^-]$ of 9.1×10^{-10} mol/L. Find the concentration of hydrogen ions $[H^+]$ in this solution.

9. A solution of 0.2 N acid is known to be 95% ionized. Find $[H^+]$, the hydrogen ion concentration.

10. A solution of 0.3 N acid is known to be 75% ionized. Find $[H^+]$, the hydrogen ion concentration.

11. A solution of 1.5 N acid is known to be 20% ionized. Find $[H^+]$, the hydrogen ion concentration.

12. A solution of 2 N acid is known to be 1% ionized. Find $[H^+]$, the hydrogen ion concentration.

13. Assume that acetic acid is 1% ionized. Find $[H^+]$ of a 1.8 N acetic acid solution.

14. Assume that acetic acid is 1% ionized. Find $[H^+]$ of a 0.05 N acetic acid solution.

15. Assume that HCl is 100% ionized. Find $[H^+]$ of a 0.08 N HCl solution.

16. Assume that HCl is 100% ionized. Find $[H^+]$ of a 1.1 N HCl solution.

SECTION 8.3   USING LOGARITHMS TO CALCULATE pH AND pOH

The acidity of a solution is a result of the concentration of hydrogen ions in the solution. However, the use of ion concentrations to express the acidity or alkalinity of solutions is often inconvenient. In 1909, the Swedish chemist S. P. L. Sørensen developed a logarithmic scale to define acidity based on the concentration of hydrogen ions in solutions. He called the scale **pH** since it measures what he called the potential or potency of the hydrogen ions in a solution. He defined pH to be the logarithm of the reciprocal of the concentration of hydrogen ions in a solution, $[H^+]$. Another way to express the same idea is that pH is the negative logarithm of $[H^+]$. Although the concept of alkalinity is much less commonly used, **pOH** is defined as the logarithm of the reciprocal of the concentration of hydroxyl in a solution, $[OH^-]$. The following formulas defining both pH and pOH will be very useful:

Important Formulas

$$pH = \log\left(\frac{1}{[H^+]}\right) = -\log[H^+]$$

$$pOH = \log\left(\frac{1}{[OH^-]}\right) = -\log[OH^-]$$

Recall that the concentration of hydrogen and hydroxyl ions in water at equilibrium is 1×10^{-14} moles per liter (M). Because water dissociates equally into hydrogen and hydroxyl, the hydrogen ion concentration of pure water is 1×10^{-7} M. We can use the log formula ($pH = -\log (1 \times 10^{-7})$) to determine that the pH of water is 7, indicating a neutral solution. The pH scale includes the numbers from 0 to 14. Numbers lower than 7.0 have higher concentrations of hydrogen ions and therefore are more acidic. Numbers higher than 7.0 have lower concentrations of hydrogen ions and therefore are less acidic and more alkaline or basic.

EXAMPLE 10: Calculating pH Using Logarithms

The hydrogen ion concentration of a certain solution is known to be 2.5×10^{-6}. What is the pH of this solution?

Solution

$$pH = -\log[H^+]$$
$$pH = -[\log(2.5 \times 10^{-6})]$$
$$pH = -(-5.6)$$

Therefore, pH = 5.6. This solution is more acidic since its pH < 7.

Most biological fluids with the exception of stomach acid have a pH between 6 and 8. Each 1-point difference in the pH scale represents a tenfold difference in the hydrogen ion concentration since these numbers are logarithms or exponents whose base is 10. Therefore, a solution with a pH of 6 is not twice as acidic as a solution with a pH of 8, but 10^2, or 100, times as acidic. Your small intestine has a pH of 9. Look at Figure 8-1 for the location of some other common items on the pH scale.

The majority of living cells have an internal pH close to 7.0. Even a minor change in the pH can be extremely harmful because the chemical processes of the cell are sensitive to the concentration of hydrogen and hydroxide ions. Biological fluids resist change to their own pH when acids and bases are introduced because of the presence of buffers. For example, buffers in human blood maintain the blood pH very close to 7.4. A person cannot survive if the pH of the blood drops to 7.0 or rises to 7.8. Under normal circumstances, the buffering capacity of the blood prevents major changes in the pH level.

Because the concentration of hydrogen and hydroxyl is in equilibrium at 1×10^{-14}, we can define a useful relationship between pH and pOH with the equation pH + pOH = 14. Therefore, a solution whose pH is 1.5 has a pOH of 14 − 1.5, or 12.5. Conversely, a solution whose pOH is 5.5 has a pH of 14 − 5.5 = 8.5.

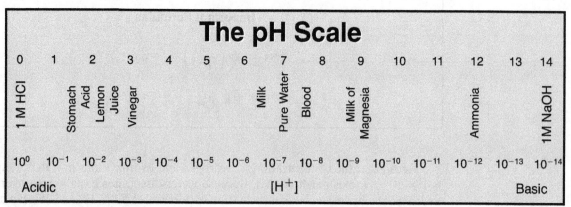

Figure 8.1 The pH Scale

## Chapter 8

EXAMPLE 11: Calculating the pH and pOH of an Ionic Solution

A solution of 0.12 N acid is known to be 20% ionized. Find each of the following:

    a. $[H^+]$

    b. $[OH^-]$

    c. pH

    d. pOH

Solution

    a. $N \times \%$ ionization $= [H^+]$

$$(0.12 \text{ N})(0.20) = [H^+]$$

$$[H^+] = 0.024 \text{ mol } H^+/L \text{ (or } 2.4 \times 10^{-2} \text{ g } H^+/L)$$

Note: The $[H^+]$ concentration has been expressed as mol/L and then as the same number of g/L. This is true because 1 mole of hydrogen has a gram molecular weight of 1 gram.

    b. $[H^+] \times [OH^-] = 1 \times 10^{-14}$

$$(2.4 \times 10^{-2})([OH^-]) = 1 \times 10^{-14}$$

$$[OH^-] = \frac{1 \times 10^{-14}}{2.4 \times 10^{-2}}$$

$$[OH^-] = 4.17 \times 10^{-13} \text{ mol } OH^-/L$$

    c.   pH $= -\log[H^+]$

         pH $= -\log(2.4 \times 10^{-2})$

         pH $= -(-1.6)$

         pH $= 1.6$

    d. pH $+$ pOH $= 14$

        $1.6 +$ pOH $= 14$

              pOH $= 14 - 1.6$

              pOH $= 12.4$

In order to calculate the concentration of hydrogen ions in a solution from the pH number, we will need to use the *antilogarithm* function. This function will reverse the process used to calculate the pH number. The pH formula gives positive values for the pH scale, but we see from the molar concentrations of these solutions that the exponents were originally negative (pH $= 6.0$ means $[H^+] = 10^{-6}$). When reversing the process, we must keep this in mind. Look at the following relationships.

Important Formulas

$[H^+] = \text{antilog}(-pH)$

$[OH^-] = \text{antilog}(-pOH)$

EXAMPLE 12: Calculating the Hydrogen Concentration from pH

An acid solution has a pH of 1.5. Find the hydrogen ion concentration of this solution.

Solution

$$[H^+] = antilog(-pH)$$
$$[H^+] = antilog(-1.5)$$
$$[H^+] = 0.00501 \text{ mol } H^+/L$$

PRACTICE PROBLEM SET 8.3

Solve each of the following problems.

1. In seawater, the concentration of hydrogen ions is 1×10^{-8}. What is the pH of seawater?
2. Find the pH of milk if $[H^+] = 1.77 \times 10^{-8}$.
3. Find $[H^+]$ for saliva with pH = 7.4.
4. Find $[H^+]$ for normal rain with pH = 5.6.
5. A certain hair conditioner has a pH of 6.1. What is the hydrogen ion concentration of the conditioner?
6. Find the hydrogen ion concentration if the pH of a glass of tomato juice is 4.1.
7. If the pH of baking soda is 9, then what is its pOH?
8. If the pOH of a soapy water is 2, what is the pH of that solution?
9. What is the pOH of a solution having $[H^+] = 3.2 \times 10^{-6}$?
10. What is the pOH of a solution having $[H^+] = 5.3 \times 10^{-9}$?
11. The most acidic fluid in the body is gastric juice with $[H^+]$ of 0.13 M. What is its pH?
12. The most alkaline body fluid is pancreatic juice. What is the pH of pancreatic juice if $[H^+] = 3.01 \times 10^{-8}$ M?
13. What is the range of hydrogen ion concentrations for whole blood if it has a slightly alkaline pH between 7.35 and 7.45?
14. If the pH of a solution is 3.25, what is the $[OH^-]$ of this solution?
15. What is the pH of a solution with $[H^+] = 1.5 \times 10^{-7}$ mol H^+/L?
16. What is the pH of a solution with $[OH^-] = 4.2 \times 10^{-8}$ mol OH^-/L?
17. In a certain solution, $[H^+] = 6.1 \times 10^{-2}$. What is its (a) pH and (b) $[OH^-]$?
18. A solution has $[OH^-] = 2.5 \times 10^{-8}$. What is its (a) $[H^+]$ and (b) pH?
19. A solution of 1.2 N acid is known to be 10% ionized. Find:
    a. $[H^+]$
    b. $[OH^-]$
    c. pH
    d. pOH

20. A certain acid dissociates slightly in solution (1% ionization). If the acid is 0.45 N, find each of the following:
    a. $[H^+]$
    b. pH
    c. pOH
    d. $[OH^-]$

Chapter Summary

In this chapter, we have given a brief introduction to logarithms and antilogarithms and their uses to measure the acidity of a solution using the pH scale. The pH scale is derived by taking the negative logarithm of the hydrogen ion concentration of a solution. The pOH scale measures the alkalinity of a solution and is the negative logarithm of the hydroxyl concentration of that solution. If we are given the pH of a solution, we can use the antilogarithm function to calculate the hydrogen ion concentration of that solution.

Important Rules and Terms

acid, base, and salt

antilogarithm, antilog

common logarithm

degree of dissociation

dissociate

equivalent weight

exponent

ionize

log

logarithm

molarity

mole

normality

pH

pOH

Important Equations

$$[H^+] \times [OH^-] = 1 \times 10^{-14}$$

$$pH = -\log[H^+]$$

$$N \times \% \text{ ionization} = [H^+]$$

$$pOH = -\log[OH^-]$$

$$pH + pOH = 14$$

Chapter Review Problems

Calculate each of the following values.

1. $\log 500$
2. $\log 0.001$
3. $\log^{-1} 1.857$
4. $\text{antilog}(-3.5)$

Solve each of the following for x.

5. $\log x = -5$
6. $\log 0.00001 = x$
7. $\log x = -2$
8. $\text{antilog}(-2.5) = x$
9. What is the pH of a solution where $[H^+] = 5.2 \times 10^{-4}$? What is the $[OH^-]$ of this solution?
10. What is the pH of a solution with a $[H^+] = 1.53 \times 10^{-7}$? What is the $[OH^-]$ of this solution?
11. If a certain solution has a pOH $= 6.4$, what is its pH? Is this solution acidic or basic (alkaline)?
12. If the pH of a solution is 2.9, the pOH $=$ _____ .

13. If the pH of a solution is 9.1, the solution is more _____ (acidic or basic). The concentration of the hydroxyl ions in this solution would be _____ .

14. Find the concentration of hydrogen ions in an apple if its pH = 3.1.

15. A 1.2 N acid solution is only 45% ionized. Calculate each of the following values for this solution (round pH and pOH to 1 decimal place and concentrations to 3 significant figures).

    a. $[H^+]$
    b. $[OH^-]$
    c. pH
    d. pOH

16. A 0.015 N acid solution is 100% ionized. Give the following (round pH and pOH to 1 decimal place and concentrations to 3 significant figures).

    a. $[H^+]$
    b. $[OH^-]$
    c. pH
    d. pOH

Chapter Test

Calculate each of the following values.

1. log 138
2. $\log^{-1} 2.7$
3. antilog(−7.5)

Solve each of the following for x.

4. log 0.01 = x
5. log x = −1.8
6. What is the pH of a solution where $[H^+]$ = 1.8 × 10^{-3}? What is the $[OH^-]$ of this solution?
7. If a glass of lemonade has a pH of 2.8, what is its pOH? Is this solution acidic or basic (alkaline)?
8. If the pH of an ammonia solution is 11.1, the solution is more _____ (acidic or basic). The concentration of the hydroxyl ions in this solution would be _____ .
9. Find the concentration of hydrogen ions in an apple if its pH = 3.1.
10. A 3.2 N acid solution is 75% ionized. Calculate each of the following values for this solution (round pH and pOH to 1 decimal place and concentrations to 3 significant figures).

    a. $[H^+]$
    b. $[OH^-]$
    c. pH
    d. pOH

Appendix A

COMMONLY USED CALCULATOR KEYS

Key	Function*
SHIFT or 2nd	Allows access to calculator functions printed above the keys
+/– or (–)	Used to change the sign of a number or enter a negative number into the calculator
$\sqrt{x}$	Used to take the square root of a number
x^2	Used to raise a number to the second power (square a number): Enter 10^2 as: 10 x^2
y^x x^y or $\wedge$	Used to raise a number to an exponential power: Enter 5^3 as: 5 y^x 3 =
EXP or EE	Used to enter a number written in scientific notation into the calculator: Enter 3×10^2 as: 3 EE 2
d/c	Used to change a mixed fraction to an improper fraction.
a^b/$_c$	Used to enter a fraction into the calculator: Enter $\frac{1}{2}$ as: 1 a^b/$_c$ 2
$\frac{1}{x}$ or x^{-1}	Used to find the reciprocal of a number
$\bar{x}$	Gives the arithmetic mean of a set of data when the calculator is in the statistics mode
δ_n or s	Gives the sample standard deviation for a set of data when the calculator is in the statistics mode
10^x	Used to find the antilogarithm of a number
log	Used to find the common logarithm of a number (base 10)

---

* The keystrokes and keys on individual calculators vary according to brands. This list is a general resource to help you quickly find an explanation of certain keys. For complete information, consult the manual that accompanied your particular calculator.

Appendix B

ADULT BSA NOMOGRAM

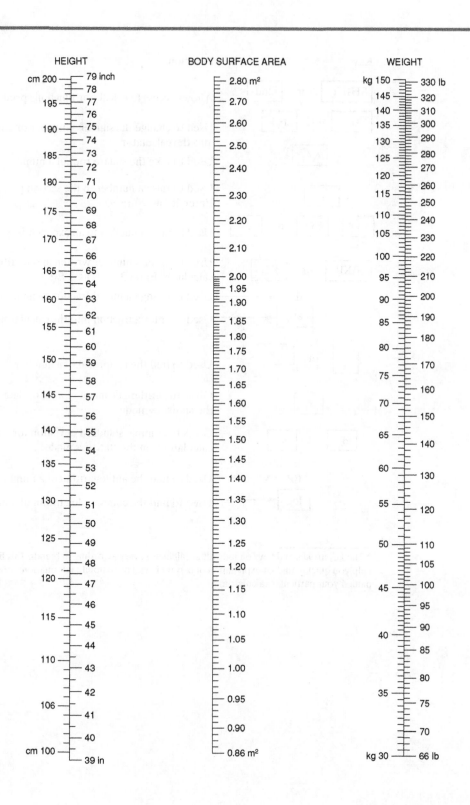

HEIGHT | BODY SURFACE AREA | WEIGHT

Appendix C

COMMON ABBREVIATIONS

Abbreviations Prohibited by JACHO

Abbreviation or Symbol	Potential Problem	Use Instead
U (unit)	mistaken for the numbers 0 or 4 or cc	write "unit"
IU (International Unit)	mistaken for IV (intravenous) or the number 10	write "International Unit"
Q.D., QD, q.d., qd (daily) Q.O.D., QOD, q.o.d., qod (every other day)	mistaken for each other; the period after the Q mistaken for "l" and the "O" mistaken for "l"	write "daily" write "every other day"
trailing zero (X.0 mg)	decimal point is missed	write "X mg" unless the trailing zero is required to show the level of precision
lack of leading zero (.X mg)	decimal point is missed	write "0.X mg"
MS	can mean morphine sulfate or magnesium sulfate	write "morphine sulfate" or "magnesium sulfate"
MSO_4 and $MgSO_4$	confused with one another	write "morphine sulfate" or "magnesium sulfate"

Abbreviations and Symbols Still in Use BUT Scheduled for Possible Future Elimination

Abbreviation or Symbol	Potential Problem	Use Instead
> (greater than) < (less than)	misinterpreted as the number 7 or the letter "L" and confused with one another	write "greater than" write "less than"
abbreviations for drug names	misinterpreted due to similar abbreviations for multiple drugs	write drug names in full
apothecary units	unfamiliar to many practitioners and confused with metric units	use metric units
@	mistaken for the number 2	write "at"
cc	mistaken for U (units) when poorly written	write "ml" or "milliliters"
µg	mistaken for mg (milligrams) resulting in a 1000-fold overdose	write "mcg" or "micrograms"

Routes of Drug Administration

Abbreviation	Meaning
a.d.	right ear (dexter ear)
a.s	left ear (sinister ear)
a.u.	both ears
buc. or buccal	inside the cheek
IM	intramuscular, into the muscle
inj.	injection
IV	into a vein
IVP	intravenous push
IVPB	intravenous piggy back
ID	beneath the skin
o.d.	right eye (dexter eye)
o.l. or o.s.	left eye (sinister eye)
o.u. or o_2	both eyes
p.o.	by mouth
R or p.r.	rectal
subL or SL	sunlingual, under the tongue
Sub-Q or subQ	into the subcutaneous tissue
top	topically (on the skin)
V or p.v. or vag	vaginal (in the vagina)

Abbreviations Referring to Time and/or Frequency of Administration

Abbreviation	Meaning
a.c.	before meals
ad	up to
ad lib	at your pleasure or freely
a.m.	morning
ATC	around the clock
b.i.d.	twice a day
d.	day
disc or D.C.	discontinue
e.m.p.	as directed
h or hr	hour
HS or hs	at bedtime (hour of sleep)
noct	night
p.c.	after meals

(Continued)

Appendix C

Abbreviation	Meaning
p.m.	afternoon
p.r.n.	as needed
qh	every hour
q2h, q3h, q4h	every 2, 3, or 4 hours
qid	four times a day
s.o.s.	if there is need
stat	immediately
tid	three times a day
T.I.W.	three times a week

Abbreviations Related to Amounts

Abbreviation	Meaning
aa	of each
amp	ampule or ampoule
c.	with
cc	cubic centimeter
cap.	capsule
dil.	dilute
div.	divide
g. or GM or g	gram
gr.	grain
gtt.	drop
HS	half strength
mcg or μg	microgram
mg	milligram
mL or ml	milliliter
NMT	not more than
O	pint
qs	a sufficient quantity
qs ad	a sufficient quantity to make
ss	one-half
t	teaspoon
T	tablespoon
x	times
w/	with
w/o or s.	without

Miscellaneous Commonly Used Medical Abbreviations

Abbreviation	Meaning
aq.	water
ASA	aspirin
BM	bowel movement
BP	blood pressure
BS	blood sugar
BSA	body surface area
CHF	congestive heart failure
comp.	compound
disp.	dispense
DW	distilled water
D5W	dextrose 5% in water
TPN	total parenteral nutrition
tr.	tincture
ung.	ointment
URI	upper respiratory infection
USP	United States Pharmacopedia
UTI	urinary tract infection
VS	vital signs
WBC	white blood cell count

CONVERSION FACTORS

Common Metric Equivalents and Symbols

Equivalents for Liquid Volumes
1 mL (or ml, one milliliter) = 1 cc (or cm³, one cubic centimeter)
1000 mL = 1 L (liter)
1000 cc = 1 L (liter)
Equivalents for Weights (Masses)
1 kg (kilogram) = 1000 g (grams)
1 g (gram) = 1000 mg (milligrams)
1 mg (milligram) = 1000 mcg (μg or micrograms)

Equivalents and Symbols for Household Units

Liquid Volume Equivalents
1 glass = 8 oz (ounces)
1 measuring cup = 8 oz (ounces)
1 oz (ounce) = 2 T (tablespoons)
1 T (tablespoon) = 3 t (teaspoons)
1 t (teaspoon) = 60 gtt (drops)
Weight Equivalents
1 lb (pound) = 16 oz (ounces)

Equivalents and Symbols for the Apothecary System

Liquid Volume Equivalents
1 quart = qt 1 = 2 pints = pt 2 = pt ii
qt 1 = 32 fluid ounces = floz 32 = fl℥ 32 = fl℥ XXXII
pt 1 = 16 fluid ounces = floz 16 = fl℥ 16 = fl℥ xvi
fl℥ 1 = floz 1 = 8 fluid drams = fldr 8 = flℨ 8 = flℨ viii
fldr 1 = flℨ 1 = 60 minims = min 60 = m 60 = m LX
Weight Equivalents
oz 1 = ℥ 1 = 8 drams = ℨ 8 = ℨ viii
1 dram = ℨ 1 = 60 grains = gr 60 = gr LX

Metric	Apothecary	Household
Liquid Volumes	**Liquid Volumes**	**Liquid Volumes**
30 or 32 mL (30 mL is used most)	fl ℥1 = fl ʒ 8	2 T
4 or 5 mL (5 mL is used most)	fl ʒ 1 = min 60	1 t = 60 gtt
	min 1	1 gtt
15 mL	fl ʒ 4	1 T
1 mL = 1 cc	min 15 or 16	15 or 16 gtt
Weights	**Weights**	**Weights**
60 mg	gr 1	
1 g	gr 15	
1 kg	gr 15,000 = oz 35.2	2.2 lb
0.45 kg	oz 16	1 lb
Lengths	**Lengths**	**Lengths**
2.54 cm	None	1 in

Temperature Conversion Formulas

$$T_C = \frac{T_F - 32}{1.8} \qquad T_F = 1.8T_C + 32 \qquad T_K = T_C + 273$$

ANSWERS TO ODD-NUMBERED PROBLEMS

Chapter 1

Practice Problem Set 1.1

1. 18
3. $12\frac{1}{2}$
5. 15
7. 4
9. 28
11. 24
13. 40
15. 400
17. 57
19. 72
21. 2600
23. $1609\frac{1}{2}$
25. 189
27. viii
29. xii
31. iiiss
33. xix
35. LXIX
37. XXIX
39. XL
41. XCIX
43. CXLVI
45. CDL
47. CCCXC
49. MDCXXVI
51. 2085 mL
53. 300 cc
55. 540 cc
57. 120 cc more output than input
59. 2703 used; 2179 should be ordered; 9 boxes
61. 672; 2 bottles of 250, 1 bottle of 100, and 3 bottles of 25
63. 1269; 731
65. Ray—1982, Nancy—1820, John—1874

Practice Problem Set 1.2

1. $\frac{3}{4}$
3. $\frac{3}{7}$
5. $1\frac{1}{19}$
7. $3\frac{1}{9}$
9. 25
11. 10
13. 30
15. $\frac{1}{2}, \frac{1}{3}, \frac{1}{6}$
17. $\frac{2}{3}, \frac{2}{5}, \frac{3}{10}$
19. $\frac{3}{4}, \frac{3}{5}, \frac{1}{2}, \frac{1}{8}$
21. $1\frac{9}{40}$
23. $1\frac{7}{24}$
25. $13\frac{5}{6}$
27. $10\frac{13}{18}$
29. $13\frac{13}{20}$
31. $\frac{1}{4}$
33. $\frac{17}{30}$
35. $3\frac{1}{4}$
37. $6\frac{53}{120}$
39. $\frac{1}{3}$
41. $18\frac{3}{8}$
43. $4\frac{1}{2}$
45. $1\frac{3}{7}$
47. $\frac{1}{8}$
49. $\frac{39}{50}$
51. $\frac{4}{5}$
53. $\frac{3}{625}$
55. 75
57. $93\frac{3}{4}$
59. 20 oz
61. 11 oz; 330 cc
63. $13\frac{1}{2}$ cups
65. 7 t
67. $225\frac{3}{4}$ lb
69. 687,500

Practice Problem Set 1.3

1. $\frac{2}{5}$
3. $\frac{3}{20}$
5. $\frac{113}{1000}$
7. $\frac{33}{40}$
9. $\frac{1}{400}$
11. $16\frac{1}{8}$
13. $3\frac{1}{10,000}$
15. 6.755
17. 35.1452
19. 13.53
21. 15.647
23. 7.5225
25. 8.785
27. 0.24
29. 4.2
31. 5.2
33. 0.03

35. 60.126
37. 11
39. 2.0
41. <
43. >
45. >
47. >
49. >
51. deposit: $674.31; balance: $2817.88
53. 9.5 million gallons
55. 2 tablets
57. 0.7 g
59. 7.5 mg

Practice Problem Set 1.4
1. $\frac{7}{20}$

3. $\frac{1}{20}$

5. $\frac{7}{200}$
7. 0.06
9. 0.75
11. 0.0004
13. 0.000012
15. 0.015
17. 1.45
19. 62.5%
21. 33.33%
23. 125%
25. 20%
27. 37.5%
29. 0.125%
31. 150%
33. 12.5%
35. 0.1%
37. 3.33%
39. 0.05%
41. 15%
43. 40%
45. 3.33%
47. 5%

Practice Problem Set 1.5
1. $\frac{7}{8}$; 87.5%
3. 0.4; 40%
5. $\frac{7}{200}$; 0.035

7. $\frac{1}{50}$; 2%
9. 0.5; 50%
11. $\frac{9}{100}$; 0.09

13. $\frac{1}{10,000}$; 0.01%

15. 0.333 . . . ; $33\frac{1}{3}$%

17. $\frac{1}{500}$; 0.002
19. 2.25; 225%
21. $\frac{5}{8}$
23. 0.125
25. 0.5
27. $\frac{7}{400}$; 0.0175

29. $\frac{9}{1000}$; 0.009

Chapter 1 Review
1. 27
2. 14
3. $26\frac{1}{2}$
4. 45
5. 134
6. XLVI
7. xix
8. xxxviii
9. CL
10. ixss

11. $\frac{2}{7}$

12. $\frac{3}{8}$

13. $\frac{1}{25}$

14. $5\frac{5}{6}$

15. $\frac{1}{3}, \frac{1}{4}, \frac{1}{6}$

16. $\frac{1}{3}, \frac{1}{6}, \frac{1}{8}$

17. $\frac{2}{3}, \frac{2}{5}, \frac{3}{10}$

18. $1\frac{7}{30}$

19. $5\frac{11}{12}$

20. $\frac{2}{3}$

21. $15\frac{5}{12}$

22. $16\frac{11}{12}$

23. $\frac{1}{5}$

24. $5\frac{7}{36}$

25. $\frac{3}{5}$
26. 4500
27. $\frac{1}{8}$

28. $\frac{3}{50}$

29. $\frac{3}{2000}$

30. $\frac{1}{100,000}$

31. 7.5855
32. 29.291
33. 5.497
34. 2.945
35. 0.01845
36. 5.995
37. 0.43
38. 0.2099
39. 255.25
40. 38.2
41. 0.027
42. 0.01
43. <
44. >

45. $\frac{11}{20}$

46. $\frac{13}{200}$

47. $\frac{1}{20,000}$

Answers to Odd-Numbered Problems

48. 0.025
49. 0.0009
50. 0.05
51. 12.5%
52. 12%
53. $66\frac{2}{3}\%$
54. 0.3%
55. 57.5%
56. 15%
57. 35%
58. 35%
59. $\frac{1}{200}$; 0.5%
60. $\frac{1}{40}$; 0.025
61. 0.8; 80%
62. 345 cc more output
63. 1750; 2475; 10 boxes
64. 9 in.
65. less
66. 12
67. 825 calories
68. 37 in.
69. 3 tablets
70. $822; $8967.57
71. 8%
72. 14.7%
73. $\frac{29}{100}$; $\frac{71}{100}$
74. 36%; 0.36; $\frac{9}{25}$
75. 44%; $\frac{11}{25}$; 0.44
76. Yes, that would be 6.7%, which is higher than average of 3%

Chapter 1 Test
1. 18
2. $14\frac{1}{2}$
3. 95
4. 1221
5. ivss
6. xxix
7. $\frac{5}{6}, \frac{3}{4}, \frac{1}{5}$
8. $\frac{7}{10}, \frac{5}{12}, \frac{1}{3}$
9. $1\frac{1}{2}$
10. $9\frac{7}{12}$
11. $2\frac{79}{100}$
12. $\frac{7}{10}$
13. 36
14. $1\frac{1}{2}$
15. $\frac{1}{84}$
16. 4.875
17. 15.8475
18. 8.82
19. 0.0033
20. 0.75
21. 24.0
22. 0.2152, 0.2, 0.152, 0.1, 0.015
23. 15%

24. $\frac{9}{1000}$; 0.009
25. 1/40; 2.5%
26. 0.833...; $83\frac{1}{3}\%$
27. 1007; 4 bottles of 250 and 1 bottle of 25
28. 60 doses
29. 4 days
30. 0.46; $\frac{23}{50}$

Chapter 2
Practice Problem Set 2.1
1. 3
3. −1360
5. 0
7. undefined
9. $-\frac{11}{24}$
11. $-2\frac{1}{12}$
13. 9.6
15. 0.06
17. −5
19. −9
21. −10
23. 0
25. 13
27. $1\frac{1}{4}$
29. $2\frac{3}{8}$
31. −6
33. 27.75
35. 80.4
37. 0
39. 5

Practice Problem Set 2.2
1. $x = 2$
3. $k = 73.42$
5. $x = \frac{1}{4}$
7. $x = -3$
9. $x = -3.5$
11. $a = 36$
13. $x = -\frac{3}{5}$
15. $x = -7$
17. $x = 10$
19. $x = 45$
21. $x = 2\frac{2}{21}$
23. $x = -45$
25. $x = 1$
27. $d = 2$
29. $x = -3$
31. $x = -4$
33. $x = -1$
35. $x = -1$
37. $x = 5$
39. $x = -\frac{1}{3}$
41. $a = -2.5$
43. $x = -6$
45. $x = 12$
47. $x = -4$
49. $x = 0$

Practice Problem Set 2.3

1. T
3. T
5. T
7. 6
9. 9
11. $1\frac{1}{3}$
13. 75
15. 0.005
17. 0.2
19. 6 capsules
21. 1.25 mL
23. 0.4 mL
25. 1050 mg
27. 3 tablets
29. 0.875 cc
31. 0.1 mL
33. $3\frac{1}{3}$ cc
35. 6.5 mg
37. 980 mg
39. 135 g
41. 360 calories
43. 4.5 T
45. 136.66 . . . , or 137 g
47. 88 children
49. 8.625, or 9 infant deaths

Practice Problem Set 2.4

1. 12.75
3. 102
5. 35%
7. 190
9. 50%
11. 102
13. 59
15. 3%
17. 600
19. 3.5%
21. +20%
23. −10%
25. −9.1%
27. −2.55%
29. 28.75 lb
31. 149.4 lb
33. 118 (117.6) to 137 (137.2)
35. 6%
37. 32%
39. 1 g
41. 3.6 mL
43. 2.5 g
45. 0.53 mL
47. 5% increase
49. $7\frac{1}{3}$% gain

Practice Problem Set 2.5

1. 20°C
3. 212°F
5. 3.3 mg
7. gr 2.2
9. 0.5 t
11. 10.4, or about 10 drops per minute

13. 16.6, or about 17 drops per minute
15. 20.1 normal
17. 27.0 overweight
19. 22.13 normal
21. $g = \dfrac{H}{1.36\,s}$
23. $F = \dfrac{9}{5}C + 32$
25. $W = \dfrac{(BMI) \cdot H^2}{703}$
27. 0.407 mg
29. 3264.16, or 3264 cc
31. 1462.05, or 1462 calories
33. 2137.35, or 2137 calories
35. 2094 calories
37. 2797.75, or 2798 calories
39. 100 mL
41. 300 mL
43. 60%
45. 140 lb

Practice Problem Set 2.6

1. a. As a person ages, blood flow decreases. b. 70%
3. 3 mg
5. 16.67 mg
7. 1.5 mL
9. 0.015 mg
11. two 8-mg tablets
13. 200 mL
15. Can't make a stronger solution from a weaker stock solution
17. 9%
19. 2.25%
21. 20 mL of 9%
23. $49.51
25. $67.27
27. $10.97
29. $11.94
31. $y = 65,000 + 3.50x$; $152,500

Chapter 2 Review

1. 5
2. −15
3. 3.6
4. 28
5. $-\frac{1}{2}$
6. 5
7. −19
8. 3.95
9. 20.26
10. $\frac{1}{5}$
11. $y = 4.15$
12. $x = 0.125$, or $\frac{1}{8}$
13. $a = -15$
14. $x = 15$
15. $x = 12.375$
16. $x = 6$
17. $d = -5$
18. $x = 11$
19. $x = -2$
20. $x = -10$

21. $a = -4$
22. $s = 1$
23. $x = 1$
24. $x = 3$
25. $x = -16$
26. $C_1 = \dfrac{V_2 C_2}{V_1}$

27. $m = \dfrac{150p}{A}$

28. 50
29. 5
30. 0.0133 . . .
31. 0.75
32. 10 mL
33. 2.5 mL
34. 375 mg
35. 22.5 mg
36. 3 tablets
37. 1.125 cc
38. 12 mL
39. 480 mg
40. 510 calories
41. 360 calories
42. 60 g
43. 3.75
44. 5100
45. 1.67%
46. 1440
47. 35%
48. 15
49. 42
50. 5.5%
51. +4%
52. −7% (6.99)
53. −2.54%
54. +320%
55. 10%
56. 4 g
57. 0.01857, or 1.9%
58. 118.25, or 118 people
59. 0.2%
60. 245
61. 0.085714, or 8.6%
62. 3247.61 or 3248 cc
63. −25°C
64. 6.6 mg
65. 0.5866, or 0.6 t
66. 2 mg
67. 39.8% decrease
68. 238.71, or 239 students
69. 160 mL
70. 15%
71. 4.125%
72. $52.50

Chapter 2 Test
1. 28
2. 3.95
3. 20.26
4. $\frac{1}{3}$

5. $a = -8$
6. $x = -31.5$
7. $x = 6$
8. $x = 5$
9. $x = -9$
10. $x = 1$
11. 5
12. 2 mL
13. 1.5 tablets
14. 136.67, or 137 calories
15. 0.028
16. 480
17. 7.5%
18. 1.125 g
19. $3\frac{1}{3}\%$
20. 134.75, or 135 people
21. 61.625, or 62 babies
22. 0.69%
23. 6% increase
24. 23°F
25. 16.67 mL

Chapter 3
Practice Problem Set 3.1
1. 0400 h
3. 1500 h
5. 1435 h
7. 0000 h or 2400 h
9. 0015 h
11. 8:00 A.M.
13. 11:45 A.M.
15. 6:20 P.M.
17. midnight
19. 12:15 A.M.

Practice Problem Set 3.2
1. 8×10^3
3. 6.8×10^{-3}
5. 2.34×10^{11}
7. 2.366584×10^2
9. 2.005×10^{-1}
11. 4.65×10^0
13. 5×10^6
15. 4.58×10^2
17. 3.045×10^{-2}
19. $\frac{3}{4} = 0.75 = 7.5 \times 10^{-1}$
21. 0.85
23. 4,250,000
25. 7,000
27. 0.00008
29. 4.52
31. 645.7
33. 21.5
35. 8.208×10^6
37. 9.118×10^9
39. 1.2744×10^{-4}
41. $3.37894737 \times 10^{-5}$
43. 2×10^0
45. 1.8×10^{-5}
47. 1×10^0

49. 7×10^2

51. 2.3698×10^{-1} g, 2.1567×10^{-1} g, 2.2514×10^{-1} g

53. 2.5×10^{-7} g/tablet

55. $2^{20} = 1,048,576 = 1.048576 \times 10^6$

Practice Problem Set 3.3

1. 2
3. 2
5. 1
7. 4
9. 5
11. 4
13. 2
15. 3
17. 1
19. 1
21. 4
23. 2
25. 3
27. 3
29. 6
31. 0.326 m
33. 200. mg, or $20\overline{0}$ mg
35. 169,000 mcL
37. 0.00290 mcg
39. 800. g, or $80\overline{0}$ g
41. $3672 \text{ m}^2 = 3700 \text{ m}^2$
43. $2.75862069 \ldots$ mL/min = 2.8 mL/min
45. 25.6411 cm = 25.6 cm
47. 74 m = 70 m
49. $31.6906 \text{ cm}^2 = 31.7 \text{ cm}^2$
51. exact
53. approximate
55. 18.165 in. = 18.17 in.
57. $110.784 \text{ cm}^2 = 111 \text{ cm}^2$
59. 27 mL = 27.0 mL

Practice Problem Set 3.4

1. 5.698 m
3. 0.565 kL
5. 7400 mg
7. 6.85 mL
9. 0.00007 g
11. 0.76 mL
13. 3 dL
15. Cannot be converted—different base units
17. 4500 mg/L
19. 0.05 L/min
21. 0.7575 L = 0.76 L
23. $28.35 \text{ mm}^2 = 28 \text{ mm}^2$
25. 55.98167 g = 56.0 g
27. 12 mL/min = 10 mL/min
29. 0.026885559 cm = 0.0269 cm
31. two 500-cc cases

Practice Set 3.5

1. 3 T
3. $2\frac{1}{4}$ cups
5. 5 gtt
7. 1 oz
9. $4\frac{1}{2}$ t

11. $\frac{1}{2}$ oz
13. 40 T
15. $1\frac{1}{3}$ T
17. 6 t
19. 16 T
21. 30 gtt
23. $\frac{1}{4}$ t
25. 2 oz
27. $1\frac{1}{2}$ glass
29. 270 gtt
31. $\frac{1}{6}$ T
33. $3\frac{1}{3}$ oz
35. $\frac{1}{9}$ oz
37. 3 lb
39. 32 oz
41. 1.5 oz
43. 3 T
45. 0.367 oz = 2.2 t
47. 132 gtt

Practice Problem Set 3.6

1. gr $5\frac{1}{2}$
3. min 5
5. dr 4 = ʒ 4
7. fldr 4 = fʒ 4
9. floz 14 = fl ℥ 14
11. gr $\frac{1}{15}$
13. qt $3\frac{1}{2}$
15. pt 7
17. fl ℥ 5 $\frac{25}{100}$
19. ℥ 75
21. fʒ 12
23. fʒ 1792
25. fl ℥ 80
27. ʒ 3.5
29. fʒ $\frac{1}{4}$
31. fʒ 3840
33. fl ℥ $1\frac{1}{2}$
35. gr 120
37. pt $\frac{1}{2}$
39. min 960

Practice Problem Set 3.7

1. 45 mg
3. fl ℥ 1.33
5. 30 mL
7. 2 t
9. 2.5 mL
11. gr 0.000146
13. 8 gtt
15. 660 mL
17. 25 mL
19. fʒ 10
21. fʒ 20

23. fl ʒ 20
25. min 7680 = 7680 gtt
27. fl ʒ $\frac{3}{4}$
29. gr 1687.5 = gr 1700
31. 0.3125 cups
33. 60 cc
35. min 54
37. 90 kg
39. gr 7.5

Practice Problem Set 3.8
1. 31.7°C
3. 388 K
5. 77°F
7. −15.6°C
9. −40°C
11. −269°C
13. 5°F
15. 1472°F
17. 37°C = 310 K
19. −73°C = −99.4°F
21. 98.6°F
23. 98.4°F
25. 99.2
27. 99.4°F

Chapter 3 Review Problems
1. 5.67×10^{-3}
2. 5.5×10^{5}
3. 1×10^{2}
4. 7×10^{-9}
5. 4.6×10^{0}
6. 8.9×10^{3} L
7. 6×10^{-6} g
8. 4.500×10^{2} mL
9. 6.0×10^{0} m
10. 5.600×10^{-3} mg
11. 0.0000000679
12. 0.002843
13. 92,300
14. 2.9
15. 0.8
16. 4
17. 4
18. 6
19. 3
20. 2
21. micrograms
22. ounces
23. fluid drams
24. minims
25. milliliter
26. grain
27. degree
28. nanoliter
29. teaspoon
30. drop
31. An exact number contains no possible error.
32. Accuracy refers to the closeness of a measurement to the "real" value; precision refers to the

tolerance of the measurement instrument and its reliability.
33. No, 45 mL contains 2 sig. fig. and 45.0 mL contains 3 sig. fig.
34. Because there are a variety of measurement systems in current use in the United States.
35. They indicate the accuracy of the measuring instrument used.
36. fl ʒ 10
37. Can't answer—dry ounces ≠ fluid ounces.
38. 15 gtt
39. 8 oz
40. 750 cc
41. 1450 mL
42. 0.076 mg
43. ʒ 768
44. min 180
45. 4 gtt
46. 24 t
47. 760 g
48. gr 16.7
49. 40 mL
50. 90 gtt
51. 3.75 kg
52. 2 t
53. 120 gtt
54. 29.3 g
55. 465 mL
56. 149°F
57. 195 K
58. 42.2°C
59. −22.2°C
60. They are all the same.
61. 5.3698×10^{-1} g, 5.5567×10^{-1} g, 5.2574×10^{-1} g
62. 3.053×10^{-2} g
63. 18.75 mL = 18.8 mL
64. 4 of the 250-cc cases
65. 0.467 oz = 2.8 t
66. 168 gtt

Chapter 3 Test
1. 7.65×10^{8}
2. 6.7×10^{-7}
3. 9.45×10^{0}
4. 6.098
5. 0.0000793
6. 349,700,000
7. 56,900 mg
8. 0.00678 L
9. 50.0 m
10. 17 m^2
11. 35.6 g
12. 98.0 mL
13. 1050 mg
14. 0.00678 L
15. 315 gtt
16. 200 mcg
17. fl ʒ 90
18. 15 gtt
19. 0.24 g

20. 270 gtt
21. 98.6°F
22. 213 K
23. −23.3°C
24. gr 0.002
25. fl℥ 160

26. 3.63 cm^2
27. 1.25 mL
28. 7.2 t
29. 2.4 T
30. fl℥ 9.6

Chapter 4

Practice Problem Set 4.1

#	(a) Manufacturer	(b) Brand Name	(c) Generic Name	(d) Admin. Route	(e) Total Amount of Drug	(f) Amt. of Drug per tab, mL
1	Abbott Labs.	Biaxin Filmtab	clarithromycin	p.o.	60 tab.	250 mg/tab.
3	GlaxoSmithKline	Zovirax	acyclovir	p.o.	473 mL	200 mg/5 mL or 200 mg/t
5	Roxane	Diazepam	diazepam	p.o.	500 mL	1 mg/mL
7	Eli Lilly	Zyprexa	olanzapine	p.o.	60 tab.	7.5 mg/mL
9	Pharmacia	Vantin	cefpodoxime proxetil	p.o.	100 tab.	200 mg/tab.
11	Pharmacia	Atgam	lymphocyte immune globulin	IV	5 mL	50 mg/mL
13	Pharmacia	Azulfidine	sulfasalazine	p.o.	100 tab.	500 mg/tab.
15	Pfizer	Diflucan	fluconazole	p.o.	35 mL	40 mg/mL
17	Pfizer	Zithromax	azithromycin	p.o.	30 mL when mixed	40 mg/mL
19	Eli Lilly	Ceclor	cefaclor	p.o.	100 mL when mixed	75 mg/mL

Practice Problem Set 4.2

1. by mouth
3. R or p.r.
5. before meals
7. p.r.n.
9. microgram
11. tr.
13. body surface area

15. ss
17. twice a day
19. IV
21. into the vagina
23. at your pleasure or freely
25. every four hours

Practice Problem Set 4.3

#	(a) Admin. Route	(b) One Dose Amount	(c) Daily Dose Amount	(d) Total to Fill Prescription
1	by mouth	gr 6 = 1 tab.	6 tab.	30 tab.
3	by mouth	2 tab.	2 tab.	30 tab.
5	intramuscular inj.	gr $\frac{1}{4}$ = 15 mg = 1 mL	single dose	single dose
7	by mouth	2 cap.	8 cap.	40 cap.
9	by mouth	0.4 mL	single dose	single dose
11	by mouth	1 tab.	6 tab.	30 tab.
13	intramuscular inj.	0.8 mL	4.8 mL (6 vials)	14.4 mL (15 vials)
15	intramuscular inj.	2.0 mL	6.0 mL	24.0 mL
17	by mouth	1 tab.	2 tab.	8 tab.
19	by mouth	5 mL	5 mL	25 mL

Answers to Odd-Numbered Problems

Practice Problem Set 4.4

1. false (1.0 mL max)
3. false (larger dia. = smaller gauge number)
5. false (calibrated in tenths of a cc)
7. 1.0-mL tuberculin syringe; the nearest hundredth of a cc equals 0.83 mL.

9. 3-cc syringe; the nearest tenth of a cc is 1.6 cc (mL).
11. 3-cc syringe; the nearest tenth of a cc is 1.2 cc (mL).
13. 20-cc syringe; the nearest whole cc is 11 cc.
15. 3-cc syringe; the nearest tenth of a cc is 1.2 cc (mL).

Chapter 4 Review Problems

#	(a) Manufacturer	(b) Brand Name	(c) Generic Name	(d) Admin. Route	(e) Total Amount of Drug	(f) Amt. of Drug per tab., mL
1	Pharmacia	Vantin	cefpodoxime proxtil	p.o.	20 tab.	200 mg/tab.
2	Pharmacia	Provera	medroxyprogesterone acetate	p.o.	30 tab.	10 mg/tab.
3	Eli Lilly	Ceclor	cefaclor	p.o.	100 mL when mixed	375 mL/5mL
4	Pharmacia	Detrol LA	tolterodine tartrate	p.o.	90 cap.	2 mg/cap.
5	Roxane	Intensol	alprazolam	p.o.	30 mL	1 mg/mL
6	Pharmacia	Azulfidine	sulfasalazine	p.o.	300 tab.	500 mg/tab.

7. p.o.
8. npo
9. capsule
10. suspension

11. three times a week
12. q8h
13. s.o.s.
14. vaginally

#	(a) Admin. Route	(b) One Dose Amount	(c) Daily Dose Amount	(d) Total to Fill Prescription
15	by mouth	3 tab.	18 tab.	54 tab.
16	under the tongue	1 tab.	single dose	single dose
17	by mouth	1 mL	4 mL	40 mL
18	subcutaneous inj.	2 mL	4 mL	8 mL
19	intramuscular inj.	2 mL	single dose	single dose

20. 20-cc syringe; the nearest whole cc is 11 cc (mL).
21. 0.5-mL syringe, give 0.5 mL.

22. 5-cc syringe; the nearest fifth of a cc is 4.4 cc (mL).
23. 3-cc syringe; the nearest tenth of a cc is 1.3 cc (mL).

Chapter 4 Practice Test

#	(a) Manufacturer	(b) Brand Name	(c) Generic Name	(d) Admin. Route	(e) Total Amount of Drug	(f) Amt. of Drug per tab., mL
1	Pharmacia	Provera	medroxyprogesterone acetate	p.o.	500 tab.	10 mg/tab
2	Abbott	Biaxin	clarithromycin	p.o.	60 tab.	250 mg/tab
3	Eli Lilly	Evista	raloxifene HCl	p.o.	100 tab.	60 mg/tab
4	Pharmacia	Vantin	cefpodoxime proxetil	p.o.	50 mL when mixed	10 mg/mL
5	Pharmacia	Detrol LA	tolterodine tartrate	p.o.	30 cap.	2 mg/cap.

6. water
7. intravenous piggy back
8. subcutaneously
9. one-half

10. gtt
11. ID
12. a.c.
13. stat

#	(a) Admin. Route	(b) One Dose Amount	(c) Daily Dose Amount	(d) Total to Fill Prescription
14	by mouth	2 cap.	8 cap.	80 cap.
15	by mouth	2 tab.	12 tab	unknown
16	by mouth	3.0 mL	single dose	single dose
17	by mouth	2 tab.	4 tab.	12 tab.

18. 3-cc syringe; the nearest tenth of a cc is 1.5 cc (mL).
19. 0.5-cc syringe; the nearest hundredth of a cc is 0.25 cc (mL).
20. 10-cc syringe; the nearest fifth of a cc is 7.4 (or 7.6) cc (mL).

21. 1.0-mL tuberculin syringe; the nearest hundredth of a mL is 0.83 mL.
22. 1.0-mL tuberculin syringe; the nearest hundredth of a mL is 0.80 mL.

Chapter 5

Practice Problem Set 5.2
1. 7.5 mL or 1.5 t
3. 3 tab.; no; enteric coated
5. 1800. mg = 1.8 g
7. 1 tab.
9. 1 tab.
11. 10 mL
13. 1 cap.
15. 30 mL/day
17. 5 mL initial dose; 2.5 mL last 4 doses

19. 187 mg/dose
21. 1.3 tab.
23. 50 mg
25. 500 mg
27. 3 mg
29. 750 mg
31. 210 mg; 8.4 mL
33. 2700 mg/day; 675 mg/dose
35. no
37. yes

Practice Problem Set 5.3
1. 0.7 mL
3. 3 mL
5. 25 mL
7. 25 mL; 5 t
9. 1 tab.
11. approx. 55 g; approx. 5 mL
13. 125 mg/dose; 0.75 mL/dose
15. no

17. yes
19. yes; 0.5 t = 2.5 mL
21. 0.55 m^2
23. 2.14 m^2
25. 3 cap.
27. 1 tab.
29. 96.2 mg

Practice Problem Set 5.4
1. milliamperes; electric current
3. distance from the focus of the x-ray machine to the x-ray film surface
5. distance between the object being x-rayed and the film surface
7. 4.50 mA
9. 0.900 s
11. 39.7 cm
13. 0.450 s
15. 17.8 mA
17. 200. mA

19. 8.16 cm
21. There should be no complications (8.33 cm).
23. 8.52 cm
25. Like light rays, which spread out as they pass through a magnifying glass, x-rays spread out as they leave the x-ray machine. After they pass through the object (person) being x-rayed, they continue to spread until they hit the x-ray film. This produces an image that is slightly larger than the object the x-ray just passed through.

Practice Problem Set 5.5

1. decreases
3. inversely
5. 400.0 mL
7. 114.2 mmHg
9. 893.9 mmHg
11. 53.1°C
13. 1213 K = 939.5°C
15. 251.5 mL
17. 1102 mmHg
19. 23.2 mL
21. −190°C

Practice Problem Set 5.6

1. solute, solvent
3. 0.5 L
5. 56.25% alcohol, 43.75% water
7. 2.5%$^{w/v}$ NaCl
9. 90 cc
11. 180 mL
13. 4000 mL
15. 4%$^{w/v}$ NaOH
17. 200 mL
19. a. 75 g
    b. 7.5 g
    c. 6 g
21. 10 tab.
23. 15 tab.
25. 3.75 g iodine crystals ↑ 75 mL with alcohol → 75 mL, 5%$^{w/v}$ tincture of iodine
27. 5 L
29. Add 333 cc water.
31. Cannot be done since you cannot increase concentration (8% up to 15%) by dilution.

Practice Problem Set 5.7

1. 30°
3. 7°
5. 90°
7. 6°
9. 174°

11.

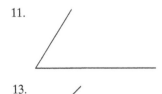

13.

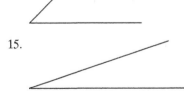

15.

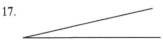

17.

19.

Chapter 5 Review Problems

1. 2 tab.
2. 20 mL
3. 2 tab.
4. 3000 mg = 3 g
5. 4 tab./day
6. 10 mL; 2 t
7. 100 mg
8. 93.5 mg
9. 4 tab./day
10. 0.4 mL
11. 2 cap.
12. 1000 mg
13. 800 mg given in two 400-mg doses
14. 204 mg/day to 408 mg/day; 102 mg/dose to 204 mg/dose; yes
15. 0.8 mL
16. 2.5 mL
17. 1 t
18. 50 mg/dose; 7 mL/dose
19. 600 mg/dose; 2 tab./dose
20. 170 mg per dose, administer 1 mL
21. no
22. yes
23. yes; 1.6 mL
24. yes; 2.5 mL = 0.5 t
25. 0.48 m^2
26. 0.87 m^2
27. 1.83 m^2
28. 2.68 m^2
29. 2 cap.
30. 221 mcg
31. 10.7 mA
32. 9 s
33. 39.5 cm
34. 0.27 s
35. 18 mA
36. 150 mA
37. 7.5 cm
38. There should be no complication in delivery (7.93 cm).
39. There should be no complication in delivery (7.95 cm).
40. V_2 = 600 mL
41. P_2 = 153.8 mmHg
42. P_2 = 765.2 mmHg
43. T_2 = −49.5°C
44. T_2 = 137.7°C
45. V_2 = 393.6 mL
46. P_2 = 1052 mmHg
47. P_2 = 214 mmHg
48. T_2 = 15°C
49. 40%$^{v/v}$ alcohol; 60%$^{v/v}$ water
50. 1.3%$^{w/v}$
51. 150 mL alcohol
52. 250 mL alcohol

53. 2500 mL
54. 3.3% $^{w/v}$
55. 1200 mL
56. 24 g
57. 12 tab.
58. 12 tab.
59. 6.25 g iodine crystals ↑ 250 mL with alcohol → 250 mL, 2.5% $^{w/v}$ tincture of iodine
60. 6 L
61. Add 375 cc of water.
62. 75 mL, 40% stock ↑ 750 mL → 750 mL, 4%
63. 24.2 mL, 75% ↑ 550 mL → 550 mL, 1:30
64. 10 T
65. 60°
66. 138°
67. 16°
68. 25°
69.

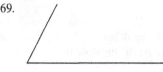

70.

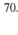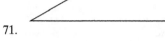

71.

72.

Chapter 5 Practice Test
1. 10 mL; 2 t
2. 1 tab.; no; enteric coated
3. 18 mg
4. 450 mg
5. 570 mg/day; 285 mg/dose
6. 0.8 mL
7. 40 mg/dose; 4 mL
8. yes; 2.5 mL = 0.5 t
9. 1.90 m^2
10. 2 cap.
11. 11.1 mA
12. 0.4 s
13. There should be no complications (8.23 cm).
14. 311 mmHg
15. 854 mmHg
16. 959 mmHg
17. 33.3% $^{v/v}$ alcohol, 67.7% $^{v/v}$ water
18. 1% $^{w/v}$
19. 2000 mL
20. 2.7% $^{w/v}$
21. 3 L
22. Add 75 cc water.
23. 100 mL 40% alcohol ↑ 1000 mL → 1 L, 4% alcohol
24. 27.5 mL 50% stock ↑ 550 mL → 550 mL, 1:40 (2.5%)
25. You cannot increase concentration (from 10% to 15%) by dilution.

26. 25°
27. 140°

28.

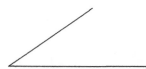

Chapter 6
Practice Problem Set 6.1
1. 5% dextrose and Ringer's Lactate Solution
3. 5% dextrose and 0.22% normal saline
5. 2.5% dextrose and water
7. 5% dextrose and 0.9% normal saline
9. 20% dextrose and water
11. 25 g dextrose
13. 100 g dextrose
15. 9 g salt
17. 12.5 g dextrose, 0.55 g salt
19. 25 g dextrose and 2.25 g salt
21. 75 g dextrose

Practice Problem Set 6.2
1. yes
3. approx. 11 gtt
5. approx. 4 gtt
7. 31.25 = 31 gtt/min
9. 10 gtt/min
11. 62.5 = 63 gtt/min
13. 20.83 = 21 gtt/min
15. 66.7 = 67 gtt/min
17. 62.5 = 63 gtt/min
19. 20.83 = 21 gtt/min
21. 125 mL/hr
23. 200 mL/hr
25. 11 gtt/min
27. 65 mL/hr
29. 96 mL/hr

Practice Problem Set 6.3
1. 25 hr
3. 6 hr
5. 3 A.M.
7. 7:30 P.M.
9. 10 hours; 10 P.M.
11. 1 hr
13. 6 hr 40 min
15. 7 P.M.
17. 5:25 P.M.
19. 9:10 P.M.

Chapter 6 Review Problems
1. 5% dextrose and 0.22% normal saline
2. 5% dextrose and Ringer's Lactate
3. 25 g dextrose
4. 50 g dextrose; 2.2 g salt
5. yes
6. 4–5 gtt every 15 s
7. 33.3 = 33 gtt/min
8. 25 gtt/min
9. 13.9 = 14 gtt/min

10. 16.7 = 17 gtt/min
11. 144 mL/hr
12. 200 mL/hr
13. 24 hr
14. 10.56 = 11 gtt/min
15. 100 gtt/min
16. 100 mL/hr
17. 16.7 = 17 gtt/min
18. 100 mL/hr
19. 86.4 mL/hr
20. 37.5 = 38 gtt/min
21. 4 hr
22. approximately 29 h 25 min
23. approximately 4 hr 44 min
24. 4:20 P.M.
25. approximately 11:57 P.M.

Chapter 6 Practice Test
1. 5% dextrose and half strength (0.45%) normal saline
2. 25 g dextrose; 2.25 g salt
3. 8–9 gtt per 15 s
4. 16.7 = 17 gtt/min
5. 37.5 = 38 gtt/min
6. 25 gtt /min
7. 62.5 = 63 mL/hr
8. 83.3 = 83 mL/hr
9. 26 gtt/min
10. 104 mL/hr
11. 36 gtt/min
12. 49.5 = 50 mL/hr
13. 9 hr 48 min
14. 2 hr 49 min
15. 12:57 A.M.

Chapter 7

Practice Problem Set 7.1
1. Statistics is the area of mathematics that is involved with the collection, summary, classification, and presentation of data that has been collected.
3. A population is a complete set of data, whereas a sample is a subset of data drawn from a population.
5. Various answers are possible.
7. quantitative
9. qualitative
11. quantitative
13. qualitative
15. quantitative
17. quantitative
19. qualitative
21. Arizona's climate is good for people with breathing problems. Therefore, there are probably more people with asthma in Arizona than in other states.
23. By saying 4 out of 5, you have no idea how many were actually polled. If only 5 were polled, this may not be an accurate statement.
25. The average is a measure of center, which means about half make more than this and half will make less. This is probably not a good indicator of a beginning nurse's salary if it is the average salary of all nurses regardless of experience.
27. Many people are out late on Saturday night and many may have been drinking. Therefore, with this combination, there may be more accidents on Saturday night.
29. Even though there is no cholesterol, there are other ingredients that affect health. Eating a large quantity may result in weight gain because of the calories in the chips. This would not be healthy.

Practice Problem Set 7.2

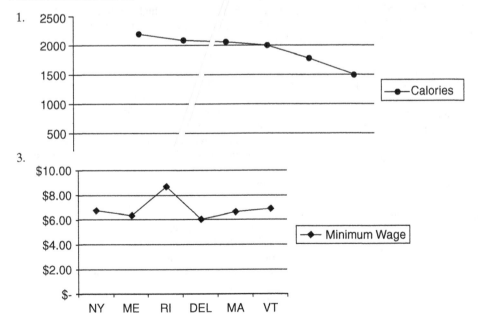

5.

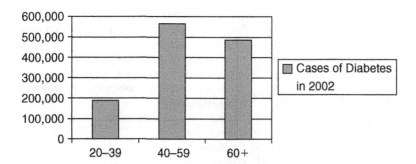

7.

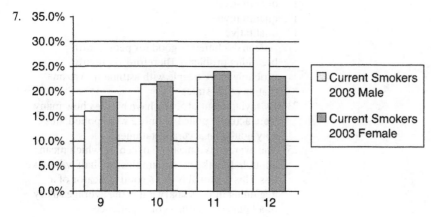

9. May
11. April, May, June, September
13. 2003
15. 3 years
17. highways
19. $255,500
21. 20.25%; $506,250
23. car maintenance and gas
25. $1470
27. house payment = $1225; food = $700; car payment = $350; utilities = $525; entertainment = $175; savings = $245; car maintenance and gas = $70; miscellaneous = $210

Practice Problem Set 7.3
1. Mode is the data item that occurs most often. It is very appropriate when dealing with qualitative data.
3. The mean is the arithmetic average—add the data and divide by the number of data items. It is appropriate for data that does not have any, or very few, outliers.
5. mode = 2 oz; median = 3.5 oz; mean = 4.6 oz; midrange = 5.5 oz
7. mode = none; median = 132.5 lb; mean = 156.5 lb; midrange = 188.5
9. mode = none; median = 1850; mean = 1875; midrange = 1875
11. mode = $7.70; median = $7.08; mean = $7.72; midrange = $9.50
13. mode = 300 cc; median = 300 cc; mean = 287.5 cc; midrange = 275 cc
15. mean = 200.75; midrange = 198; very close in value
17. mode

19. mean
21. median
23. mode
25. mean
27. mean = 4.3, median = 4, mode = 4, midrange = 5; mean and midrange are affected by the change (mean = 5.9 and midrange = 10.5).
29. mode
31. median
33. Half of the states have a higher percentage of smokers and half have a lower percentage.
35. $45,500
37. Answers will vary.

Practice Problem Set 7.4
1. There is no deviation in the data—all items are identical.
3. John's are more consistently close to the mean of 128 mg/dL because of the low SD.
5. The standard deviation is the same for both sets because the differences among data items are the same.
7. mean = 4.5, range = 9, s = 3.03
9. mean = 8.4, range = 18, s = 6.95
11. mean = 7, range = 9, s = 3.35
13. mean = 5, range = 12, s = 3.56
15. You want a low standard deviation so that results are consistently close to the mean.
17. Brand X because it is more reliable.
19. The mean increases by $50 but the standard deviation does not change.
21. 3.2%
23. 3.4%

Practice Problem Set 7.5

1. The class with the highest frequency is 215–234. There are 33 values of 195 and above.

Cholesterol	Frequency
135–154	7
155–174	2
175–194	8
195–214	8
215–234	10
235–254	4
255–274	2
275–294	1
295–314	1
315–334	6
335–354	1

3.

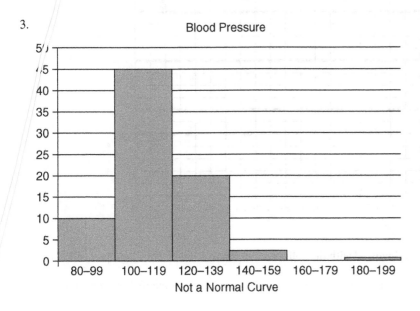

Blood Pressure

Not a Normal Curve

5.

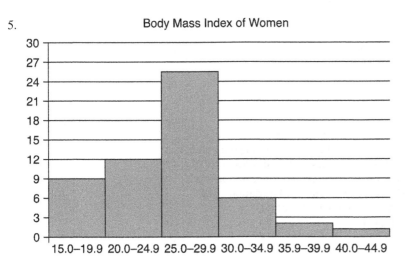

Body Mass Index of Women

7. 7.8 mmol/L upper limit and 7.4 mmol/L lower limit
9. 148 mg/dL upper limit and 76 mg/dL lower limit

11.

Blood Glucose	Frequency
97	1
98	1
99	4
100	3
101	2
102	2
103	2

13. mean = 100.2, median = 100, mode = 99, range = 6, standard deviation = 1.8, CV = 1.8%

15.

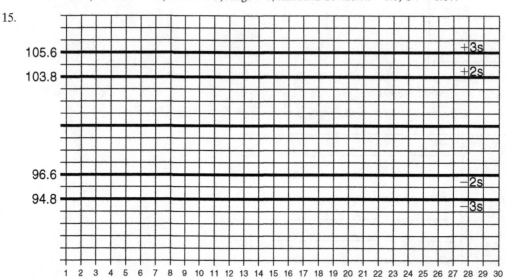

Chapter 7 Review Problems
 1. Statistics is the area of mathematics that is involved with the collection, summary, classification, and presentation of data that has been collected.
 2. Descriptive statistics gathers, charts and presents data; inferential statistics uses sample data to draw conclusions about a population of data.
 3. A population is a complete set of data, whereas a sample is a subset of a population.
 4. Quantitative data is numerical data that represents a count or amount; qualitative data is data that is categorical or descriptive.
 5. Sample sizes too small, exaggerated graphs, biased questions on a survey, biased sample chosen, misuse of percentages and very precise numbers, vague questions or definitions
 6. quantitative
 7. qualitative
 8. qualitative
 9. quantitative
10. If this is the median cost, then half of the houses sell for less than this number.
11. Set B has the highest deviation since there are larger differences among the numbers.
12. mean = 36.5 lb, median = 36, mode = 36 lb, range = 12, standard deviation = 3.9
13. mean = 15.7, median = 16.2, mode = none, range = 33.6, standard deviation = 11.1
14. mean = 108.9, median = 106, mode = 115, range = 46, standard deviation = 14.6
15. mean = $8, median = $8, mode = $8, range = 0, standard deviation = 0
16. mean = 168.25; median = 177; median is higher
17. median
18. mean

19. mode
20. 6.9%
21. mean = 156.1, median = 140, mode = none, s = 63.0, CV = 40.4%

25. Trend is downward; 4.04% decrease.

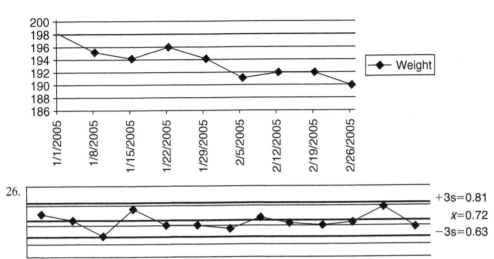

26.

22. individual income taxes
23. $219.2 billion, or $219,200,000,000
24. $723.36 billion, or $723,360,000,000

Chapter 7 Practice Test
1. Data is numerical facts or categorical information that is collected through experimentation or research.
2. Qualitative; it is the person's name in numbers.
3. Quantitative; it measures a quantity.
4. median
5. An outlier is an extreme value (either high or low) in the data set. It will skew the mean average.
6. mode
7. mean
8. s = 4.5; that is a large deviation for an average of 100 so they need improvement.
9. mean = 23.7, median = 25, mode = 12, midrange = 29, range = 34, s = 11.0
10. mean = $5.98, median = $6.13, mode = $5.15, midrange = $5.95, range = $1.60, s = $0.72
11. mean = 1.96375, median = 1.96, mode = none, midrange = 1.65, range = 3.2, s = 0.998
12. Data set A has the largest standard deviation because the differences among the data items is larger in set A.
13. mean = 203.5; range = 32
14. 7.3%
15. mean = 145.8, median = 161.5, mode = 168, s = 47.8, CV = 32.8%
16. Social Security
17. $240,000,000,000
18. $140,000,000,000
19.

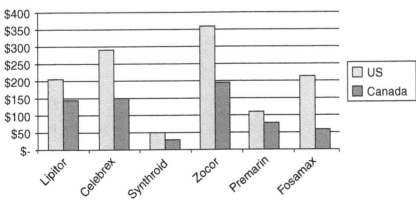

20. Yes, three are above the upper limit and one is below the lower limit (upper limit is 1.5 and lower limit is 0.9).

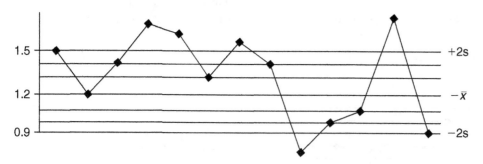

Chapter 8

Practice Problem Set 8.1

1. 1
3. −2
5. 5
7. 1.544
9. Negative numbers do not have logs.
11. −1.921
13. 4.740
15. −0.426
17. 2.807
19. −7
21. 4.544
23. 100
25. 0.891
27. 2.371
29. 100
31. 22.387
33. 0.01
35. 10
37. 338.844
39. 0.00316

Practice Problem Set 8.2

1. 2.0×10^{-14} mol/L
3. 7.69×10^{-10} mol/L
5. 5×10^{-11} mol/L
7. 5.714×10^{-8} mol/L
9. 0.19 mol/L
11. 0.3 mol/L
13. 0.018 mol/L
15. 0.08 mol/L

Practice Problem Set 8.3

1. 8
3. 3.981×10^{-8} mol/L
5. 7.943×10^{-7} mol/L
7. 5
9. 8.5 mL
11. 0.9
13. from 4.467×10^{-8} mol/L to 3.548×10^{-8} mol/L
15. 6.8
17. a. 1.2
    b. 1.639×10^{-13}

19. a. 0.12 mol/L
    b. 8.333×10^{-14} mol/L
    c. 0.9
    d. 13.1

Chapter 8 Review Problems

1. 2.699
2. −3
3. 71.945
4. 0.000316
5. 0.00001
6. −5
7. 0.01
8. 0.00316
9. 3.3, 1.923×10^{-11} mol/L
10. 6.8, 6.536×10^{-8} mol/L
11. 7.6, basic
12. 11.1
13. basic, 1.259×10^{-5} mol/L
14. 7.943×10^{-4} mol/L
15. a. .540 mol/L
    b. 1.85×10^{-14} mol/L
    c. 0.3
    d. 13.7
16. a. 0.015 mol/L
    b. 6.67×10^{-13} mol/L
    c. 1.8
    d. 12.2

Chapter 8 Practice Test

1. 2.140
2. 501.187
3. 0.0000000316
4. −2
5. 0.0158
6. 2.7, 5.556×10^{-12} mol/L
7. 11.2, acidic
8. basic, 1.26×10^{-3} mol/L
9. 7.943×10^{-4} mol/L
10. a. 2.40 mol/L
    b. 4.17×10^{-15} mol/L
    c. −0.380 (*Note:* This unusual answer is due to the incomplete ionization of the acid.)
    d. 14.380 (*Note:* This unusual answer is due to the incomplete ionization of the acid.)

INDEX